Hydra: Research Methods

Hydra: Research Methods

Edited by
Howard M. Lenhoff
University of California
Irvine, California

SPRINGER SCIENCE+BUSINESS MEDIA, LLC

Library of Congress Cataloging in Publication Data

Main entry under title:

Hydra: research methods.

Includes bibliographical references and index.
1. Hydra. I. Lenhoff, Howard M.
QL377.H9H93 1982   593.7'1   82-24648
ISBN 978-1-4757-0598-0   ISBN 978-1-4757-0596-6 (eBook)
DOI 10.1007/978-1-4757-0596-6

Cover photo courtesy of
Regula Bänninger and Prof. Pierre Tardent,
Zoological Institute, University of Zurich, Switzerland.

Contributors

Richard S. Blanquet, Department of Biology, Georgetown University, Washington, D.C. 20057

Hans R. Bode, Developmental Biology Center and Department of Developmental and Cell Biology, University of California, Irvine, California 92717

Patricia M. Bode, Developmental Biology Center and Department of Developmental and Cell Biology, University of California, Irvine, California 92717

Richard D. Campbell, Department of Developmental and Cell Biology, University of California, Irvine, California 92717

Jean Danner, Biochemistry Section, NIOSH, Morgantown, West Virginia 26505

Charles N. David, Department of Molecular Biology, Albert Einstein College of Medicine, Bronx, New York 10461

Robert M. Day, Department of Developmental and Cell Biology, University of California, Irvine, California 92717

John F. Dunne, Developmental Biology Center, University of California, Irvine, California 92717

Kristine M. Flick, Developmental Biology Center and Department of Developmental and Cell Biology, University of California, Irvine, California 92717

Cheng-Mei Fradkin, Department of Developmental and Cell Biology, University of California, Irvine, California 92717

Cornelius J. P. Grimmelikhuijzen, Max-Planck-Institut für medizinische Forschung, Abteilung Biophysik, 6900 Heidelberg, Federal Republic of Germany

Wyrta Heagy, Department of Microbiology, University of Massachusetts, Amherst, Massachusetts 01003

David A. Hessinger, Department of Physiology and Pharmacology, School of Medicine, Loma Linda University, Loma Linda, California 92350

Jeanne Ivy, Department of Developmental and Cell Biology, University of California, Irvine California 92717

Robert K. Josephson, School of Biological Science, University of California, Irvine, California 92717

Edward S. Kline, Department of Biochemistry, Medical College of Virginia, Virginia Commonwealth University, Richmond, Virginia 23298

Howard M. Lenhoff, Department of Developmental and Cell Biology, University of California, Irvine, California 92717

Georgia E. Lesh-Laurie, Department of Biology, Cleveland State University, Cleveland, Ohio 44115

C. Lynne Littlefield, Developmental Biology Center, University of California, Irvine, California 92717

Stephen S. Macintyre, Department of Anatomy, Case Western Reserve University, Cleveland, Ohio 44106

Harry K. MacWilliams, Department of Anatomy, University of Massachusetts Medical Center, Worcester, Massachusetts 01605

Beverly A. Marcum, Department of Biological Sciences, California State University, Chico, California, 95929

L. Muscatine, Department of Biology, University of California, Los Angeles, California 90024

That T. Ngo, Department of Developmental and Cell Biology, University of California, Irvine, California 92717

Patricia Novak, Department of Developmental and Cell Biology, University of California, Irvine, California 92717

Joann J. Otto, Department of Biological Sciences, Purdue University, West Lafayette, Indiana 47907

R. L. Pardy, School of Life Sciences, University of Nebraska, Lincoln, Nebraska 68588

Donald W. Phipps, Jr., School of Life Sciences, University of Nebraska, Lincoln, Nebraska 68588

M. Rahat, Department of Zoology, The Hebrew University of Jerusalem, Israel

Vanda Reich, Department of Zoology, The Hebrew University of Jerusalem, Israel

Norman Rushforth, Department of Biology, Case Western Reserve University, Cleveland, Ohio 44106

Charles L. Rutherford, Biology Department, Virginia Polytechnic Institute and State University, Blacksburg, Virginia 24061

H. Chica Schaller, Max-Planck-Institut für medizinsche Forschung, Abteilung Biophysik, 6900 Heidelberg, Federal Republic of Germany

Tobias Schmidt, Max-Planck-Institut für medizinsche Forschung, Abteilung Biophysik, 6900 Heidelberg, Federal Republic of Germany

G. Scott Smith, Developmental Biology Center and Department of Developmental and Cell Biology, University of California, Irvine, California 92717

Alan E. Stiven, Department of Biology 046A, University of North Carolina, Chapel Hill, North Carolina 27514

Tsutomu Sugiyama, National Institute of Genetics, Mishima, Shizuoka-ken 411, Japan

Joseph R. Voland, Department of Pathology, University of California, San Diego, La Jolla, California

Nancy Wanek, Developmental Biology Center and Department of Developmental and Cell Biology, University of California, Irvine, California 92717. Current address: Department of Biology and Health Science, Chapman College, Orange, California 92666.

Vaman S. Waravdekar, Microbiological Associates, Bethesda, Maryland 20016

Richard L. Wood, Department of Anatomy, University of Southern California, School of Medicine, Los Angeles, California 90007

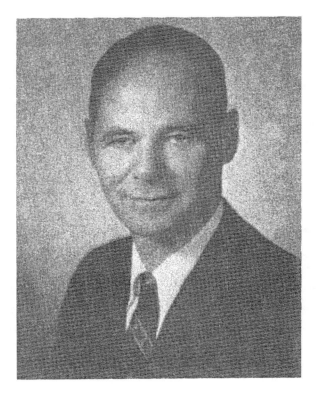

William Farnsworth Loomis
(1914–1973)

The fall of 1973 saw the passing of a unique scientist and individual who more than anyone was responsible for the current renaissance in the use of hydra as an experimental animal in biological research; he introduced the precision, quantification, and methodology of the physical sciences to the study of this simple invertebrate. I refer, of course, to William Farnsworth Loomis, "Farnie" as he liked to be called by his friends—scientist, explorer, philanthropist, and philosopher. It is fitting that this book be dedicated to him, for Loomis believed that the large advances in biology had their origin with the concomitant development of quantitative methods.

For example, when he was demonstrating for the first time that mitochondrial particles (called "cyclophorase" then) respire (Green *et al.*, 1948) and the dinitrophenol uncoupled oxidation from phosphorylation (Loomis and Lipmann, 1948), he developed a quick and simple way to calibrate the Warburg respirometer (Loomis, 1949), the major apparatus used in those classic studies. In his research with hydra he is best known for developing methods for culturing the animals *en masse*, methods which opened the door wide for future generations of biologists to have an ample and continuous supply of this animal in their laboratories. But Loomis did more than simply develop a method for growing the animal; he developed a simple, reliable, repeatable assay for quantifying the logarithmic growth rate of growing cultures of hydra (Loomis, 1954). This assay allowed him to determine the extent to which such physicochemical factors as pH, oxygen tension, and ionic strength affected their rate of growth. As a last example of his respect for good methods, when he was concerned about whether the partial pressure of either oxygen or carbon dioxide affected the differentiation of hydra, he developed sensitive micromethods for measuring small amounts of these two gases in fresh water (Loomis, 1954, 1956, 1958).

In the ensuing pages I will try to paint a portrait of the man, drawing mostly from recollections of my experiences and conversations with him and also from a few of our letters. I first heard him speak in the winter of 1953 in a seminar at Johns Hopkins University. I was a graduate student in biochemistry at the time, working in the laboratory of Professor Nathan O. Kaplan. Loomis, a friend of Kaplan while both were postdoctoral students in the laboratory of Nobel Laureate Fritz Lipmann at Massachusetts General Hospital, was invited to Johns Hopkins to present the first seminar on his new research—the developmental biology of hydra. I remember so well his first slide, a homemade one impressed on cellophane from carbon paper. It was a drawing of a coin with arrows to the side indicating that when considering any problem, "there are two sides to every coin." He was concerned with the problem of cancer—which, according to his son, Professor William F. Loomis, Jr., of the University of California, San Diego, was his long-term interest.

On one side of the coin were listed properties of normally developing cells and on the other, properties of cancerous cells. Loomis believed that to understand abnormal development we first had to be firmly grounded in knowledge of the development and differentiation of normal cells. His second slide was that of a hydra, because he said that in order to study development he wanted to examine a simple biological system. Not being trained in invertebrate biology, Loomis thumbed through Ralph Buchsbaum's classic *Animals Without Backbones* (1948), played around with the idea of using sponges, only to find them too difficult to work with, and settled upon the next example of lower invertebrates described by Buchsbaum—hydra.

Most of us know the scientific works of Loomis, but few know the man. What kind of person was he? What forces shaped his life? What motivated him? To answer these and other questions, we have to go back three generations, because Farnie Loomis was part of a dynasty of well-to-do, public-spirited scientists. His laboratory in Greenwich, Connecticut, called the Loomis Laboratory, was actually the fourth Loomis Laboratory.

The first Loomis Laboratory was established by Farnie's great-grandfather, Alfred Loomis. The elder Alfred Loomis, son of a Vermont farmer and a self-made man, had two medical crises in his life—both of which he turned around to help advance American medicine. The first crisis concerned his wife, who was extremely ill. Because at that time, the second part of the nineteenth century, the best physicians were in Europe, Alfred Loomis and his wife moved to Germany in order to get the best care available. Mrs. Loomis' recovery was a long one. In the meantime, her husband became fascinated with medicine, especially the advances in the new field of microbiology initiated by Pasteur. Loomis studied medicine while in Europe, and by the time his wife was ready to return to America, he had obtained a medical degree.

The elder Alfred Loomis proceeded to establish himself as a significant factor in American medicine, author of a number of medical books, and frequent antagonist in medical controversies with the famous Welsch of Johns Hopkins. But perhaps the most significant contribution coming from his entry into medicine was the establishment in the Harkness Pavilion of Columbia University of the first Loomis Laboratories—purported to be one of the first (if not the first) clinical laboratories in the United States, one equipped to diagnose some illnesses of microbiological origin.

The second medical crisis in the life of the elder Alfred Loomis was his own contraction of tuberculosis. Although I do not have all the details, it is my understanding that Loomis and his friend Edward Trudeau, also diseased with tuberculosis, decided that a healthy, open air and rigorous life-style would do much to relieve them of the symptoms of tuberculosis. This approach worked for them and they established what later became known as the Trudeau Institute in upstate New York so that others could experience a similar cure. The Trudeau Institute functioned continuously until the mid-twentieth century, when the rise of the new antituberculin drugs became widespread.

The son of Alfred Loomis, and grandfather of Farnie, Henry Patterson Loomis, died young and therefore never had the chance to achieve the distinction of either his father, Alfred Labaeus Loomis, or his son, Alfred

Lee. Nonetheless, he was a successful physician who continued the Loomis tradition by running the second Loomis Laboratory, also at the Harkness Pavilion of Columbia, where he was professor of clinical medicine.

Farnie's father, Alfred Lee Loomis, was another case—a great man in his own right and a major force in the development of young Farnie. Alfred Lee Loomis was a success in government, business, and science. He had three sons, one a successful financier and deep-sea sailor (Alfred Lee Loomis, Jr.), one in government and former president of Voice of America and the Public Broadcast System (Henry Loomis), and one a scientist— Farnie. Some admirers of Alfred Lee Loomis say that he was a greater success in all three areas than each of the sons was in his chosen profession. Without debating that remark, unquestionably Alfred Lee Loomis was a giant and he must have been a stimulus to his boys.

Father Loomis was a prelaw student at Yale majoring in mathematics. Influenced by his cousin, Henry Stimson, former Secretary of War under Roosevelt, Alfred Loomis went to law school. After law school he and his brother-in-law, Landon Thorne, started a partnership on Wall Street in New York. Loomis, always interested in science, became intrigued with the work on population growth of Raymond Pearl of Johns Hopkins. If the laws of population growth, i.e., lag phase, logarithmic growth, and stationary phase, apply to all organisms, he thought, why not to businesses as well? I remember so clearly Alfred Lee Loomis telling me this story one of the times he visited Farnie's laboratory in Greenwich, Connecticut. "I simply made a number of drawings of typical growth curves and plotted the rate of growth of various industries. It was soon apparent to me that railroads, for example, were in the stationary phase (no pun intended) in 1916, whereas the automobile industry was just getting out of the lag phase." And apparently Loomis purchased stocks in the correct automobile and other companies and his fortune increased many fold. He and Thorne also formed and owned New England Power and Light. Around 1928 he saw a pattern developing whereby the logarithmic growth of industries was not going to continue indefinitely. Before the crash of 1929 he sold most of his holdings, except for some utility stocks, and it is rumored that he was one of the few men of wealth not seriously hurt by the collapse of the market.

I tell you this story only to point out that Alfred Lee Loomis was a financial wizard, and not to suggest that his life was obsessed with making money. On the contrary, Loomis's obsession was science. In fact, he liked to be called "an amateur of science" because amateur is derived from *amator*, meaning "lover." Not only did he give money for research to scientists he recognized as having great talent, such as Ernest Orlando Lawrence, physicist Robert William Wood, biochemist Fritz Lipmann, and microbiologist C. B. Van Niel, but he was actively involved in research himself. At his home in Tuxedo Park, New York, Alfred Lee Loomis sponsored the third Loomis Laboratory. And it is in this type of environment that young Farnie Loomis grew up.

Alfred Lee Loomis initiated and participated in many research projects during his years (1928–1941) at Tuxedo Park. Coming immediately to mind are his pioneering works on brain waves and the effects of sound waves and neutron irradiation on biological tissue. Although the effects of neutron irradiation may excite some interest today because of current talk of a neutron bomb, it was his pioneering work on brain waves that aroused the interest of the public. I remember Fritz Goro, the famous photographer for *Life* magazine, and better known to this audience as father of the late coral biologist, Thomas Goreau, telling me that his first assignment in America after escaping from the Nazis was to do a feature on Alfred Lee Loomis and his work on brain waves.

To invertebrate biologists, Alfred Lee Loomis is best known for his work with E. Newton Harvey and Ethel Browne Harvey on the separation of light and heavy components of the sea urchin egg. It was A. L. Loomis (Harvey and Loomis, 1930) who designed and built the instrument that allowed the centrifuging eggs to be photographed while separating into the nuclear and anuclear components.

His laboratory was a beehive of activity, having many visitors and guest resident scientists. While looking through his guest book, I saw the signature of such giants as Marconi, Einstein, and Bohr and a host of other notables who visited the Tuxedo Park laboratory.

Most of the work mentioned above occurred between the two World Wars. In both wars, A. L. Loomis served the U.S. government. In World War I, he was a major administrator at the Aberdeen Proving Grounds in Maryland in charge of experimental research on exterior ballistics. He told me of the time he requested fifty Ph.D.s from the army personnel office. He got them all right—Ph.D.s in French, sociology, literature, etc. But it was in the Second World War that A. L. Loomis made his greatest contributions to the war effort. He closed his laboratory at Tuxedo Park and moved to the Massachusetts Institute of Technology in Cambridge, Massachusetts. There he was instrumental in setting up the Lincoln Laboratories, best known for the development of GCA (Ground Control Approach "for landing airplanes in bad weather") and LORAN (Long Range Navigation)—methods that played such an important role in winning the Battle of Britain in World War II and in airplane navigation in general. Both of these ideas grew out of Alfred Loomis' obsession with understanding the nature of time. Farnie told me of an anecdote in which his father, while on a commercial airplane, was invited into the cockpit by the crew. "And this," said the pilot, "is LORAN," and he started to explain what it did. Alfred Lee interrupted and said, "Yes, I know. I have the patent on it" (Loomis, 1959). (For more on Alfred Loomis, see Alvarez, 1980.)

Alfred Lee Loomis, outstanding in business, government, and science, never received a formal Ph.D. He was honored, however, with numerous honorary doctorates, and served on the board of trustees of many leading institutions such as M.I.T. and the Carnegie Institution of Washington. But, my story is about his son, William Farnsworth. Farnie once told me that a person does not really mature until after his father dies. Fate did not have it that way because Farnie died two years before his father. The rest of this story, thus, is about the maturing and genius of William Farnsworth Loomis.

I will begin with his college years at Harvard in the mid-thirties. Already an accomplished mountain climber and skier, Loomis took off his junior year and became "a prime mover in one of the finest expeditions of the century" (Roberts, 1981). Loomis organized the climb of the Himalayan mountain Nanda Devi. His expedition succeeded in climbing the highest mountain (25,645 feet) ever climbed by man until then—a record held for fourteen years until Annapurna was climbed by the French after World War II.

Although Loomis became ill at the last station before the final ascent, which he personally did not make, he took great pride in the accomplishment of his colleagues and his role in it. Climbing Nanda Devi was not just a fluke. Throughout his adult life he enjoyed mountain climbing. Once, upon returning from climbing a mountain in California, he reported back to the ranger station so that they would know he returned. When he told them that he climbed it from the eastern approach, they exclaimed that he was the first man to have ever made the ascent alone from that extremely difficult side. And that was the way it was with Loomis in his science too; whether the obstacles were known, as in Nanda Devi, or unknown, as in the California mountain, he would barrel on ahead to achieve his goal. But, as I will point out later, he preferred not be informed of obstacles, even if they were known. He believed that man's ingenuity would find the way.

After receiving his bachelor's degree, Loomis went on, like his grandfather before him, to study medicine at Harvard Medical School. That Loomis received an M.D. and not a Ph.D. may surprise some who know Loomis for his accomplishments in biochemistry and hydra biology. As was true for a number of scientists of his generation and before, medical schools were about the only places to receive training in the new emerging fields of biochemistry and microbiology. "Medical school was an excellent place to get an appreciation of life," Loomis told me. "It was quite a sobering experience because my 'first patient'—the cadaver for anatomy class—was a dead one."

But it was biochemistry, not anatomy, that fascinated young Loomis. Paradoxically, "I learned more biochemistry while I was in the army than I did in medical school," he said as he told me a revealing tale. "During the war, I was a medic in the ski corps and spent a great deal of time in Burma and China." (I later learned that he was an OSS physician and parachuted into China behind Japanese lines.) "I spent much time between assignments, however, sitting around docks waiting to be transferred. It was there that I studied biochemistry. I wrote to mother to send me my biochemistry books. Because war-time regulations wouldn't allow her to send books by mail, she used to rip out pages and chapters and send them to me bits and pieces at a time in her letters."

Although Farnie claims that is how he learned biochemistry, there is no doubt that his experience during the years immediately following the war in the laboratories of the two scientific giants—David E. Green and Fritz Lipmann—greatly shaped his career.

It was at Green's laboratory at Columbia as a National Research Council Fellow that Loomis participated in and coauthored the first of Green's pioneering papers on "cyclophorase," the name they applied to the cellular oxidative system of mitochondria (Green, *et al.*, 1948). This research was a major advance in biochemistry, as it marked a change in biochemical research from investigating *soluble* single enzymes carrying out a *single reaction* to that of *particulate* complexes of enzymes carrying out *a host of related sequential reactions*.

After this immediate success, Loomis decided, as he told me, "to hand in my pipets," and to move on to a different laboratory. He went next to the laboratory of Fritz Lipmann, a recent refugee from Germany, who was working as a research associate in the basement of Massachusetts General Hospital of Harvard University. It was there, while Lipmann was doing his work on coenzyme A which later brought him the Nobel Prize, that Loomis rubbed shoulders with a group of young postdoctorals and students, such as Nathan Kaplan and David Novelli, men who later became leaders in biochemistry during the fifties and sixties. Kaplan, my Ph.D. mentor, told me that Loomis then was so excited about his research that he barely took time to eat. "I remember," Kaplan said, "that Farnie used to eat his lunch while going through the cafeteria line, so that by the time he got to the cashier, he was finished eating and ready to go back to the lab."

At "Mass General" Loomis did not work on the coenzyme A project, but instead used his experience with respiring mitochondria to demonstrate for the first time the phenomenon of "uncoupling" of phosphorylation from oxidation using dinitrophenol (Loomis and Lipmann, 1948). "After repeating the experiment numerous times under all sorts of conditions, I thought it would be nice to publish my first uncoupling experiment," he told me—and he did. Loomis continued this line of research even after he left Mass General and demonstrated that the antibiotic aureomycin and the respiration inhibitor azide also uncoupled phosphorylation from oxidation. Delving further into methodology, he developed a means for stabilizing mitochondria by vitrification (Loomis, 1950).

He then devoted much time to a new interest—semantics. Loomis was greatly influenced by the writings of the quantitative semanticist Alfred Korzybski. While studying Korzybski's tome *Science and Sanity* (1948), Loomis felt he had to write a paper on semantics so he would be certain that he had his own clear ideas as to what semantics meant. He later presented this paper, actually a short book, at a national meeting of the Semantics Society in Colorado, and for it he was given one of their awards. The main lesson Loomis drew from his excursion into semantics was that with clear thinking, one could do almost anything. And clear thinking to Loomis began with clear writing. He put his new credo to test by his next move, from research to academic teaching.

In 1948 Loomis joined the biology department of M.I.T., where he applied his semantic principles to developing a course in embryology, a subject he never studied formally. According to his former chairman, Professor F. O. Schmitt, and former students of the course, Loomis taught a course which, rather than simply covering traditional descriptive embryology, introduced the students to the dynamic and experimental aspects of developmental biology. This approach is now considered standard practice at today's universities, but in the forties, it was, to say the least, not customary. This experience in developmental biology later influenced the direction his research was to take.

By 1950 Loomis, although pleased with his university experience, was not satisfied intellectually, nor was he sure of the branch of science toward which he would devote the next decade of his life. His decision to enter a new research field was delayed for a few years when he left the safe and sure paths of academia to take advantage of a unique opportunity at the Rockefeller Foundation. There, working under the well-known scientific administrator Warren Weaver, Loomis became a traveling administrator whose major job was to visit and investigate the laboratories of those scientists applying to the Rockefeller Foundation for research funds. It was this experience in the days before Sputnik and huge government funding of research that took Loomis to the doorsteps of some of the greatest scientists of that time. But not everyone would have gained from these site visits as Loomis did. It was his voracious appetite for scientific information and his demand for clarity and simplicity nurtured by his study of semantics, that allowed Loomis to sift ideas from these great minds so that he could formulate the research directions he would pursue in the future.

His method of visiting these laboratories is instructive. "Before I would visit a laboratory," he told me, "I would ask them to send me reprints of their published research. Then I would take a train rather than an airplane to visit them so I would have ample time to study those reprints thoroughly. When I visited their laboratories, I would question the applicants mostly on what they had already accomplished and less about what they hoped to do. So many ideas never work out when put to the test. I wanted to learn about those experiments that worked, about their successes."

Loomis took accurate notes and kept a careful diary of his visits with the scientists who shaped one of the greatest eras of modern biology. While I was a postdoctoral student at Loomis' laboratory, he would occasionally give me the treat of peaking into his accounts of those giants of the fifties.

His brief stint as an administrator served him well. In 1952 he informed Warren Weaver that he finally had made his decision. He would set up his own laboratory, the fourth Loomis Laboratory, and would devote his next years to a biochemical investigation of developmental biology—a decision he made one year before Watson and Crick published their classic paper on DNA structure.

Loomis, living "across the street from David Rockefeller" in Greenwich, Connecticut, a conservative suburb of New York inhabited mostly by the very wealthy, tore up his tennis court (which today I find unconscionable) and in its place built his laboratory. He went to a nearby pond, found his first hydra, and started his research. After he gave his first talk at Johns Hopkins, he asked his close friend from Mass General days, Nathan Kaplan, who was then a budding star at Hopkins, if he knew of a student trained in biochemistry but interested in biology who might want to spend a few postdoctoral years working in his laboratory. A few days after Loomis' visit, Kaplan, who as my Ph.D. mentor knew of my interest in biology, suggested that I speak to Loomis. The thought of leaving the university environment to work alone on a suburban estate came as a mild shock to me, still a third-year graduate student just into my Ph.D. research, but Loomis's seminar was appealing to me and I agreed to talk with him. That spring I met Loomis at the meeting of the Federation of Experimental Biologists in Chicago, and he invited me, before I made any decision, to spend a week in Greenwich to see how I would like the work and the isolation of his laboratory. I visited the laboratory in June 1953, and in September 1954 I started what proved to be two memorable years of tutelage under a remarkable man, and years of friendship that ended only with his death twenty years later.

One of my first exercises at the Loomis Laboratory was to repeat his experiments on the logarithmic clonal growth of hydra. I asked him how he had made this discovery and how he had developed the first artificial solution in which to grow hydra.

"To grow hydra in the laboratory," he told me, "I had to overcome two obstacles. For one, the hydra needed a source of live food, and two, they needed to live in a solution that was similar to pond water in composition. I solved both problems quickly. As for the food, I couldn't see growing *Daphnia* in the standard magical broths of boiled lettuce and sheep dung. Much too chancy and uncontrolled. Father suggested hatching brine shrimp eggs; they were cheap, stable and reliable."

"But the culture solution was more of a problem," he continued. "I deduced that I needed a solution which had fixed amounts of most salts, and which was fairly well defined. Sea water seemed the answer; so I grabbed a gallon cider bottle and trotted down to Long Island Sound to get some. To my great pleasure I found that hydra fed daily and maintained in five percent sea water grew at a constant logarithmic rate doubling about every two days. Now I could grow hydra and was ready to work. I sent off a note to *Science* and began my experiments."

"Wait a minute," I commented. "Your *Science* paper (Loomis, 1953) describes a culture solution requiring Ca^{++} and says nothing about dilute sea water."

"You are right," Loomis replied. "After my paper was accepted I started to test hydra for growth on the various ions making up sea water, and soon found the Ca^{++} alone added to distilled water was sufficient to support growth of hydra fed on brine shrimp. But then I found a dilemma. *Science* sent me the page proofs of the sea water paper. I decided to rewrite the entire paper with the new information even though *Science*'s policy was to charge five dollars a word for any changes over 10% of the article."

From this practical advance, Loomis went on to show how ions and various physical factors affected the growth characteristics of hydra (Loomis, 1954) and to describe the first method for growing mass cultures of hydra (Loomis and Lenhoff, 1956). Now hydra could be grown in most any laboratory, or as Loomis might say, "hydra was tamed," and the stage was set for the current renaissance of research using this animal.

Despite his many startling discoveries on the growth of hydra (Loomis, 1954), the glutathione control of the feeding response (Loomis, 1955) and the control of sexual differentiation by P_{CO_2} (Loomis, 1957), Loomis still was not accepted by the descriptive biologists, the "old guard." The legendary Libbie Hyman, for one, never seemed to be able to accept that good experiments could be done on hydra reared in the laboratory. When she visited Loomis' laboratory once at his invitation, he asked her to identify the hydra he had collected from a nearby pond. At first she was dumbfounded to see tens of thousands of hydra growing well in neatly stacked Pyrex cake dishes. She said that she couldn't identify them because she needed sexually differentiated animals to examine the theca of their embryos. "And besides," she told him, "this is the wrong season for hydra to develop gonads." "She nearly flipped," Loomis told me with a wide grin, "when I gave her a tray of five thousand hydra with spermaries, and another of five thousand female hydra with eggs." "What happened?" I asked. "She said they were *Hydra littoralis*," Loomis chuckled (Loomis, 1954).

Farnie was very proud of his laboratory (Fig. 1), which he designed and outfitted himself. It was a pioneering experience to leave the world of academia and group research to set out as a "lone wolf," as the now defunct New York *Herald Tribune* called him, to tackle tough scientific problems. But he had good examples. His father was a lone wolf. His mentors David Green and Fritz Lipmann began as lone wolves, and so were most of the scientists he investigated for the Rockefeller Foundation.

Loomis firmly believed, however, that many scientists were shackled to satisfying others, such as department heads and granting agencies. He felt if scientists had the freedom to do what they pleased, they would make creative discoveries rather than follow the fads. Although he was blessed with financial independence and had the luxury to do what he wanted, he and his father also felt that other scientists less fortunate than they also needed such financial independence. Together they ran the Loomis Institute for Scientific Research. Many times just a friendly visit by one of them to a scientist's laboratory convinced them to support that scientist. "How much do you need," they would ask. And, after a week or so, without lengthy bureaucratic grant applications, a check would arrive.

In the same vein, Farnie was one of the first to propose the idea of Career Awards to granting agencies. He made this proposal in 1955 to one of

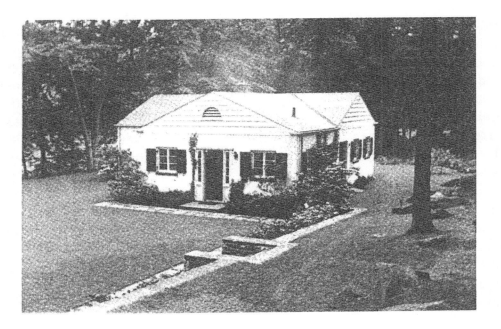

FIGURE 1. Fourth Loomis Laboratory. Greenwich. Connecticut. 1954.

the numerous organizations that he advised. In essence he suggested that the agencies guarantee support to a scientist for extended periods ranging from five to twenty-five years. "Such financial independence," Loomis said, "will give them the freedom to try out their wildest ideas."

Once hs served on the "Visiting Committee" consisting of Harvard University alumni to review the program of its Museum of Comparative Zoology (MCZ). In his report he aroused the consternation of a number of the MCZ's National Academy members when he criticized them for not having one laboratory for experimental research. He remarked that "Louis Agassiz would turn over in his grave if he were to return and see that the MCZ had not kept pace with modern biology."

He had some laboratory habits that I thought were strange. He washed all his own glassware. "Can't take any chances of an experiment going wrong," he said. "Besides it gives me time to think." He didn't believe in hiring technicians. "Takes too much time to tell them what to do. Besides, why should they have all the fun!"

He believed that if a piece of equipment were available, then the scientist would find some way to use it. Thus, his laboratory was fairly well stocked. Nonetheless, he said his stock room was Fisher Scientific Co., which was "just a telephone call away." On the other hand, every six months I would find his waste basket full of hardly touched books, some of which I greedily retrieved and still possess today. "If I haven't opened a book in five years, I toss it out because I'll probably never use it. Besides, they take up too much space."

As I was his only colleague, we interacted a great deal. There was hardly a day that we did not discuss some matter in depth. He had strong—but original—views on approaches to science. First of all, as I have already pointed out, there was his great concern for technique. Regarding "reading the literature," on the other hand, he had less concern. "I don't want to become prejudiced by their results," he said. "In biology, so much of the literature is wrong, that I prefer not to read the papers. Instead, I'd rather just do experiments. At worst, I would repeat and confirm someone else's results. But more than likely I will get closer to the truth by taking an unbiased fresh approach." And his results shows that usually he did.

Secondly, his "addiction" to the Oriental game of Go (he was recognized as one of the best players in the United States) showed in his approach to research. "Western thinking is not conducive to carrying out research with whole animals," he told me. We usually think in terms of shades of black and white, of going from point A to point B in a straight line. You can't solve biological problems that way. It is more like the game of Go. Rather than reach your goal by going from one side of the board to the other, as in getting king in checkers, or queen in chess, in Go you can move in any which direction so long as at the end you encompass the entire problem. So it is in biology too. You can't move in only one direction, but must sidestep, branch out, divert and encircle in order to get answers to the complex problems posed." To Loomis, these were not mere words, but were reality as he skipped from research on culture solutions, to work on the feeding response and on sexual differentiation as he established hydra as an animal to be used for experimental research.

Thirdly, I recall that during my first three months at his laboratory, while I was still writing my thesis, I fell easy prey to Loomis' almost missionary semantic zeal for promoting clear and precise writing. Although I advise all students to complete writing their theses before leaving their universities, I did not. I had the unique good fortune, however, to fall into the hands of Loomis. Every morning we went over every word and nuance of my thesis until it was comprehensible to biochemists not specializing in my field and contained not a single superfluous word, or at least we thought it did not. Much to the agony of my own graduate students, I continue this ritual and consider it a most valuable part of graduate education.

We did, however, feel the need for outside intellectual stimulation, which we tried to fill by periodic visits to Columbia University, one hour away by automobile, or to the New York Enzyme Club meetings attended by some of the leading biochemists of the time.

But few scientists then appreciated Loomis's attempts to bring the rigors of biochemistry to the study of whole animals. Thus, we tried to assemble biologists working with hydra to review the field and to discuss mutual problems. Our first such attempt to meet found Loomis, Helen Park of NIH, and I meeting at his laboratory, while the late Al Burnett never made it as his car broke down en route to our conference. Nonetheless, from this meeting the seeds were planted for the first symposium on hydra, to be held in Miami in the spring of 1961.

This meeting was finally arranged when I was at the Howard Hughes Medical Institute in Miami and Loomis was on the faculty of the Graduate Department of Biochemistry at Brandeis University in Waltham, Massachusetts. Finally, at a meeting at Captain Kidd's bar at Woods Hole, Massachusetts, Loomis told me to organize a symposium centered around hydra and to invite "our friends," and not necessarily everyone working with hydra and coelenterates. The expenses would be paid by the Loomis Institute for Scientific Research.

The results of the meeting are now history. Biologists from a variety of disciplines—natural history, taxonomy, ecology, physiology, biochemistry, pharmacology, gerontology, developmental biology, and electron microscopy—all met in Miami to share their ideas on research on "Hydra and Some Other Coelenterates." The results of that symposium, published 6 months after its conclusion (Lenhoff and Loomis, 1961), paved the way and posed many of the questions for the next two decades of research on hydra. As Loomis (and I) wrote (1961): "Much of the work presented at this symposium is in an early stage. At times we have thought that perhaps these results are too preliminary and should only be compiled after more data have been accumulated. The situation is analogous to constructing a new building. At times we might feel that all such work should proceed behind walls marked 'Work in Progress. No Admittance.' At other times we are intrigued with the very smell of sawdust and of wet paint. It is in this latter spirit that the volume was compiled, for these efforts, given time, may well show that hydra are particularly favorable material for the investigation of cellular and intercellular problems. History at least supports this view, because it was in hydroid material that asexual reproduction and regeneration were first discovered over two hundred years ago."

The economics of the symposium and book were rather unusual and deserve to be told. All expenses of the participants were paid by the Loomis Institute. The book was published by the University of Miami Press under the following arrangement: All publishing costs were to be borne by the Loomis Institute. The book was to be sold at $4.50, which was a bargain even in 1961. In fact, the book cost $4.75 per volume to produce, but Loomis wanted it to be low enough in price for graduate students to be able to afford it. The University of Miami Press would oversee all sales and handling expenses. During the first two years, any income on the book, minus the University of Miami Press's expenses, would be returned to the Loomis Institute. Finally, income on the book during subsequent years would go directly to the university press.

Loomis did something unique with the "income" from the book (which, of course, never covered its cost). He turned the proceeds over to the Laboratory of Quantative Biology of the University of Miami, which I directed. With those funds we commissioned a talented student in Russian to translate the volume on hydra by the Russian biologist I. I. Kanaev into English. One hundred copies of the typescript of that volume were published in 1969, with fifty going to established investigators of hydra and the rest to major libraries throughout the world. So in a sense, one book fed another. This was the Loomis way: There were no precedents—nor to my knowledge, have any followed this example!

Another book was spun from the daily discussions Farnie and I had at his laboratory. It so happened that at that time we were each independently involved in deep inner searches about the place of religion in our lives. Loomis was of Protestant background and I was Jewish. Both of us had been through agnostic and atheistic stages, and both were searching for a rational, nonmagical understanding of the nature of man and of our universe. Loomis, however, was an unusual individual, whose responses to such common experiences were often unique. Thus, to articulate his search, he wrote and published a book—*The God$_B$ Within* (1967)—in which he applied his semantic reasoning and inner emotions to come up with his own view of religions, a view about which theologian Bishop James A. Pike wrote, "[Dr. Loomis] has modestly told me that he is not a theologian. . . . But in terms of capacity to contribute to the present theological dialogue he has more to offer theology, right at this point [of rapid theological transition], by the very fact that he is a scientist and philosopher of science. . . . [It] is evident that *The God Within* appears at a most important time in the theological revolution. It does not of itself entirely provide a viable view of God in these times; but certainly no view of God is viable which does not take into account the story which [Dr. Loomis] so magnificently tells and the pointers to meaning which he supplies in the course of its telling."

In 1956 I left the Loomis Laboratory to begin a trek taking me to the U.S. Air Force at the Armed Forces Institute of Pathology at Walter Reed Medical Center, the Department of Terrestrial Magnetism of the Carnegie Institution of Washington, the Howard Hughes Medical Institute, and the University of Miami in Florida, and now the University of California at Irvine.

Loomis, troubled by a number of personal tragedies, also started a number of moves that ended with his own death in 1973. In 1963, he closed the fourth Loomis Laboratory and joined the biochemistry faculty at Brandeis University. He went to Brandeis because, as he told his son, Prof. W. F. Loomis, Jr., "it is not good for a scientist to work in isolation for a long time." At Brandeis he never seemed to get seriously back into his research with hydra, but created a stir with his research on Vitamin D (Loomis, 1970).

In the late sixties he decided to leave the university to move to England to "a secluded manor house," where he would have time to think and write a number of books that he had on his mind. He did not stay long in England, but returned to Massachusetts, where he embarked at age 55 on an internship in psychiatry.

During our respective perigrinations, Farnie and I always kept contact with each other, either by letter or phone. I last spoke to him in the fall of 1973 just before I left for Israel for a six-month sabbatical leave. A few months after I returned, one of my colleagues asked me if I knew that Loomis was dead. I had not heard, and to this day I still find it hard to believe—he was such an intensely alive human being.

Because I was one of the privileged few to have experienced intimately the genius of this unique individual who has influenced biology in America in so many ways, and who has completely altered the path of my life for the better, I share these recollections with you. Science progresses through individuals, but we tend to remember only their discoveries. I cannot and will not forget William Farnsworth Loomis the person, nor should you.

Howard M. Lenhoff

REFERENCES

Alvarez, L. W. 1980. Alfred Lee Loomis. Biographical memories. *Natl. Acad. Sci. U.S.A.* **51**:309–341.

Buchsbaum, T. 1948. *Animals Without Backbones*, 2nd ed. University of Chicago Press, Chicago.

Green, D. E., Loomis, W. F., and Auerbach, V. H. 1948. Studies on the cyclophorose system. I. The complete oxidation of pyruvic acid to carbon dioxide and water. *J. Biol. Chem.* **172**:389–403.

Harvey, E. N., and Loomis, A. L. 1930. A microscope-centrifuge. *Science* **72**:42–44.

Kanaev, I. I. 1969. *Hydra: Essays on the Biology of Fresh Water Polyps*. Translated by E. T. Burrows and H. M. Lenhoff. Edited and published by H. M. Lenhoff. [Moscow: Soviet Academy of Science, 1952.]

Korzybski, A. 1948. *Science and Sanity: An Introduction to Non-Aristotelian Systems and General Semantics*, 3rd ed. International Non-Aristotelian Library, Lakeville, Conn.

Lenhoff, H. M., and Loomis, W. F. 1961. *The Biology of Hydra and of Some Other Coelenterates*. University of Miami Press, Coral Gables, Fla.

Loomis, W. F. 1949. A convenient and rapid method for calibrating working Warberg manometers. *Science* **109**:491–492.

Loomis, W. F. 1950. Stabilization of mitochondrial activity by vitrification. *Arch. Biochem.* **26**:355–357.

Loomis, W. F. 1953. The cultivation of *Hydra* under controlled conditions. *Science* **117**:565–566.

Loomis, W. F. 1954a. Environmental factors controlling growth in hydra. *J. Exp. Zool.* **126**:223–234.

Loomis, W. F. 1954b. Rapid microcolorimetric determination of dissolved oxygen. *Anal. Chem.* **26**:402–404.

Loomis, W. F. 1955. Glutathione control of the specific feeding reactions of hydra. *Ann. N.Y. Acad. Sci.* **62**:209–228.

Loomis, W. F. 1956. Improved rapid colorimetric microdetermination of dissolved oxygen. *Anal. Chem.* **28**:1347–1349.

Loomis, W. F. 1957. Sexual differentiation in hydra: Control by carbon dioxide tension. *Science* **126**:735–739.

Loomis, W. F. 1958. Direct method of determining carbon dioxide tension. *Anal. Chem.* **30**:1865–1868.

Loomis, W. F. 1967. *The God$_B$ Within*. October House, New York.

Loomis, W. F. 1970. Rickets. *Sci. Am.* **223**:76–91.

Loomis, W. F., and Lenhoff, H. M. 1956. Growth and sexual differentiation of hydra in mass culture. *J. Exp. Zool.* **132**:555–574.

Loomis, W. F., and Lipmann, F. 1948. Reversible inhibition of the coupling between phosphorylation and oxidation. *J. Biol. Chem.* **173**:807–808.

Roberts, D. 1981. Five who made it to the top. *Harvard Magazine* **83**:31–40.

Contents

Introduction 1
    Howard M. Lenhoff

1. Terminology for Morphology and Cell Types 5
    Richard D. Campbell and Hans R. Bode

I.   *Culture and Handling*

2. Collecting Hydra 17
    Richard D. Campbell

3. Identifying Hydra Species 19
    Richard D. Campbell

4. Water, Culture Solutions, and Buffers 29
    Howard M. Lenhoff

5. Visual Monitoring of pH in Solutions with Phenol Red 35
    M. Rahat and Vanda Reich

6. Hatching Brine Shrimp Larvae Axenically and/or
in a Range of Quantities 39
    Howard M. Lenhoff

7. Determining Growth Rates of Groups of Hydra and
   Budding Rates of Individual Hydra 47
      Howard M. Lenhoff

8. Culturing Large Numbers of Hydra 53
      Howard M. Lenhoff

9. Turbidimetric and Pipetimetric Measurements of
   Number of Hydra 63
      Howard M. Lenhoff

10. Culturing Hydra of the Same Species but of
    Different Sizes 67
      Richard D. Campbell and Joann J. Otto

11. Culturing Sexually Differentiated Hydra 71
      Charles L. Rutherford, David Hessinger, and
      Howard M. Lenhoff

12. Preparing Axenic Hydra 79
      M. Rahat and Vanda Reich

II. Histology

13. Preparing Hydra for Transmission Electron Microscopy 87
      Richard L. Wood

14. Preparing Hydra for Scanning Electron Microscopy 95
      Richard L. Wood

15. Preparing Hydra for Freeze-Fracture and Freeze-Etching 105
      Richard L. Wood

16. Whole Mounts for Light Microscopy 117
      Richard D. Campbell

17. Preparing Histological Sections for Light Microscopy 121
      Richard D. Campbell

18. Vital Staining: Fluorescent and Immunofluorescent,
    and Review of Nonfluorescent Dyes...................... 131
    John F. Dunne and C. Lynne Littlefield

III. Macrophotography

19. Macrophotography................................. 143
    Richard D. Campbell

IV. Quantitative Cytology

20. Dissociating Hydra Tissue into Single Cells by the
    Maceration Technique................................. 153
    Charles N. David

21. Cell Cycle Analysis of Hydra Cells...................... 157
    Charles N. David

22. Mitotic Index 165
    Richard D. Campbell

23. Measuring Numbers of Nematoblasts, Nematocytes,
    and Nematocysts 169
    Hans R. Bode, G. Scott Smith, and Patricia M. Bode

24. Marking Epithelial Cells in Living Hydra
    with Indian Ink..................................... 183
    Joann J. Otto and Richard D. Campbell

V. Techniques Using Isotopes

25. Incorporating [^{3}H]Thymidine into Hydra by
    Microinjection...................................... 189
    Charles N. David

26. Labeling with Gaseous $^{14}CO_2$ or by Feeding Hydra on

Radioactive Tissues.. 193
      Howard M. Lenhoff

27. Fractionating Small Amounts of Radioactive Tissue.......... 197
      Howard M. Lenhoff

28. Rapid Whole-Mount Radioautography..................... 205
      Howard M. Lenhoff

VI. Isolating Hydra Mutants by Sexual Inbreeding

29. Isolating Hydra Mutants by Sexual Inbreeding 211
      Tsutomu Sugiyama

VII. Manipulating Tissue Organization

30. Grafting: A Rapid Method for Transplanting Tissue.......... 225
      Harry K. MacWilliams

31. Quantitative Interpretation of Transplantation
      Phenomena 233
      Harry K. MacWilliams

32. Dissociated Tissues into Cells and the Development of
      Hydra from Aggregated Cells 251
      Kristine M. Flick and Hans R. Bode

33. Culturing Interstitial Stem Cells in Hydra Aggregates......... 261
      Charles N. David

34. Separating Viable Tissue Layers.......................... 267
      Georgia E. Lesh-Laurie

35. Preparing Ectoderm/Endoderm Chimeras.................. 273
      Nancy Wanek

Contents   xxix

VIII. Manipulating Cellular Composition in Vivo

36. Eliminating All Nonepithelial Cells Using Colchicine......... 281
        Beverly A. Marcum and Richard D. Campbell

37. Culturing Epithelial Hydra............................. 287
        Beverly A. Marcum

38. Reducing Populations of Interstitial Cells and
    Nematoblasts with Hydroxyurea......................... 291
        Hans R. Bode

39. Preparing *Hydra viridis* with Nerve Cells and No
    Interstitial Cells, or with Neither of These
    Cell Types... 295
        Patricia Novak

40. Eliminating Interstitial Cells with Nitrogen Mustard.......... 299
        Charles N. David

41. Altering Cell Population Levels by Gamma Irradiation 303
        Cheng-Mei Fradkin

42. Reducing Number of Nematocytes in the Tentacles 305
        G. Scott Smith and Hans R. Bode

*IX. Assay and Isolation of Substances Controlling
    Morphogenesis in Hydra*

43. Assay and Isolation of Substances Controlling
    Morphogenesis in Hydra............................. 311
        H. Chica Schaller, Cornelis J. P. Grimmelikhuijzen,
        and Tobias Schmidt

*X. Isolation and/or Properties of Acellular Mesoglea
    and Nematocysts*

44. Isolating Mesolamellae................................. 327
        Robert M. Day and Howard M. Lenhoff

45. Isolating Undischarged and Discharged Nematocysts
     from Acontiate Sea Anemones 331
        Richard S. Blanquet

46. Dissolving the Nematocyst Capsule Wall and Identifying
     Its Protein Component(s)............................... 335
        Richard S. Blanquet

47. Purifying an Inhibitor of Succinoxidase Activity from
     Hydra littoralis 341
        Edward S. Kline and Vaman S. Waravdekar

48. Assays for Activities of Nematocyst Venoms and
     Their Components...................................... 347
        David A. Hessinger

XI. *Analytical Procedures*

49. Special Techniques for Weighing Microgram Quantities
     of Tissue and Assaying Them for Enzyme Activities 361
        Charles L. Rutherford

50. Extracting and Characterizing Hydra RNA: Modifications
     to Allow Extraction of Undegraded Material in the
     Presence of High Levels of Degradative Enzymes............ 373
        Georgia E. Lesh-Laurie, Joseph R. Voland, and
        Stephen S. Macintyre

51. Colorimetric Analysis for Protein of Hydra 379
        Howard M. Lenhoff

52. Determining Respiration and Oxygen Evolution of Green
     Hydra with the Rank Brothers Oxygen Electrode............. 383
        Donald W. Phipps, Jr.

XII. Symbiotic Relationships

53. Isolating Endosymbiotic Algae from *Hydra viridis* 391
    L. Muscatine

54. Preparing Aposymbiotic Hydra 393
    R. L. Pardy

55. Introducing Symbiotic Algae into Aposymbiotic Hydra 399
    R. L. Pardy

56. Measuring Number of Algal Symbionts in *Hydra viridis* 401
    R. L. Pardy

57. Measuring *in Vivo* Translocation of Reduced Organic
    Carbon Compounds from Endosymbiotic Algae to
    Hydra 407
    L. Muscatine

58. Spectrophotometric Assay for Maltose 411
    That T. Ngo, Jeanne Ivy, and Howard M. Lenhoff

XIII. Methods for Epizootilogical Research with Hydra

59. Methods for Epizootilogical Research with Hydra 417
    Alan E. Stiven

XIV. Electrophysiology and Behavior

60. Recording Electrical Activity 429
    Robert K. Josephson and Norman B. Rushforth

61. Bioassay for, and Characterization of, Activators and
    Inhibitors of the Feeding Response 443
    Howard M. Lenhoff, Wyrta Heagy, and Jean Danner

Index 453

Introduction

This little creature . . . revealed to me facts so unusual, so contrary to the customary opinions on the nature of animals, that to accept them required the clearest proofs. More than once haste and predilection for the fantastic have induced naturalists into error, and have concealed matters from them that otherwise they could have identified with ease. It is not enough to say, therefore, that one has seen such and such a thing. This has no meaning unless, at the same time, the observer indicates how the reported facts were seen, and allows the reader to evaluate the manner of their observation.
As for me, I need to adhere to this rule as strictly, and more strictly, than anyone. The facts I report are too extraordinary to demand that anyone should believe me at my word. I shall therefore expose as clearly as possible every consideration that guided me, and every precaution I took to avoid self-deception.

> From the first page *Mémoires pour servir à l'histoire naturelle d'un genre de polype d'eau douce à bras en forme de cornes*, by Abraham Trembley (Leyden, 1744). Translated by Sylvia G. Lenhoff.

Simple freshwater hydra not only have long delighted students and teachers of biology, but also have served research biologists in their experiments since the early 18th century. Many notable scientific "firsts" were achieved using hydra from the time they were discovered in 1702 up to the present.

To cite but a few such instances, Anton van Leeuwenhoek, while publishing in 1702 the first description of hydra, also sketched the first instance of asexual reproduction (budding) ever observed in animals. Even more noteworthy were the discoveries presented by Abraham Trembley in his superb *Mémoires* in 1744. He described experiments conclusively proving asexual reproduction by budding, the first controlled experiments in animals on regeneration, the first successful animal grafts, the first study of phototaxis in animals without eyes, and the first vital staining of tissues.

In more modern times we have only to look at the field of electron microscopy to see many fundamental discoveries still being made using hydra as the research material. Septate desmosomes, which are found

1

between invertebrate cells, were first described in hydra. Microtubules, now recognized as major organelles of most cells, were first described in nematoblasts of hydra.

The popularity of hydra among biologists emanates not only from the relative simplicity of its structure and its graceful beauty and symmetry, but also from the ease with which it is possible to raise and maintain either large or small numbers of hydra in the laboratory. The modern science and art of "hydra husbandry" began with W. Farnsworth Loomis in 1953 and is no doubt the major factor accounting for the current renaissance of hydra research. *Hydra: Research Methods* is dedicated to this giant among modern experimental biologists.

Today hydra serves as a research animal for a host of biologists in many different fields. It is a favorite animal of a growing cadre of young developmental biologists, and for that reason the greatest share of the methods in this volume deal with that area of research.

Other general areas of research that employ hydra concern studies of algae–host endosymbioses, of the behavior and electrophysiology of animals having simple nervous systems, and of the nature of such cellular materials or secretions as mesoglea (basement membrane) and nematocyst capsules and toxins.

A number of reasons account for hydra's being a productive research animal. (1) Primarily because of its short doubling time of 2–3 days and the availability of *Artemia nauplii* as food and of synthetic "pond water," hydra is simple and inexpensive to grow in large numbers in the laboratory. (2) Animals grown asexually by budding are genetically alike. (3) The aqueous environment surrounding the animal can be controlled and modified by the investigator. (4) Because of its small size and lack of a hard endoskeleton, this multicellular animal is easy to dissociate into its component cells and organelles and to handle intact using many of the quantitative techniques applied to simpler systems. (5) Hydra is simply constructed at the tissue level of organization, having about 10 basic cell types arranged in two concentric cell layers. (6) Hydra tissue grafts easily, and isolated cells reaggregate to eventually form intact animals. (7) The cell composition of the animal can be artificially manipulated, and hydra can be altered to exist without the pluripotent interstitial cells (i cells) and those specialized cells derived from the i cells, such as nerve cells and nematocytes.

Hydra also present a number of disadvantages to the experimental biologist. For one thing, genetic research is difficult because it is difficult to get the animal to develop even a single egg, and because a fertilized egg takes about 3–6 weeks to hatch. Secondly, because hydra is not readily permeable to most nutrients, growing the animal on a defined liquid medium has not been possible. Current research, however, indicates that even these disadvantages may be overcome.

This book brings together in one package a wide assortment of methods from a variety of disciplines, a package that might otherwise take a researcher years to put together. The book is based on the conviction that many more basic discoveries are yet to be made using hydra, and that the methods we describe should be useful for years to come to biologists—researchers, teachers, and students.

Among researchers, especially graduate and postdoctoral students, *Hydra: Research Methods* should be particularly useful to the new generation of molecular biologists who are looking for simple metazoan systems with which to investigate intercellular phenomena. Likewise, those biologists whose approaches to research are more cellular and organismic may find here convenient and readily applicable experimental techniques normally not found in their literature.

Teachers should also find this book useful. Many of these methods are readily adaptable to use by undergraduate majors. Furthermore, hydra are inexpensive and simple to maintain, can be used to illustrate many general principles of biology, and in many ways are ideal animals to use in laboratory sections. High school teachers may enjoy using this book to help budding biologists in their special research projects.

Finally, this book may provide a guide for those biologists who use for their research other simple organisms such as slime molds, flatworms, roundworms, and a variety of marine invertebrates.

The idea for *Hydra: Research Methods* grew out of two kinds of summer programs. In one, hydra were used by the students for their research projects (University of Hawaii). In the other, the animal was used to illustrate its possibilities in enhancing the teaching of biology (Hebrew University, Jerusalem). Although short laboratory manuals have been prepared, both the students and the faculty expressed the need for a more comprehensive and detailed methods book. Later, at the University of California, Irvine, where four faculty in the School of Biological Sciences use hydra in many of their researches, the usefulness of such a methods book became a topic of discussion each time we initiated new undergraduate, graduate, and postdoctoral students into our laboratories.

I am grateful to the many contributors who suffered with me while we struggled to work out suitable formats to present methods that involve whole animals. I particularly thank Dr. Richard D. Campbell for editing my papers and for his contributions, advice, and encouragement.

Howard M. Lenhoff

Department of Developmental and Cell Biology
University of California, Irvine

Chapter 1

Terminology for Morphology and Cell Types

Richard D. Campbell and Hans R. Bode

MORPHOLOGY

Hydra exist as polyps, i.e., as sedentary forms of coelenterates. A single animal has the form of a tube, about 5–20 mm long and 0.3–1.0 mm wide, bearing a whorl of hollow tentacles near one end. Animals undergoing asexual reproduction produce buds, which arise as evaginations of the body wall. The body wall consists of two concentric epithelia, the *ectoderm* and *endoderm*, separated by a common acellular basement membrane, the *mesolamella* or *mesoglea*. This trilaminar structure extends throughout the entire body column tentacles and buds. The *ectoderm** (or *epidermis*) faces the environment, whereas the *endoderm* (or *gastrodermis*) lines the hollow cavity called the *gastric cavity* (*coelentron, gut*). In describing the morphology of hydra, the adjectives *apical* (or *distal*) and *basal* (or *proximal*) refer to the directions toward the tentacles and base, respectively.

Useful terminology for the body parts is summarized in Fig. 1. The apical end is termed the *hydranth*. It consists of the *hypostome*, which is a

---

* The terms *ectoderm* and *endoderm* were coined by Allman (see *Monograph on the Gymnoblastic or Tubularian Hydroids*, Ray Society, 1872) to designate the two lawyers of the coelenterate polyp, and thus have precedence over the terms *epidermis* and *gastrodermis*.—Ed.

Richard D. Campbell ● Department of Developmental and Cell Biology, University of California, Irvine, California.   Hans R. Bode ● Developmental Biology Center and Department of Developmental and Cell Biology, University of California, Irvine, California.

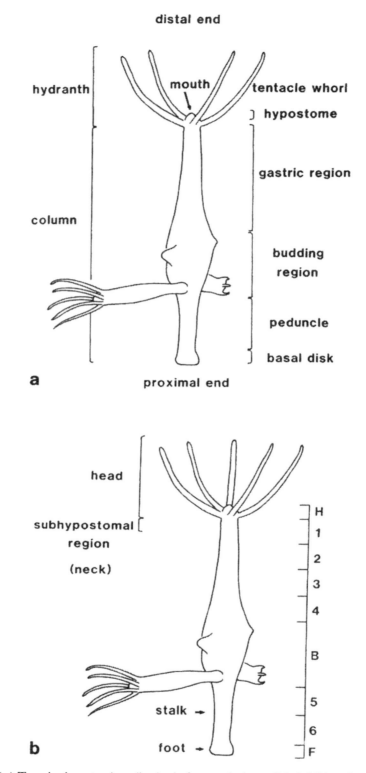

FIGURE 1. (a) Terminology to describe hydra's morphology. (b) Additional terminology.

dome-shaped or cone-shaped structure having a *mouth* at its tip, and, just beneath the hypostome, a whorl of *tentacles*. Below the hydranth, the *body column* of a budding hydra can be described as being composed of several regions (Fig. 1): The *gastric region*, between the tentacles and the most apical bud, is the largest. The *budding region (budding zone)* bears the buds which emanate in an apicobasal order of advancing stages of development. The *peduncle*, the region between the lowest bud and the basal disk, is usually narrower than the budding zone and sometimes more transparent. The *basal disk*, at the basal tip of the column, secretes a sticky material that fastens the animal to a substrate. In the center of the basal disk is an *aboral pore*.

The boundary between the gastric and budding regions is not fixed, because newer buds are initiated above older ones. Therefore, when a new bud is first recognized, the upper boundary of the budding zone "shifts" to include the level of this new bud. If a hydra has no buds, the peduncle is usually considered as the basal one-quarter to one-third of the column, and the apical part is termed the gastric region. Some authors call the zone between the peduncle and gastric region of a nonbudding animal the budding region.

Numerous vernacular and anthropomorphic terms are used to describe the overall morphology of hydra. Even Abraham Trembley (1744) described the tentacles of hydra as "arms shaped in the form of horns." The most frequently used of these terms are shown in Fig. 1b. In addition, the body may be considered to comprise the following regions: *head* (*H*), synonymous with hydranth; *regions 1–4*, forming the gastric region; *budding region* (*B*); regions 5–6, forming the peduncle; and *foot* (*F*), synonymous with basal disk. These designations are useful in describing tissue arrangements in grafting experiments. Sometimes regions 1 and 2 are referred to as the *neck* or *subhypostomal region*.

Regarding the two openings to the gastric cavity, when the mouth opens, the hypostome assumes a cylindrical shape with the edges becoming the lips. When the mouth is closed, it is undetectable except as a minute histological discontinuity in the tissue layers. The aboral pore in the center of the basal disk is sometimes visible when the hydra is freed from the substratum and the contracting column expels fluid and particles. Otherwise the pore is visible only as a minute histological discontinuity in the tissue structure.

Just before undergoing sexual reproduction, hydra develop *testes* and *ovaries* (Fig. 2). These gonads are specialized thickenings of the ectoderm, usually along the gastric region of the body column. The testes are transparent, conical or bulbous protrusions, sometimes ending in a *nipple* that serves as a sperm duct. An ovary is a low mound of distended epithelial cells

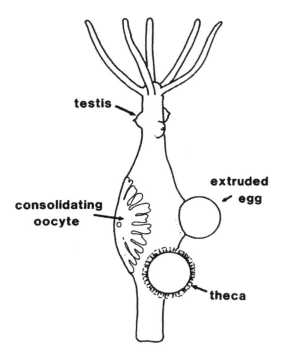

FIGURE 2. Terminology related to sexual reproduction of hydra. (Based on a monoecious species but highly diagrammatic.)

between which large numbers of interstitial cells consolidate into a single oocyte. The oocyte is extruded as an egg from the ectoderm and appears as a ball resting in a "nest" or *cushion* on the body wall. Fertilization can occur after the egg is extruded. The embryo secretes a transparent cuticle, the *embryotheca*, and detaches from the parent before or after forming the theca. In some species the theca is spherical; in others it is helmet shaped and flattens the egg against the substratum. The theca may be smooth or ornamented with spines, depending upon the species. In *hermaphroditic (monoecious)* species the testes occupy a narrow zone under the tentacles and the ovaries arise in or near the budding region. In *gonochoric (dioecious)* species the gonads may have these same locations or they may be more broadly spread along the gastric column.

Hydra contract and extend often, so that their sizes and proportions are not constant. While the lengths of hydra are often cited, there is currently no means of measuring the dimensions of a hydra in a consistent manner. Quantitative assessment of hydra's size is most reliably done in terms of cell number (Chapter 32) or dry weight (Chapter 49).

CELLS

Of the 15–20 identified cell types in hydra, most can be placed in one of three cell lineages. Each lineage contains a population of self-renewing stem cells and differentiated cells derived from those stem cells.

Epitheliomuscular Cell Lineages

The ectoderm and endoderm each contain a major epithelial cell type, called, respectively, the *ectodermal* and *endodermal epitheliomuscular cells*, or simply *epithelial cells*. These are large, vacuolated cells. Each of these cell types has muscular processes that project from the base of the cell and lie along the mesolamella. In the ectoderm the muscle processes are so long and numerous that they form a confluent mat covering the mesolamella. This sheet of parallel, adjacent processes is called the *muscle mat*. The appearances of epithelial cells in histological section are shown in Fig. 3, and in macerated tissue as viewed using phase microscopy, in Fig. 4. The cells are large, vacuolated, and usually cuboidal or columnar. At the extremities of the polyp the epithelial cells become modified in form and function and are sometimes considered as different cell types and given different names. The ectodermal epitheliomuscular cells in the tentacles develop into *battery cells* (Fig. 4b), which are more squamous than the cells of the column and do not undergo mitosis. Battery cells are characterized primarily by the cluster of nematocytes they harbor. At the basal disk the ectodermal epitheliomuscular cells transform into *basal disk gland cells* (Fig.4c). These cells are somewhat smaller than their parent cells, have much reduced vacuoles, and do not undergo mitosis. The apical portions of the gland cells are filled with small secretory granules.

The endodermal epitheliomuscular cells of the tentacles are more swollen than in the gastric region and have the shapes of helmets or wide wedges, each cell spanning one-fourth or more of the circumference around the tentacle. In the hypostome, these cells are small and tightly packed and often obscured from view by the large and numerous mucous cells. In the peduncle, the endodermal epitheliomuscular cells are very large and vacuolated and are responsible for the more or less translucent appearance of the peduncle. In the basal disk, these cells are small and rounded.

The endoderm is molded into longitudinal ridges, called *taeniolae*, that begin at the mouth and extend basally. The taeniolae give a cross section of the gastric cavity of the hypostome a star-shaped appearance and sometimes almost obliterate the cavity. At the level of the tentacle whorl, the taeniolae alternate with the bases of the tentacles. Below the tentacle whorl the

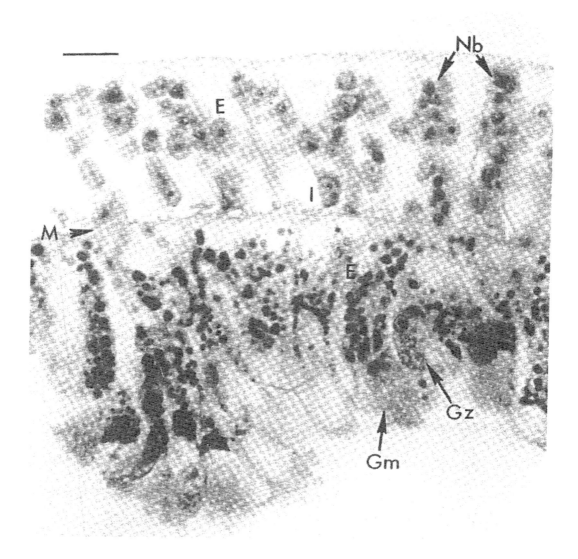

FIGURE 3. Histological cross section of the budding region of a hydra showing the ectoderm (top) and endoderm (bottom) separated by mesoglea (M). Individual labeled cells are: E, epitheliomuscular cells in both ectoderm and endoderm. The letter "E" is placed just above the nucleus of each of these cells. The large, clear space surrounding this nucleus in the ectoderm represents the large vacuole of the ectodermal epitheliomuscular cell; I, interstitial cell, situated to the right of the letter; Nb, nematoblasts in two nests, both of which have pronematocyst capsules. To the upper right of the labeled epitheliomuscular cell nucleus is a nest of young nematoblasts that do not yet have procapsules; Gz, zymogen gland cell; Gm, mucous gland cell. (*Hydra littoralis*, fixed with Lavdowsky's fixative and stained with Ehrlich's hematoxylin as described in Chapter 17.) Scale bar: 20 μm.

taeniolae become irregular in height and grade into the numerous *endodermal villi* that are borne by the endoderm of the gastric column. Taeniolae and endodermal villi are regions where the epithelial cells are particularly tall and therefore project, as a cluster or ridge, into the gastric cavity. However, all of the cells rest on the mesolamella.

Interstitial Cell Lineages

In the ectoderm, many cells are found wedged into the interstices between epithelial cells. These cells make up the interstitial cell lineage and include multipotent stem cells as well as several classes of differentiated ones. The names given to these cells have been inconsistent in the past because the functions of some of the cells have been unclear. In particular, the term *interstitial cell* has been used in many ways. With the current state of knowledge, the following terms are most appropriate. Some types of cells, such as the precursors of nerve cells, are still not well characterized; thus some additions or revisions of these terms may be required eventually.

Interstitial cells (*i cells*) are undifferentiated cells of this lineage. They have a large, clear nucleus and a prominent nucleolus and occur either as single cells or as pairs (Figs. 4e, f). These cells are often called "big interstitial cells." Some of them are multipotent stem cells having an extensive capacity to proliferate, and some are already committed to a particular differentiation pathway. Interstitial cells are found throughout the animal except in the tentacles and basal disk.

Nematoblasts (*cnidoblasts*) include all cells intermediate between the stages of interstitial cell and mature nematocyte. They occur in nests or clusters of cells ranging from 4 to 32 cells. The cells of a nest are joined by cytoplasmic bridges that represent the remnants of incomplete cytokinesis. Nematoblasts in nests of 4 cells (Fig. 4g) resemble small interstitial cells and can divide further. In nests of 8, 16, or 32 the cells are conspicuously smaller; when isolated and viewed with phase microscopy they have a granular appearance and an inconspicuous nucleolus (Fig. 4h). These cells (8–32 nest stages) have often been called "little interstitial cells" or "dividing nematoblasts." All the cells within a nest divide and differentiate synchronously.

Nematocyte differentiation is characterized by the development of an intracellular nematocyst that passes through stages of, first, a small round vesicle called the *pronematocyst vesicle* (Fig. 4i), then a large vesicle with the characteristic shape of the nematocyst, and finally a fully formed *capsule* containing visible spines and coiled tubule (Fig. 4j). Nests of nematoblasts are found throughout the body column but not in the hypostome, basal disk, or tentacles.

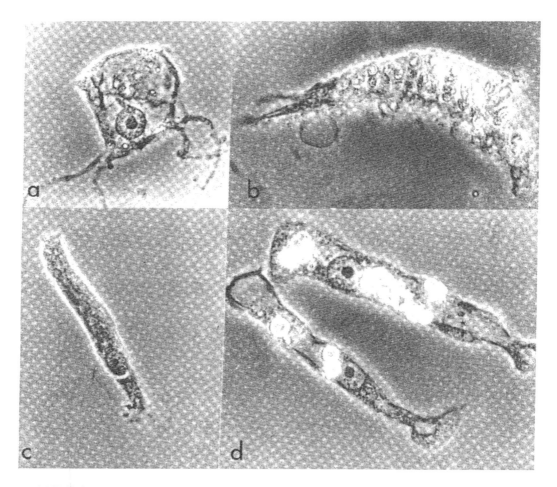

FIGURE 4. Isolated cells from macerated hydra tissue as viewed using phase microscopy. The cell types illustrated are: a, ectodermal epitheliomuscular cell from body column; b, battery cell of tentacle, harboring numerous poised nematocytes; c, basal disk gland cell; d, endodermal epitheliomuscular cells; e, single interstitial cell; f, interstitial cells in nest of two; g, nematoblasts in nest of four; h, nest of nematoblasts that do not contain pronematocyst capsules (clear vesicles); i, nest of nematoblasts containing pronematocyst capsules; j, nearly mature stenotele nematoblasts; k, neuron of body column; l, sensory cell; m, neuron of basal disk; n, zymogen cell; and o, mucous cells. All photographs are at the magnification indicated by the scale bar in Fig. 4n, which represents 20μm. (*Hydra attenuata.* See Chapter 20 for method of tissue maceration.)

Nematocytes (*cnidocytes*) contain fully developed *nematocysts* (*cnidae*) and occur singly. There are four types of nematocytes, each chacterized by a distinct type of nematocyst: the *stenotele* (penetrant), the *holotrichous isorhiza* (*streptoline glutinant*), *atrichous isorhiza* (*stereoline glutinant*), and *desmoneme* (*volvent*). These are illustrated in Chapter 3 and 23. Individual migrating nematocytes are found at the base of the ectoderm, along the surface of the muscle processes; poised nematocytes are found within chambers within the ectodermal epitheliomuscular cells.

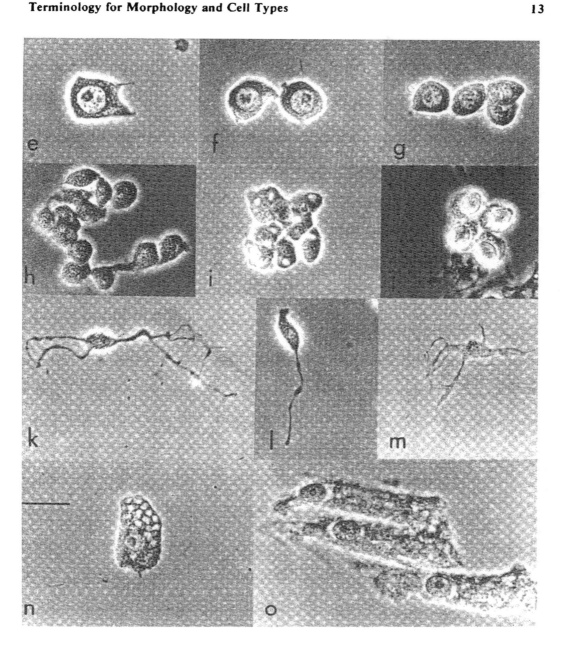

FIGURE 4. (*continued*)

   Nerve cells (*neurons*) are small cells with about two to five slender processes emanating from the cell body (Fig. 4k,m). The nucleus of a nerve cell is condensed, and the cell body has little cytoplasm. In the basal disk the nerve cells have a characteristically stubby appearance (Fig. 4m). Some nerve cells are bipolar and one end bears a flagellum; these are termed *sensory neurons* (Fig. 4l). These cells are wedged between epithelial cells of both the ectoderm and endoderm with the flagellum at the surface of the epithelium. The other neurons exhibit diverse appearances. It is not known whether they constitute a single cell type having neurosecretory, ganglionic, and sensory functions simultaneously, or whether they exist as a number of more specialized cell types. Tardent and Weber (1976) have proposed a set of terms to apply to the different classes of neurons that one can distinguish in macerated tissue. Most of the nerve cells form a *nerve net* in the interstitial spaces just above the mat of ectodermal muscle processes.

Spermatozoa and *ova* and their precursors occur only in hydra undergoing sexual differentiation. Cells in the two pathways of gamete differentiation include *mitotic gonial cells* (*spermatogonia* and *oogonia*), *meiotic gonocytes* (*primary* and *secondary spermatocytes* and *oocytes*), and *postmitotic spermatids*. These cells are found in the testes and ovaries, respectively. The very early stages cannot, on the basis of descriptions in the literature, be distinguished from interstitial cells.

Other Endodermal Cells

There are four cell types in the endoderm for which the lineage relationships to other cells are not known. One is the *basal cell* (*basal reserve cell*), which resembles an interstitial cell and is found near the mesoglea primarily in the gastric region. The other three cell types are *gland cells*, which fall into two classes: *zymogen cells* and *mucous cells*. The zymogen cell is characterized by its large (about 2 μm in diameter), dense secretory vesicles (Fig. 4n). Zymogen cells occur throughout the body column but not in the hypostome or basal disk. Mucous cells are present as two types, a *foamy* ("*spumeuse*") type and a *granular* ("*spheruleuse*") type. The foamy one (Fig. 4o) is filled with vesicles 1–2 μm in diameter that often appear to be partially fused into a reticulum. The granular mucous cell is filled with discrete, small granules (less than 1 μm in diameter). Mucous cells are found chiefly in the hypostome.

REFERENCES

(This article has not attempted to trace the origins of each term. The article cited below offers additional terminology regarding nerve cells of hydra.)

Tardent, P., and C. Weber, 1976. A qualitative and quantitative inventory of nervous cells in *Hydra attentuata* Pall. In: *Coelenterate Ecology and Behavior* (G. O. Mackie, ed.), Plenum Press, New York, pp. 501–512.

Part I

Culture and Handling

Chapter 2

Collecting Hydra

Richard D. Campbell

PURPOSE

To find hydra in, and collect them from their natural habitats.

INTRODUCTION

Hydra occur in most permanent bodies of fresh water. They are usually more abundant in quiet water than in swiftly moving water. They are often abundant on water plants at all levels of a pond or lake. When plants are not abundant, hydra are most numerous on the undersides of sticks and leaves on the bottom. At lake shores where there is wave action, they are most abundant on the undersides of stones. In swift streams and rivers they are usually found only on the undersides of stones and sticks on the bottom, especially below exits from lakes or below falls. Hydra are often abundant in quiet arms of rapid streams.

MATERIALS

Large white enamel or plastic tray several inches deep or wide-mouthed gallon jars; Pasteur pipets; magnifying glass.

Richard D. Campbell ● Department of Developmental and Cell Biology, University of California, Irvine, California.

PROCEDURES

There are two basic methods for collecting hydra.

1. Fill the tray or large jar with water from a pond, lake, or stream. Include moderate amounts of pondweeds, sticks, and stones. Set the vessel in a well-lighted room or on a window sill. After 2 hr examine the sides and surface for hydra. In a tray the colored hydra will stand out against the white surface. In a jar set so the light is coming from behind, hydra will appear as silhouettes against the bright background. Pipet them out into a culture vessel. Reexamine the tray or jar again 24 or 48 hr later, as more hydra may appear.

2. Bend over a pond or stream and examine materials such as leaves, sticks, and weeds in the water. Because hydra are usually on the undersides of substrates, turn over the material to see the polyps. Do these movements very slowly to avoid stimulating the hydra to contract. Hydra will show up dark or bright according to the background. If it is too awkward to look directly into the water, lift the substrate materials into a wide tray for examination. Allow a few minutes for the polyps to relax and stretch out.

Method 1 is simpler and is suitable for collecting at one or two sites. It may take a day or two, however, to find hydra, if at all. Method 2 is best for sampling a number of different localities. It can also be more thorough since one can continue sampling as long as desired. However, it requires more experience to recognize hydra in the field.

PRECAUTIONS

Hydra may undergo "depression" when transferred from their natural habitat to laboratory conditions. Therefore, keep them at a low temperature (10–15°C) and unfed; it also helps to flush out their gastric cavities daily (see Chapter 37).

Hydra often have parasites and/or ectocommensals. These may overgrow the hydra in the laboratory. There are three common parasites or commensals of hydra: an amoeba, *Hydramoeba*; a ciliated protozoa, *Kerona*; and a cladoceran, *Anchistropus* (see Chapter 59). Clean the infested hydra by brushing them, or by picking off parasites individually using a mouth pipet with a fine capillary tip just large enough to admit one parasite at a time. Repeat the cleaning twice a day for 2 or 3 days.

If a collection is being made as a survey of species present, take care to look for inconspicuous types. Large, bright hydra with long tentacles (such as *Pelmatohydra oligactis*) are so much more conspicuous than some smaller species, however, that they may capture one's attention to the exclusion of other species.

Chapter 3

Identifying Hydra Species

Richard D. Campbell

PURPOSE

Hydra species differ in morphology, development, physiology, and ecology. Repeatability of experiments therefore will depend upon correct identification. I outline a procedure for distinguishing between the types of hydra used most frequently in research. Three major criteria are used: (1) presence or absence of symbiotic algae, (2) arrangement of tentacles on buds, and (3) shape of the holotrichous isorhiza nematocyst.

INTRODUCTION

Hydra systematics are in an unsettled state. No doubt the partial evolutionary isolation of hydra in separate bodies of water and the preponderance of asexual reproduction result in a great number of hydra types that may show wide ranges of variation in morphology. In addition, only a few reliable characteristics of the polyp are suitable for identification purposes, and some of these, such as those involving several reproductive structures, may not be present when one wishes to classify them. Thus, traditional taxonomic methods may not be easily applied to hydra.

By this method, there are four hydra groups to which polyps may be referred when specific determinations are impossible. Each group contains several species that may be distinguished from one another only with

Richard D. Campbell ● Department of Developmental and Cell Biology, University of California, Irvine, California.

19

difficulty. In identifying a hydra it is most useful to first assign the hydra to one of the four groups, and then, if possible, to assign it to a species or species cluster within the group.

I do not cover all species of hydra, but focus on those adequately described North American species and on other species of the world that are being used in laboratories.

The most important literature on hydra systematics is Schulze (1917), Hyman (1929), Ewer (1948), Semal-van Gansen (1954), Forrest (1963), Grayson (1971), and the review of Kanaev (1969).

MATERIALS

To observe general morphology, place hydra in a dish of pond water or culture solution, and use a magnifying glass or dissecting microscope, a pipet, and a dissection probe.

To observe nematocysts, use a bright-field compound microscope with objectives of 40 and 100 (oil immersion) powers. Also needed are a microscope slide and cover slip; petroleum jelly or silicone stopcock grease in a 1- to 5-ml syringe without a needle; a small scalpel; small squares of filter paper; hydra in a dish, preferably a plastic Petri dish; a Pasteur pipet; and a compound microscope with a calibrated ocular reticle.

Use hydra only when they are healthy, preferably those which are freshly collected or which are actively budding in the laboratory.

PROCEDURES

Preparing Tissue for Examining Nematocysts

1. Isolate the hydranth of a hydra with a cut immediately under the ringlet of tentacles.

2. Transfer the hydranth to a microscope slide in a large drop of pond or culture water.

3. Place a tiny drop (about 1 mm across) of silicone grease or petroleum jelly on the underside of each corner of a cover glass and set the cover slip over the hydranth. The grease should hold the glass above the hydranth.

4. Place the slide in a microscope and focus on a tentacle base using a 40× objective.

5. Using a needle, slowly press the cover slip down on the four corners and absorb any water expressed with filter paper. Stop pressing when the tentacles are flattened to about twice their original diameters. Flattening the

tentacles immobilizes the tentacles and reorients most of the nematocysts so that their long axes are horizontal. Do not flatten the tentacles too much or the nematocysts will break.

Examining Undischarged Holotrichous Isorhiza Nematocysts

1. Search along the tentacle length for holotrichous isorhiza nematocysts by a process of elimination using Fig. 1 as a guide.

2. First, locate the two most distinctive nematocyst types: the abundant desmoneme with a single internal coil and the large, pear-shaped stenotele with the conspicuous axial barbs and transverse loops. More searching may be required to find the holotrichous isorhiza and the other remaining type, the atrichous isorhiza. The holotrichous isorhiza is the larger of these two and the only one of the two in which individual coils of the inverted tube are clearly visible. If holotrichous isorhizas cannot be located on the tentacles, they may be located (along with stenoteles) at the surface of the body column ectoderm in the peduncle.

3. Measure the maximum length and maximum width of five holotrichous isorhizas and from these obtain an average length and an average width.

Note: For some identifications, measurements of the lengths of other nematocysts will also be necessary.

Determining the Origin of Tentacles on Buds

Examine the order in which tentacles arise on young buds. Use a dissecting microscope. Note whether the tentacles arise simultaneously (or

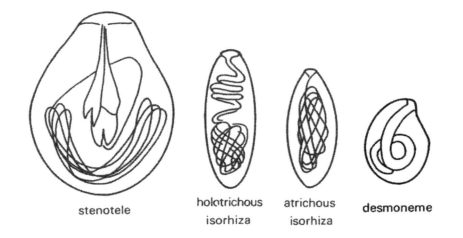

FIGURE 1. The four types of hydra nematocysts.

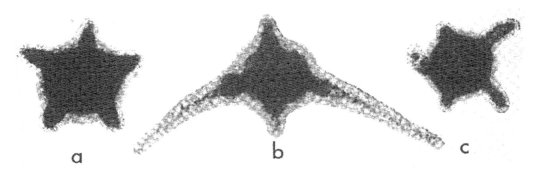

FIGURE 2. Comparison of tentacle origin on buds as viewed toward the hypostome of the bud: (a) tentacles arising simultaneously (*H. hymanae*); (b) lateral tentacles arising conspicuously early (*H. oligactis*); (c) tentacles arising in slightly staggered sequence (*H. attenuata*). Scale bar: 0.2 mm.

slightly staggered) or whether two lateral tentacles arise and take on a slender shape before the other tentacles appear (Fig. 2). Tentacles arising in a slightly staggered sequence appear to be the same length when a bud is nearly complete (stages 8–9 in Otto and Campbell, 1977); in species where two lateral tentacles arise early, these two tentacles are conspicuously longer during bud development.

Assigning Hydra to One of the Four Groups

Using Key I, determine which of the four groups is represented by your specimen.

Specific Identification within Subgroups

Viridissima Group

Species of this group are sometimes referred to the genus *Chlorohydra*. They include *Hydra viridissima* (Pallas, 1766),* *Hydra hadleyi*, and several other poorly known species. Hydra of these species almost always harbor numerous symbiotic algae in the endodermal cells, and other hydra with green color lose the color during laboratory culture. Hence, a green color retained during laboratory culture is almost always diagnostic for natural specimens of these species (see Goetsch, 1924, for one exception).

---

* Pallas (1766) gave the name *H. viridissima* to the green hydra 1 year before Linnaeus (1767) named the species *Hydra viridis*; therefore, according to the International Code of Zoological Nomenclature, the name *H. viridissima* has priority. [In deference to current usage, *H. viridis* is used throughout the rest of this volume—Ed.]

KEY I. The four major hydra groups, with names of common American species

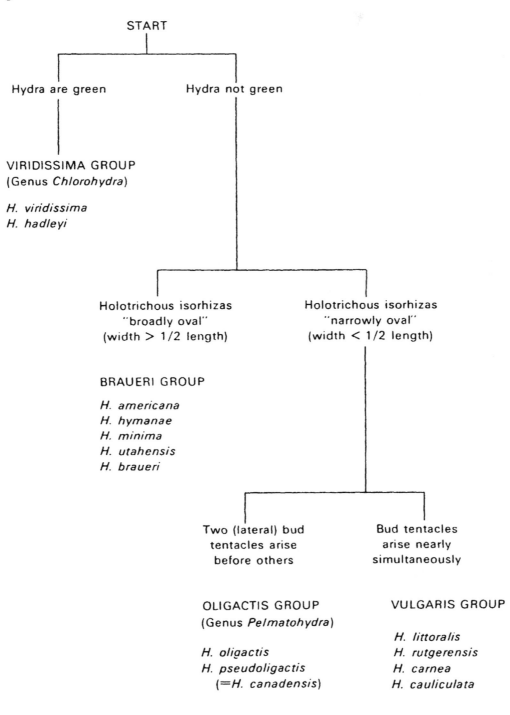

START

Hydra are green

Hydra not green

VIRIDISSIMA GROUP
(Genus *Chlorohydra*)

H. viridissima
H. hadleyi

Holotrichous isorhizas
"broadly oval"
(width > 1/2 length)

Holotrichous isorhizas
"narrowly oval"
(width < 1/2 length)

BRAUERI GROUP

H. americana
H. hymanae
H. minima
H. utahensis
H. braueri

Two (lateral) bud
tentacles arise
before others

Bud tentacles
arise nearly
simultaneously

OLIGACTIS GROUP
(Genus *Pelmatohydra*)

H. oligactis
H. pseudoligactis
  (=*H. canadensis*)

VULGARIS GROUP

H. littoralis
H. rutgerensis
H. carnea
H. cauliculata

Laboratory cultures of aposymbiotic hydra of the *viridissima* group can be recognized on the basis of the small nematocyst sizes (see Fig. 3, for nematocyst sizes.) Hydra of the *viridissima* group are monoecious.

Of the two species of green hydra used in laboratory, systematic distinction is drawn on the basis of embryotheca structure. The embryo attached to a polyp of *H. hadleyi* is underlain by an empty, secondary chamber which is absent in *H. viridissima* (although the validity of this character is questioned by Grayson, 1971). *H. viridissima* is moderate in size and described from Europe, while *H. hadleyi* is a smaller hydra and is described from North America (see Forrest, 1963). Laboratory cultures of green hydra from different localities exhibit physiological and developmental differences.

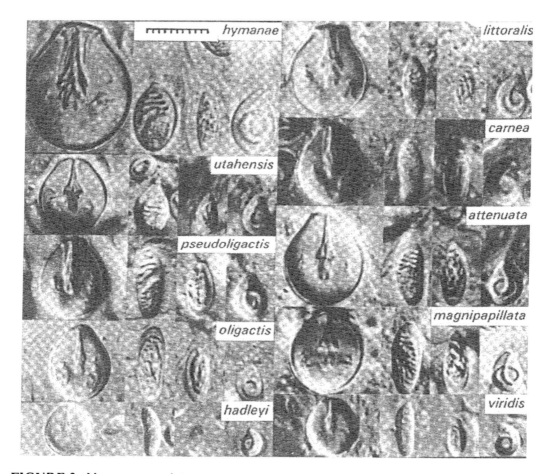

FIGURE 3. Nematocysts of the commonly used laboratory hydra species. Nematocysts in a single hydra vary in size and shape, so these illustrations can only be used as guides. Scale bar: 10 μm.

Braueri Group

These species, rarely cultured in the laboratory, include *Hydra circumcincta* (=*Hydra ovata*, =*Hydra stellata*) (Europe and Asia); *Hydra braueri* (Europe and North America); *Hydra americana, Hydra hymanae*, and *Hydra utahensis* (North America); and *Hydra parva* (Japan). The most distinctive character is the broad shape of the holotrichous isorhiza (Fig. 3). Most are small, unstalked, and monoecious. Key II may be used to distinguish between the American species of the *braueri* group.

Oligactis Group

Species of this group are sometimes referred to the genus *Pelmatohydra*. They include *Hydra oligactis* (=*Hydra fusca*) (cosmopolitan), *Hydra pseudoligactis* (=*Hydra canadensis*) (North America), and *Hydra robusta* (Japan).

KEY II. American species of the *braueri* group

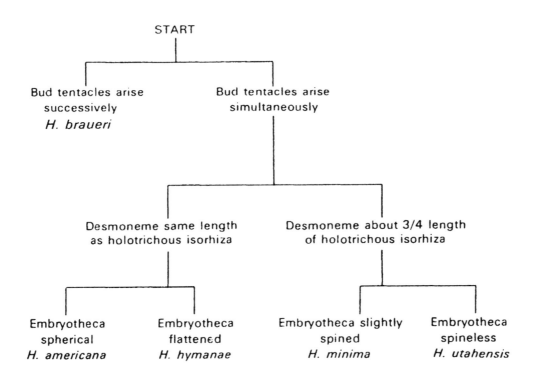

These hydra are distinctive in appearance. They have conspicuous stalks (peduncles) and long tentacles and are large. The two lateral tentacles of buds arise earlier and are longer than the other tentacles (Fig. 2b). These hydra often have a yellow-golden pigment, some of which is in the ectoderm, which under laboratory culture gives the polyps a characteristic yellowish appearance. They are strictly dioecious. Species of the *oligactis* group can be distinguished using Key III.

Vulgaris Group

These hydra are widely used in research. The group includes *Hydra littoralis* (North America), *Hydra attenuata* (=*Hydra vulgaris*) (Europe), and *Hydra magnipapillata* (Japan), all very similar species which can only be easily distinguished on the basis of their geographical origin. These three are the most frequently studied species in the *vulgaris* group. They tend to be dioecious, but hermaphroditism and sex reversals occur. Another species, *Hydra pirardi*, has also been used in research, and may be distinguished from the other three species on the basis of its larger size and its nematocysts (Brien, 1961). Its stenotele is conspicuously longer and more slender than that of the other three species mentioned. The *vulgaris* group also embraces the following North American species, which do not appear frequently in the experimental literature: *Hydra carnea, Hydra cauliculata,* and *Hydra rutgerensis*. Key IV may be used to distinguish between the American species of the *vulgaris* group.

KEY III. Species of the *oligactis* group

1. Holotrichous isorhizas with transverse coils . . . *H. pseudoligactis.*

1. Holotrichous isorhizas without transverse coils . . . Go to items 2.

2. Hydra from Japan . . . *H. robusta.*

2. Hydra from elsewhere . . . *H. oligactis.*

KEY IV. Major American species of the *vulgaris* group

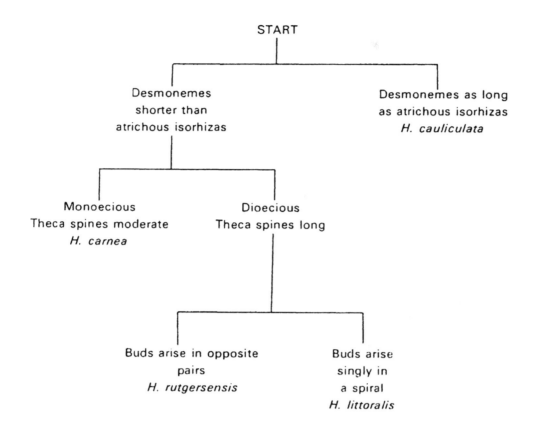

Further Identification

Numerous other characters, particularly the nature of the embryotheca, shapes and sizes of all nematocysts, and body form, are used in hydra taxonomy. For descriptions of these characters, and for identifying species not treated here, consult the references. To find the authors and locations of the descriptions of these species, as well as some of the ambiguities of the names, see Ewer (1948) and Grayson (1971).

REFERENCES

Brien, P. 1961. Étude d'*Hydra pirardi* (nov. spec). Origine et répartition des nématocystes, gamétogénèse, involution postgamétique, évolution réversible des cellules interstitielles. *Bull. Biol. Fr. Belg.* **95**:301–364.

Ewer, R. E. 1948. A review of the Hydridae and two new species of hydra from Natal. *Proc. Zool. Soc. London* **118**:226–244.

Forrest, Helen. 1963. Taxonomic studies on the hydras of North America. VIII. Descriptions of two new species, with new records and a key to the North American hydras. *Trans. Am. Microsc. Soc.* **82**:6–17.

Goetsch, W. 1924. Die Symbiose der Süsswasser-Hydroiden und ihre künstliche Beeinflussung. *Z. Morphol. Oekol. Tiere* **1**:660–751.

Grayson, Robin F. 1971. The freshwater hydras of Europe. I. A review of the European species. *Arch. Hydrobiol.* **68**:436–449.

Hadley, Charles E., and Forrest, Helen. 1949. Taxonomic studies on the hydras of North America. 6. Description of *Hydra hymanae. Am. Mus. Novit.* **1423**:1–14.

Hyman, L. H. 1929. Taxonomic studies of the hydras of North America. I. General remarks and description of *Hydra americana,* new species. *Trans. Am. Microsc. Soc.* **48**:242–255.

Kanaev, I. I. 1969. *Hydra: Essays on the Biology of Fresh Water Polyps.* Translated by E. T. Burrows and H. M. Lenhoff. Edited and published by H. M. Lenhoff. [Moscow: Soviet Academy of Science, 1952.]

Linnaeus, C. 1767. *Systema naturae per regna tria naturae, secundum classes, ordines, genera, species, cum characteribus, differentiis, synonymis locis* ... Editio duidecima. reformata. L. Salvii, Holmiae.

Otto, J. J., and Campbell, R. D. 1977. Budding in *Hydra attentuata*: Bud stages and fate map. *J. Exp. Zool.* **200**:417–428.

Pallas, P. S. 1766. *Elenchus zoophytorum, sistens generum adumbrationes generaliores et specierum cognitarum succinctas descriptiones cum selectis auctorum synonymis.* Petrum van Cleef, Hagae-Comitum, p. 31.

Schulze, Paul. 1917. Neue Beiträge zu einer monographie der Gattung Hydra. *Arch. Biontol.* **4**:31–119.

Semal-van Gansen, P. 1954. Etude d'une espèce: *Hydra attentuata* Pallas. *Ann. Soc. R. Zool. Belg.* **85**:187–216.

Chapter 4

Water, Culture Solutions, and Buffers

Howard M. Lenhoff

PURPOSE

To provide directions for preparing a variety of solutions in which hydra can be cultured or maintained for extended periods.

INTRODUCTION

Hydra is a naked animal, i.e., half of its epithelial cells are in direct contact with its aqueous environment, whereas the rest of its cells are only one cell layer away. Hence, the composition of that solution may affect most of the activities of the animal.

The term *culture medium*, as generally used when referring to micro-organisms, cannot be applied to hydra in the same manner. For hydra, the culture medium, or more properly, culture solution, does not supply the nutrients for growth, but rather serves as a solution in which the animal can be bathed and still carry out its vital functions properly.

One feature of this solution, and a key to culturing hydra, is the purity of the water. Many problems met with in culturing hydra can be traced to contaminants in the water. These contaminants are usually copper ions or ions of other heavy metals; procedures have to be used to protect hydra from them.

Howard M. Lenhoff ● Department of Developmental and Cell Biology, University of California, Irvine, California.

29

A second key feature is the ionic composition of the solution. Hydra require a range of specific ions in their environment. Wide variation from that range can alter the animals growth rate (Loomis, 1954; Lenhoff and Bovaird, 1960; Muscatine and Lenhoff, 1965), physiology (Lenhoff, 1965; Loomis and Lenhoff, 1957), and development (Loomis, 1953; Lenhoff and Bovaird, 1960).

MATERIALS

The salts and buffers needed to prepare the culture solutions are described in Table I. Other substances used are Na_2EDTA, histidine, imidazole, phthalate, cacodylic acid, and sodium phosphate. Also useful are calibrated liquid dispensers and a conductivity meter (ohmmeter).

Pure water may be obtained by a number of means: commercially installed reverse osmosis equipment; columns of resins to removed organics or ions (e.g., from Barnstead Still and Sterilizer Co.); a distilling apparatus (e.g., from Bellco Co.); or various combinations of the three.

PREPARING PURE WATER

PROCEDURES AND COMMENTS

You can obtain pure water by a number of methods. The most convenient ways are to have a piped source of large quantities of distilled water or water purified by reverse osmosis. Usually, however, waters produced in large volumes are not of the highest purity, and often the equipment is subject to mechanical failure. Therefore, as a backup, you should pass all mass-produced waters through a mixed-bed resin to remove final traces of contaminating ions. We routinely pass our deionized water, produced by reverse osmosis, through a large tank of mixed-bed resin that has a small light that stays lit as long as the resins are effective.

Do not pass untreated tap water directly through mixed-bed resins, because the high content of ions in tap water will deactivate most such columns within days if you use any sizeable quantities (60–100 liters/day) of water, and especially if your tap water is hard. If you plan to use hydra only occasionally, as for teaching purposes, and do not have a ready supply of pure water, you may detoxify the heavy metals present in most tap water by the use of Na_2EDTA (see below: Preparing Culture Solutions).

TABLE I. Composition of Stock and Regular Strength Culture Solutions

Culture solution	pH	Components of stock solutions	Dilution (to prepare culture solution)	Final concentration
CN	7.6	(a) 0.1 M NaHCO$_3$	1 in 1000	10^{-4} M
		(b) 1.0 M CaCl$_2$	1 in 1000	10^{-3} M
KNC	7.6	(a) 0.1 M NaHCO$_3$	1 in 1000	10^{-4} M
		0.1 M KCl		10^{-4} M
		(b) 1.0 M CaCl$_2$	1 in 1000	10^{-3} M
M	7.8	[a](a) 1.166 M tris-HCl buffer[b]	6 in 1000	10^{-3} M
		0.166 M NaHCO$_3$		10^{-3} M
		0.016 M KCl		10^{-4} M
		0.016 M MgCl$_2$		10^{-4} M
		(b) 1.0 M CaCl$_2$	1 in 1000	10^{-3} M

[a] Three liters of stock M solution (a) may be made by mixing 1000 ml 0.5 M tris-HCl buffer pH 7.6–7.8, 500 ml 1.0 M NaHCO$_3$, 50 ml 1.0 M KCl, 50 ml 1.0 M MgCl$_2$, and 1400 ml distilled water.

[b] Prepare tris-HCl buffer from a 1 M solution of tris adjusted to pH 7.6–7.8 with a mixture of equal volumes of water and concentrated HCl. Dilute the solution to almost 2 liters, check the pH and readjust it as required; then bring it to a final volume of 2 liters. Refrigerate this stock buffer when it is not being used.

PRECAUTIONS

For emergencies, keep a small reservoir of pure water available. I recommend that you maintain a distilling apparatus set up for use in emergencies. We describe elsewhere a simply operated, inexpensive, and self-regulated system for preparing and distributing large volumes of distilled–deionized water (Reasor and Lenhoff, 1968).

PREPARING CULTURE SOLUTIONS

COMMENTS

The specific cations affecting the growth and maintenance of hydra have been particularly well studied. Both calcium (Loomis, 1954) and sodium ions (Lenhoff and Bovaird, 1960; Muscatine and Lenhoff, 1965) are indispensable to *Hydra littoralis* and *Hydra viridis*. Magnesium and potassium ions, though not absolute requirements, enhance the growth rate of *H. viridis*. (Muscatine and Lenhoff, 1965). Potassium but not magnesium ions have a similar effect upon *H. littoralis* (Lenhoff, 1966). Chloride ions are usually the anions of choice for growing hydra, although hydra can grow well on others such as NO_3^- or HCO_3^-. The requirement of all ions for hydra were tested by measuring their effects on the logarithmic growth rates of the animal (Chapter 7).

I recommend that you use one of the three culture solutions listed in Table I. Solution CN is similar to Loomis' L solution (1954) developed for growing *H. littoralis*; this solution is useful in experiments, such as those involving glutathione, in which K^+ affect the animals negatively. Solution KNC is suitable for all brown hydras, whereas M solution (Muscatine and Lenhoff, 1965) prepared with either NaCl or $NaHCO_3$ works for both the green and the brown hydras. The doubling times and growth rates (see Chapter 7) in M solution of a number of species of hydras are listed in Table II.

PROCEDURES

Always use pure water. Prepare in advance liter amounts of the concentrated stock solutions, as listed in Table I. Because concentrated $CaCl_2$ and $NaHCO_3$ precipitate when mixed together, always prepare stock $CaCl_2$ separately. Keep the stock solution of tris buffer refrigerated to retard bacterial growth.

To dispense the stock solution conveniently and accurately ($\pm$ 1%), place calibrated delivery spouts on 1-liter plastic bottles containing the stock solutions. When preparing 5-liter amounts of culture solutions, we use a 30-ml dispenser on the M stock solution and a 5-ml dispenser on all others. Do not add the two stock solutions until sufficient water has been first added to

TABLE II. Doubling Times and Growth Rates of Some Hydra Species Reared in M Solution at 25°C

Hydra species	Doubling time (days) T	Growth rate constant k
Pelmatohydra pseudoligactis	2.40	0.288
Pelmatohydra oligactis	1.98	0.350
Hydra pirardi[a]	3.50	0.198
H. viridis (symb.)	1.20	0.577
H. viridis[b] (aposymb.)	1.88	0.368
H. littoralis	1.73	0.400

[a] Fed twice daily; all others were fed once daily.
[b] The aposymbiotic animals were not obtained from the symbiotized animals by glycerol treatment (Whitney. 1907), but were derived from an individual hatched from an algae-free embryo of *H. viridis* (Florida strain. 1961).

the container; otherwise precipitates of calcium carbonates may form.

To prepare large quantities of culture solution, such as 100- to 200-liter batches, dispense the stock solutions using large plastic graduated cylinders rather than the calibrated delivery spouts. Accordingly, prepare large batches of stock solutions. To prepare 8 liters of ingredient (a) of M solution (Table I), for example, add 1.8 liters distilled water, 2.7 liters 0.5 M tris buffer, 270 ml 5 M $NaHCO_3$ (or NaCl), 135 ml 1 M KCl, and 135 ml 1 M $MgCl_2$. For every 100 liters "M" solution needed, add 600 ml of that solution and 100 ml of 1 M $CaCl_2$ and stir well.

Alternate Solutions. In emergencies, or in situations in which you are not concerned about the overall composition of the culture solution as long as the hydra can survive in it, you may wish to use the bicarbonate–Versene–tap-water (BVT) solution (Loomis and Lenhoff, 1956). To prepare the stock solution, dissolve 20 g $NaHCO_3$ and 10 g Na_2EDTA in 1 liter tap water. Add 5 ml of this solution to 5 liters tap water. The Na_2EDTA chelates the toxic copper ions usually present in tap water. Most tap water has sufficient Ca^{2+} to support hydra growth; nonetheless you may wish to add 1 ml 10^{-3} M $CaCl_2$ to each liter of tap water to assure an adequate supply of Ca^{2+}.

For research experiments, however, do not use BVT. Tap water is a solution of unknown ionic composition and varies from laboratory to laboratory. Also, although the EDTA chelates toxic copper, it also chelates calcium and thus will vary its effective concentration.

There may be occasions to grow or maintain hydra under conditions of different pH values. Buffers that have been tried and found suitable for hydra are phthalate, histidine, imidazole, cacodylate, maleate, and phosphate. Do not add the phosphate directly to the $CaCl_2$ stock or they will precipitate. Do not use histidine buffer for long periods, as it supports bacterial growth.

PRECAUTIONS

Recall that hydra are freshwater animals and do not tolerate solutions of high ionic strengths (Loomis, 1954). Do not prepare any solution greater than 10 mosm. When in doubt of the ionic strength of a solution, test the conductivity with an ohmmeter.

If you place hydra in culture solutions altered by having the wrong salt mixture, unfavorable pH, or toxic components, the animal will go through a series of changes depending upon the severity of the alteration. Under mildly "toxic" conditions, the hydra may not capture or ingest food, they may fail to maintain an "erect" position, and the tentacles may become short and stubby. Under more severe conditions, the animals may actually begin to disintegrate, with the tentacles going first.

In all cases where you doubt the quality of a batch of culture solution, transfer the hydra in those solutions into a solution that you are confident is made up correctly. Dispose of all suspect solutions, including stock ones; clean all containers; and prepare fresh solutions.

For such emergencies, it is best to have a source of backup culture solution always in hand. If you do not, then remove some solution from cultures in which you are confident that the hydra are healthy. Use that solution to preserve hydra taken from faulty solutions while you prepare fresh solution.

REFERENCES

Lenhoff, H. M. 1965. Some physiochemical aspects of the macro- and microenvironments surrounding hydra during activation of their feeding behavior. *Am. Zool.* 5:515–524.

Lenhoff, H. M. 1966. Influence of monovalent cations on the growth of *Hydra littoralis. J. Exp. Zool.* 163:151–156.

Lenhoff, H. M., and Bovaird, J. 1960. The requirement of trace amounts of environmental sodium for the growth and development of *Hydra. Exp. Cell Res.* 20:384–34.

Lenhoff, H. M., and Brown, R. D. 1970. Mass culture of hydra: An improved method and its application to other aquatic invertebrates. *Lab. Anim.* 4:139–154.

Lenhoff, H. M., and Loomis, W. F. 1957. Environmental factors controlling respiration in hydra. *J. Exp. Zool.* 134:171–182.

Loomis. W. F. 1953. The cultivation of *Hydra* under controlled conditions. *Science* 117:565–566.

Loomis. W. F. 1954. Environmental factors controlling growth in hydra. *J. Exp. Zool.* 126:223–234.

Loomis. W. F., and Lenhoff, H. M. 1956. Growth and sexual differentiation of hydra in mass culture. *J. Exp. Zool.* 132:555–574.

Muscatine, L., and Lenhoff, H. M. 1965. Symbiosis of hydra and algae. I. Effects of some environmental cations on growth of symbiotic and aposymbiotic hydra. *Biol. Bull.* 128:415–424.

Reasor, H. S., and Lenhoff, H. M. Distilled-deionized water: A system for preparing and distributing large volumes. *Science* 161:277–279.

Chapter 5

Visual Monitoring of pH in Solutions with Phenol Red

M. Rahat and Vanda Reich

PURPOSE

To keep track by visual observation of the pH and pH changes of cultures and stock solutions.

INTRODUCTION

There are many reasons for wishing to have a simple means for constantly monitoring the pH of solutions and culture media. Such monitoring enables the detection of (1) some mistakes made in preparing culture and experimental solutions; (2) pH changes resulting from bacterial or other contamination in experimental or stock solutions; and (3) pH changes in long-term experiments in which the animals should not be disturbed, e.g., hydra kept in bacteria-free conditions (see Chapter 12).

This technique has been borrowed and adopted by us from tissue culture technology in which Phenol Red indicator is used in almost all media (e.g., see GIBCO nutritional media for tissue cultures, available from GIBCO, Grand Island, NY 14072). The wide use of this indicator supports the view that it is not toxic. Our experience of using Phenol Red with several species of hydra for over 2 years shows no observable detrimental effects on the animals.

M. Rahat and Vanda Reich ● Department of Zoology, The Hebrew University of Jerusalem, Israel.

Use of this method can provide virtually a constant record of solution pH, which is analogous to having the electrode of a recording pH meter continuously in your solution. Hence, with a sweep of the eye over your cultures each day, you can instantly detect any pH change. If no such change is observed, this monitoring gives confidence that at least one of the many variables that can affect hydra cultures has remained constant.

MATERIALS

Phenol Red pH indicator (pH 6.8 yellow, pH 8.4 red, pK 7.9, e.g., BDH Chemical Co., England); M solution; one 2-liter flask; eight 250-ml volumetric or Florence flasks; two 10-ml pipets; chloroform; Parafilm; 0.1 N HCL; 0.1 N NaOH.

PROCEDURES

Preparation of Reference Solutions

Prepare 2 liters M solution containing 1 mg/liter Phenol Red. Take out an aliquot of 250 ml and measure its pH with a pH meter (pH sould be about 8.2). Place the solution in a 250-ml volumetric flask. Add 1 ml chloroform to the flask to prevent bacterial growth and seal with a stopper and parafilm.

To a series of seven more volumetric flasks, add 250 ml of M solution, with each pH adjusted 0.2 units below the preceding one. This series covers the pH range of 6.8–8.4. Add chloroform and seal as above.

The solutions in these flasks serve as reference color standards for your experimental solutions. The depth of color of the solution in the neck of the flask serves as a reference for solutions in test tubes, while that in the body of the flask serves for bulk solutions.

Application

To all solutions whose pH you want to monitor, add 1 mg/liter Phenol Red. To determine pH within the above range, compare the color of the solution with those of the reference standards.

It is convenient to prepare a stock solution of 0.1% (= 1 mg/ml) Phenol Red and to add the desired volume to each solution.

PRECAUTIONS

Whenever using ingredients that are themselves colored, such as certain nutrients or antibiotics, prepare new reference standards containing those ingredients. Colorblind laboratory personnel may have difficulty using this method.

ACKNOWLEDGMENTS. We thank the United States–Israel Binational Science Foundation Fund for support (Grant No. 1827).

Chapter 6

Hatching Brine Shrimp Larvae Axenically and/or in a Range of Quantities

Howard M. Lenhoff

PURPOSE

To hatch a range of quantities of brine shrimp for feeding hydra, and to prepare axenic larvae (i.e. free of other organisms).

INTRODUCTION

Nauplii (newly hatched larvae) of the brine shrimp *Artemia salina* (Leach) are still the most convenient and suitable food for rearing hydra. The *Artemia* can be purchased as inexpensive and stable dormant cysts, which can reliably yield large numbers of nauplii on demand. When the cysts are placed in a saline solution (Croghan, 1958) at room temperature and are supplied with adequate oxygen (Clegg, 1964), live, swimming nauplii will hatch from them within 24–48 hr.

I present here methods for (1) preparing axenic nauplii, (2) preparing alternate hatching solutions, (3) hatching varying amounts of nauplii ranging from numbers required simply to maintain sparse culture of hydra to those needed to grow kilogram quantities of the animal, (4) incubating cysts, (5) harvesting nauplii, and (6) maintaining live nauplii throughout the day.

Howard M. Lenhoff ● Department of Developmental and Cell Biology, University of California, Irvine, California.

Special mention is given to the preparation of axenic nauplii because of their anticipated large-scale use in culturing and maintaining axenic hydra (see Chapter 12).

MATERIALS

Artemia cysts can be obtained in vacuum-packed cans (Brine Shrimp Sales Co., Haywood, CA 94545, and other sources). One gram contains about 100,000 cysts. The cysts lose viability slowly at room temperature. They keep well at $-20°$ C; allow them to equilibrate to room temperature a few hours before use.

Glass trays [Corning Utility Dishes #232 (1.9 liter) and #233 (2.8 liter); plastic kitchen basters; *Artemia* hatching bags (Halvin Products, Inc., Brooklyn, NY 11223]; large finger bowls; air pumps; bolting cloth nets having 125 meshes to the square inch (Carolina Biological Supply Co.); plastic container (*ca.* 5.5 × 7.5 × 4 in.) fitted with a spigot.

Prepare Antiformin solution (Nakanishi *et al.*, 1962) by dissolving 5.68 g NaOH and 3.2 g Na_2CO_3 in 100 ml 5.25% sodium hypochlorite solution. Other reagents are $NaHCO_3$, Na_2EDTA, and NaCl (either laboratory or grocery store grades).

PROCEDURES

Axenic Nauplii

Remove nonliving debris from the cysts by the following washing procedure.

1. Place about 1 liter of cysts in a 4-liter beaker and bring the volume up to 3 liters with cold 0.2 *M* NaCl. Let the slurry stand for several hours at about 4°C. Keep the temperature low to prevent premature development of cysts.

2. Aspirate off any cysts that float. Decant the remainder of the saline solution and repeat the 0.2 *M* NaCl wash (about three times) until you obtain a clear solution.

3. After the final wash, bring the volume to 4 liters with cold saturated NaCl solution. Because this treatment eventually dehydrates the cysts and thereby slows their development, carry out the remainder of this step conveniently at room temperature. In saturated NaCl, the cysts float and the heavy contaminants, particularly sand, settle out. Aspirate off these con-

taminants by inserting a glass suction tube to the bottom of the beaker. For smaller batches, use a separatory funnel for this step. Repeat the flotation procedure as many times as necessary to remove the extraneous material; two washes usually suffice.

4. As the cysts settle, draw off and discard any clear solution and store them at 4°C in the saturated NaCl solution. These osmotically dehydrated cysts will retain their viability for months.

To decontaminate the washed cysts, remove the saturated NaCl and replace it with about 3 liters cold 0.2 M NaCl containing 70 ml Antiformin solution. Stir the cyst slurry with a glass rod every 5 min for 15 min. Do not use a magnetic bar stirrer as it damages the cysts. Allow the cysts to settle and decant the resultant dark solution. The discoloration of the solution is caused by release of material from the cyst shell. Repeat this procedure, decant the Antiformin solution, and wash the cysts in four successive changes of cold 0.2 M NaCl. Store these cysts at 4°C for 3–4 days, changing the solution several times each day to assure complete removal of the Antiformin. Replace the 0.2 M NaCl solution with sterile saturated NaCl and store the treated cysts at 4°C until they are ready for use.

The Antiformin treatment removes the large bacterial and fungal population associated with the *Artemia* cysts. We have hatched such cysts in sterile bacterial culture broths and find that no microorganisms grow in them even 6 months after the nauplii die.

The cysts may also be decontaminated with thiomersal (Merthiolate) as described by Provasoli and Shiraishi (1959), but we find nauplii hatched from such cysts often toxic to hydra. The direct addition of antibiotics to hydra culture solution to retard the growth of bacteria is not recommended because of the likelihood of selecting a population of antibiotic-resistant microorganisms (but see Chapter 12).

Hatching Solutions

A number of hatching solutions have been devised, each giving varying degrees of hatching depending upon the batch of *Artemia* cysts used. Some are precisely made up; others are prepared with less rigor, but with great simplicity and less effort.

Original Loomis and Lenhoff (1956) Solution. Prepare a stock solution of saturated NaCl (360 g/liter) by dissolving 5 lb commercial table salt in a 2-gal bottle of hot water and allow it to cool. Dilute this stock solution 1/100 with water. You can use either tap or distilled water.

Fulton (1960) Modification. Prepare concentrated stock solution by dissolving 345.62 g NaCl, 9.6 g NaHCO₃, and 4.8 g Na₂EDTA in 3.2 liters hot tap water. Dilute 1/30 with tap or distilled water.

Solution for Large-Batch Method. When preparing large batches of nauplii daily, we find handling concentrated NaCl solutions expensive and inconvenient. Hence, we use commercial grocery store ice-cream-grade salt and add the dry salt directly to the water in the hatching container. Thus, to prepare 16 liters salt solution, add 200 g NaCl directly to either tap water or deionized water, whichever is convenient and gives the best hatching yield. To save time, place 200 g NaCl in a plastic beaker, mark with indelible ink the height the NaCl reaches in the beaker, and thereafter use the marked beaker as measure to simply scoop the dry NaCl from the salt container.

Hatching Methods

1. *For Occasional Use with Minimum of Care (Dr. Sears Crowell, personal communication).* Prepare a ring 10 cm in diameter from a 1-cm-diameter rubber tube sealed tightly by both ends around a short piece of glass rod. Float this ring on the surface of the hatching solution contained in a 20-cm-diameter finger bowl. Sprinkle 1/8 teaspoon of untreated *Artemia* cysts in the center of the ring, the ring will retain the floating cysts, so they will not interfere with the harvesting. Within a day, hatched nauplii will swim to the edge of the bowl, where there is the most light. As the demand requires, add more cysts to the center of the ring. Clean the bowl and change the solution only when needed, usually about once a month.

2. *Average Use, Floating Method—for 10,000–100,000 Hydra (Loomis and Lenhoff, 1956).* Pour about 500 ml of the dilute hatching solution in a 3-liter flat Corning dish. Sprinkle 3–4 ml (1/2 teaspoon) of the dry cysts on the surface of the solution and let them sit for 48 hr at room temperature. Usually one such tray of hatched *Artemia*, provides enough food for 20,000 hydra.

Be certain to seed the fluids in each dish *after* the dishes are stacked; otherwise, when you move the dishes, the cysts may adhere to the walls of the dishes, where they will not hatch.

3. *Average Use, Bubbling Method—for 10,000–200,000 Hydra (Lenhoff and Brown, 1970).* Use either sterilized or nonsterilized cysts. Set up a 2-liter conical plastic bag by hanging it from a ring stand fitted with a

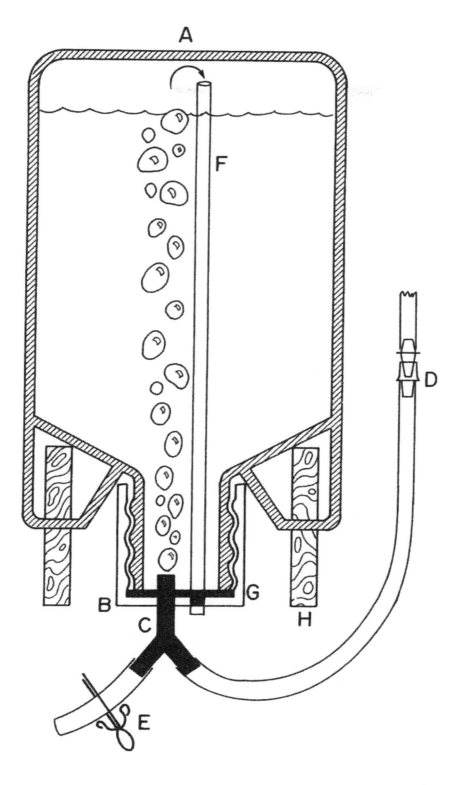

FIGURE 1. Apparatus for hatching large numbers of *Artemia* nauplii.

sidearm. Place an aeration stone, attached to a low-pressure air pump, at the bottom of the conical bag. Add 1.5 liters of hatching solution and a teaspoonful of cysts, and start the air pump. The conical shape of the bag ensures that all of the cysts will be agitated by air from the stone and will not stagnate in the absence of oxygen.

4. *Large-Batch Use, Bubbling Method—for 100,000–2,000,000 Hydra.* Instead of using a plastic bag as in the previous method, use a 20-liter polyethylene carboy (A) sitting inverted on two blocks (H) (Fig. 1). Modify the screw cap (B) as follows. Drill two holes. Into one, seal a polyethylene Y tube (C). To one arm of the Y tube, attach a tube (D); at the end of tube (D) place a joint so that it can be connected to an air pump. To the other end of the open Y tube, attach a short piece of tubing shut off with a pinch clamp [it is through this opening the nauplii can be removed (see below, Harvesting Nauplii)]. In the other hole of the screw cap (B), seal a long open tube (F) that almost reaches the "bottom" of the carboy; air exits through this tube. Insert a rubber gasket (G) between the carboy and the cap to keep the solution from leaking out.

Fill this hatching apparatus to a premarked 16-liter level with tap or deionized water; then add the sterilized or nonsterilized cysts (about 150 ml) and about 200 g dry commercial salt. Put the modified cap on the carboy, invert it, place it on the blocks (H) and attach the air pump via the joint on tube (D), and allow the solution to be aerated and agitated until you are ready for harvesting.

Incubation Conditions

The key condition to control, other than composition of the hatching solution and aeration, is the temperature of the hatching solution. Because of the constant aeration in the bubbling methods of hatching and subsequent cooling effect of evaporation, the temperature of the solution will be slightly cooler than room temperature. In general, increasing the temperature, say, from 20°C to 30°C, cuts hatching time in about half, but it also will speed up the growth of contaminating microorganisms and the consumption of oxygen. Hence, I recommend hatching the cysts at room temperature. If, for example, your cysts hatch best in 40–48 hr at room temperature, have two sets of "hatcheries" going, each seeded with new cysts on alternate days.

Harvesting Nauplii

The key features of harvesting are (1) separating the live nauplii from the unhatched cysts, shells, and dead nauplii; (2) once harvested, keeping the nauplii alive until they are used (usually during the same day); (3) just before feeding the nauplii to hydra, removing the saline from the nauplii and placing them in culture solution of the same composition in which hydra are kept.

For Finger-Bowl Ring Method (Method 1). Focus the beam from a small dissecting microscope lamp on one edge of the finger bowl. As the live nauplii swim there, remove as many as needed with an eye dropper. Rinse them through a net of 125-mesh bolting cloth with hydra culture medium, and use.

For Floating Method (Method 2). Pour the hatching solution with its contents from all the trays into one transparent container. Tilt the container by placing an object under one end and place a light at the other end. After the unhatched eggs float again, the other materials sink, and nauplii collect at the lit end, remove the live nauplii by siphoning the middle layer. Pass the clean, live nauplii through the 125-mesh net, wash in hydra culture solution, and use.

For the Conical Plastic Bag Method (Method 3). First remove the aeration stone and allow 10 min for the unhatched cysts and discarded cyst capsules to separate. Some sink to the bottom and others rise to the top. The hatched nauplii collect toward the bottom of the bag immediately above a layer of unhatched cysts. To collect these, insert into the bag a glass tube, inside diameter 0.25 in. (6.5 mm), attached to 0.6 m of plastic tubing with the end of the tube positioned within the cloud of hovering nauplii. Establish a siphon allowing the nauplii to pass through the tube and into a clear container, such as a plastic refrigerator juice container with spigot. Draw off the nauplii (with as little of the hatching solution as possible) as well as the layer of cysts at the bottom; thus the larvae that are entrapped in that layer can also be recovered. Add hydra culture solution to the plastic container holding the nauplii until it is almost overflowing. Have the container slightly inclined and positioned so that the spigot overhangs the edge of the sink and opens into a 125-mesh (0.2-mm openings) dip net fixed there. After about 10 min the unhatched cysts should sink to the bottom while the nauplii accumulate just off the bottom of the container. Take care to draw off and to collect in the new swimming nauplii only. To remove the last traces of the saline hatching solution, rinse the nauplii in the net with about 1 liter of hydra culture solution. Invert the net into a finger bowl and pour hydra culture solution through the net, thereby washing the nauplii into the dish.

For the Carboy Large-Batch Method (Method 4). After 2 days of bubbling air through the carboy, detach tube D (Fig. 1) from the joint connecting it to the pump, close the tube with a pinch clamp, and allow 5–10 min for the contents within the carboy to form a layer. Then simply open the clamp on tube F and allow the fluid with the live nauplii to collect in a bowl. Watch the existing suspension of "orange" nauplii carefully. Stop the flow if any brown debris (unhatched eggs and shells) start coming through or if too few live nauplii appear to be coming through—whichever comes first. Wash the nauplii as described in the preceding paragraph. One carboy should produce 10^8 or more nauplii per harvest.

Maintaining the Live Nauplii throughout the Day.

Seldom will you use all the nauplii as soon as you harvest them. Therefore, take your excess nauplii, pass them through the 125-mesh net, and place them into a large tray or container of hatching saline solution. If you have large numbers of excess nauplii, place a small bubbling stone in the tray to keep them aerated and moving.

Do not use the nauplii any later than 2 days after they have hatched; in that time they lose 60% of their dry weight and differ nutritionally from freshly hatched nauplii (J. S. Clegg, personal communication).

REFERENCES

Clegg, J. S. 1964. The control of emergence and metabolism by external osmotic pressure and the role of free glycerol in developing cysts of *Artemia salina. J. Exp. Biol.* **41**:879–892.

Croghan, P. C. 1958. The survival of *Artemia salina* (L.) in various media. *J. Exp. Biol.* **35**:213–218.

Fulton, C. 1960. Culture of a colonial hydroid under controlled conditions. Science **132**:473–474.

Loomis, W. F., and Lenhoff, H. M. 1956. Growth and sexual differentiation of hydra in mass culture. *J. Exp. Zool.* **132**:555–574.

Nakanishi, Y. Y., Iwasaki, T., Okigaki, T., and Kato, H. 1962. Cytological studies of *Artemia salina.* I. Embryonic development without cell multiplication after the blastula stage in encysted dry eggs. *Annot. Zool. Jpn.* **35**:223–228.

Provasoli, L., and Shiraishi, K. 1969. Axenic cultivation of the brine shrimp *Artemia salina. Biol. Bull.* **117**:347–355.

Chapter 7

Determining Growth Rates of Groups of Hydra and Budding Rates of Individual Hydra

Howard M. Lenhoff

PURPOSE

To calculate the logarithmic growth rate for groups of hydra and the linear budding rate of a single animal.

INTRODUCTION

Before initiating most laboratory investigations with hydra, the animals must be in state of "well-being." I define such hydra as animals that can multiply in laboratory solutions for a week or more at the same rate that they do in waters taken from their natural habitats. If they do not, then something is wrong with the culture solution, the food, or the technique.

The methods described in this chapter will allow you to measure two parameters of hydra's growth. These rates should be the same for a given species of hydra regardless of who measures them as long as all the conditions (pH, purity of water, ionic makeup, degree and quality of food, etc.) are the same.

Howard M. Lenhoff • Department of Developmental and Cell Biology, University of California, Irvine, California.

By being able to measure growth rate quantitatively, you will be able to evaluate the effectiveness of different culture media, their components, other environmental factors, nutrients, and various experimental reagents being tested for their ability to perturb the growth process. In addition, once you have gained proficiency in determining the conditions that allow clones of hydra to grow at their maximal rates, you should be prepared for culturing hydra in mass cultures (see Chapter 12).

MATERIALS

Typical laboratory glassware; culture solutions (see Chapter 4); *Artemia* nauplii (Chapter 6); graph paper (semilogarithmic and arithmetic); binocular dissecting microscope.

METHOD I. CLONAL GROWTH RATES (LOOMIS, 1953, 1954)

COMMENTS

The object is to feed and care for a group (or clone) of hydra until it grows at a constant logarithmic rate for 4–5 days. The clonal growth rates and doubling times measured should represent the growth characteristics of that clone under those conditions at which the animals were grown. It is best, but not necessary, to start with animals taken from a clone derived from a single hydra by budding. In this way you will be sure that the animals are all of the same genetic makeup. Although these directions are for determining growth rates under conditions at which the hydra are fed maximally, they can be modified accordingly for measuring growth rates under other conditions of feeding.

PROCEDURES

The late afternoon before taking your first measurement, place five hydra of about the same size, each having one bud just beginning to show, into a 9- to 10-cm-diameter Petri dish (glass or plastic) containing 30 ml culture solution. By the next morning the hydra should have fixed their basal disks to the bottom of the Petri dish. Once the animals adhere, it is much simpler to feed and clean them.

On the morning of the first measurement (about 8–9 A.M.), count the number of *hydranths* in the dish using a dissecting microscope. A hydranth is defined as the feeding portion ("head") of a coelenterate. Count even the smallest visual indication of a bud as a hydranth, because once a bud is initiated, it always completes its development. Thus, count a hydra with no perceptible buds as 1 hydranth, a hydra with one bud as 2 hydranths, a hydra with one well-developed bud and one that is barely perceptible as 3 hydranths, etc. By the start of the experiment the original 5 hydra have one or more buds, because in some animals a latent bud may have started to develop during the night. Hence, the original 5 animals will be recorded as 10–15 hydranths depending upon whether one or two buds are developing on each of the 5.

After counting and recording the number of hydranths, feed each individual by gently placing a thick slurry of *Artemia* nauplii right in the center of their ringlet of tentacles. It is important that each animal ingest as many nauplii as it can. Start with the animals closest to the light; if you do not, uncaptured nauplii may swim toward the light and become captured by some unfed hydra, thereby causing the tentacles of those hydra to contract greatly so that they are unable to ingest a full portion of nauplii to allow for maximal growth.

Allow the hydra 30–45 min to ingest the nauplii; by that time their tentacles should be barren of nauplii. For each Petri dish of experimental hydra, have three finger bowls nearby. Carefully decant off the culture solution and uneaten nauplii into the first bowl. Then gently rinse off any remaining nauplii into the second bowl. Add clean culture solution to the Petri dish (30 ml) and to the third finger bowl.

Do not discard the decanted and rinsed solutions, because some hydra, especially small buds, may dislodge and be transferred to the bowls. Carefully scan the bowls for hydra; begin with the rinse bowl (#2), pick up with a pipet any free hydra with as few nauplii as possible, and transfer them to the third bowl. Then do the same with hydra in the first bowl, except that in this case transfer the hydra to the second bowl in order to "dilute" out any nauplii carried over with the hydra; after the hydra are in the second bowl, transfer them with no nauplii to the third bowl. After you are positive that you have recovered all of the dislodged hydra, pick them up with an eye dropper and transfer them back into the experimental Petri dish. You should not see a single free nauplius in the Petri dish. This whole procedure should take less than 5 min per culture of hydra.

At about 2–4 hr after you have fed the animals, they should become inflated with fluid. By 5–6 hr after their feeding they will regurgitate a pellet of solid wastes. At that time (about 4 P.M.), rinse the animals to dislodge the pellets and replace the culture solution with 30 ml fresh culture solution. Make certain to recover any hydra that dislodge during the rinsing process and put them back into the experimental Petri dish.

Record and plot your data daily after counting the hydra. The plot should be on single- (or double-) cycle semilogarithmic paper with the number of hydranths in the ordinate and the time of growth, in days, on the abscissa (e.g., Fig. 1).

Repeat the above counting, feeding, washing, recovery, and afternoon rinse procedures daily. As the hydra increase in number, the amount of work will increase. By the morning of the 5th or 6th day, your plotted data should show that a sustained logarithmic rate has been attained, as evidenced by the plot being linear with a positive slope for at least 4 days. At that time you can stop the daily manipulations and calculate the growth rate and doubling time.

Rather than only recording the number of hydranths, you may also wish to record the budding states of the animals using simple "stick figure" diagrams (T. Sugiyama, personal communication). For example, $\vdash$, $\vdash$, $\vdash$, $\vdash$, and $\vdash$ signifies that you have two hydra each with one bud and three hydra each with two buds, or a total of 13 hydranths. Although this way of recording data is slightly more involved, it is useful in interpreting experiments in which you wish to know the developmental stages of the animals in the colony.

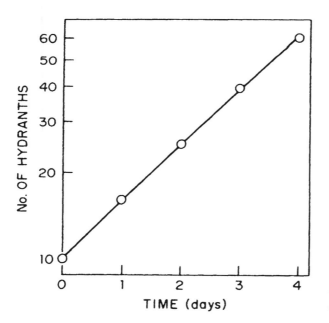

FIGURE 1. Semilogarithmic plot of the increase with time of the number of hydranths in a colony of *H. littoralis* fed daily on *Artemia* nauplii in a solution of KNC (see Chapter 4).

CALCULATIONS

To calculate the logarithmic growth rate (k), use the graph plotted from your data and the standard equation for logarithmic growth. From the graph, measure to the nearest tenth of a day the time (t) in which the number (n) of hydranths doubled; this interval is the doubling time (T). Obtain the growth rate by dividing T into 0.693 according to the integrated equation for logarithmic growth derived as follows:

$$dn/dt = kn$$

$$\ln (n/n_0) = kt$$

$$k = (\ln 2)/T = 0.693/T$$

For example, in Fig. 1 there were 20 hydranths on day 1.4, and 40 on day 3. Thus, $T = 3 - 1.4 = 1.6$, and $k = 0.693/1.6 = 0.433$. Typical growth rates and doubling times for hydra are shown in Table II of Chapter 4.

You should find that most healthy, well-fed hydra do not go through a lag phase, and that the number of hydranths will increase logarithmically within 1 day or 2 at the most. You may observe a lag period if you transfer the hydra from a favorable environment into a less favorable one at the beginning of the growth experiment, or if you start the experiment using smaller hydra that still have to grow before they start to bud at their maximal rate.

PRECAUTIONS

The most serious and most common error in growth experiments comes from lack of care in recovering dislodged animals. Failure to recover all animals, even one, can make large differences in your data, especially if the loss occurs during the first 3 days of the experiment. No harm is done, however, by not counting the hydra on one day, as long as the animals are fed and washed daily and are not lost during the cleaning procedure.

It is important to count the number of hydranths before you feed the animals, because often a bump on the side of a hydra caused by presence of ingested nauplii can be mistaken for a bud just beginning to develop.

An annoying problem is encountered when a hydra sticks to the inside of an eye dropper while being transferred. The easiest way to avoid this problem is to work fast and not dally. In the cases when such sticking occurs, do not try to force the hydra out with vigorous jets of water or you might damage the hydra and force it to regurgigate its ingested food. Instead try to dislodge the hydra using a fine Nichrome or platinum wire.

Fully fed hydra can lose the contents of their enteron if they are roughly handled, such as by dropping them on the surface of the culture medium. Therefore, when transferring hydra, especially well-fed ones, always place the tip of the eye dropper under the surface of the culture medium before releasing the hydra.

METHOD II. BUDDING RATES

There are occasions, such as when studying chimeras (see Chapter 35), when it is advantageous to measure the budding rates of individual animals. These rates are linear rather than logarithmic. For each of these measurements, place a single hydra in a Petri dish of culture solution. Every morning count and record the number of detached buds and discard them. Then feed and clean the "parent" hydra, taking care to recover any buds that may detach during those manipulations. Thus, at the end of the experimental period (usually 5–6 days) you will have in your Petri dish one large budding hydra with possibly one or two small, detached buds. Plot on linear graph paper the number of dislodged buds against time (in days); the slope of that line gives the budding rate in buds per day of that individual.

REFERENCES

Loomis, W. F. 1953. The cultivation of *Hydra* under controlled conditions. *Science* 117:565–566.

Loomis, W. F. 1954. Environmental factors controlling growth in hydra. *J. Exp. Zool.* 126:223–234.

Chapter 8

Culturing Large Numbers of Hydra

Howard M. Lenhoff

PURPOSE

To grow in the laboratory mass cultures of hydra by two methods: the tray method, which yields numbers of animals ranging from 10,000 to 100,000 at a time; and the vertical plate method, which can yield kilogram quantities (wet weight) monthly.

INTRODUCTION

The introduction by Loomis of methods for growing large numbers of hydra year-round in the laboratory opened the door for the current surge in research on hydra (Loomis, 1953, 1954; Loomis and Lenhoff, 1956). Because hydra reproduce asexually, doubling in number every 2–4 days (Chapters 4 and 7), it became possible to grow large clones of animals continuously in short periods.

Hydra are relatively undemanding laboratory animals. They will flourish in the laboratory provided they are fed regularly on live food (Chapter 6), and the culture solution (Chapter 4) is properly constituted and changed when necessary. Cultures may be left for long periods (up to about a month) without food; fasted hydra merely get smaller. Maintenance of logarithmically growing cultures, however, demands a rigorous daily schedule of feeding and cleaning that is rapid, simple, and free from error.

Howard M. Lenhoff ● Department of Developmental and Cell Biology, University of California, Irvine, California.

I describe two methods for culturing large numbers of hydra. The first, the tray method, which is similar to the original Loomis one (Loomis and Lenhoff, 1956; Lenhoff and Brown, 1970), requires no specially constructed equipment. It allows a person with a little experience to culture hundreds of thousands of animals daily with relatively little effort. It is the method used by most investigators.

The second, the vertical tray method, has not been published elsewhere. It requires the construction of some special, but inexpensive and simple, equipment. Once in operation, one person can raise kilogram quantities of hydra (wet weight) monthly. It can also be modified for culturing hydra on a smaller scale. The major operational difference between the two methods is that the vertical plate method does not require the daily changes of culture solution demanded by the tray method.

MATERIALS

In addition to materials needed to prepare culture solution (Chapter 4) and nauplii of the brine shrimp *Artemia salinas* (Chapter 5), you will need the following for the tray method: (1) Two convenient sizes of large flat glass trays; I recommend Corning Glass Pyrex Utility ("cake") Dishes, #232 (1 qt) and #233 (2 qt). (2) Finger bowls; I recommend the less expensive Pyrex casserole bowls (Corning #024, 1 qt) and custard dishes (Corning #465, 0.5). (3) Silk bolting cloth dip nets (38 mesh, 0.66-mm intervals; and 125 mesh, 0.2-mm intervals) (General Biological Supply Co., or Carolina Biological Supply Co.). (4) Plastic kitchen basters (50 ml) from hardware stores.

For the vertical plate method you will need to construct a series of culture tanks 18 X 12 X 12 in. (Fig. 1D), depending upon your needs. A commerical polyethylene tank (Nalge Sybron Corp., Rochester, NY, No. 14100-0015) is also suitable. Each tank is capable of holding up to 200,000 hydranths. At the bottom of each tank, set a standard undergravel aquarium filter (Fig. 1E) and cover it with almost 2 cm "medium course" washed aquarium gravel (Fig. 1F). Connect the tube of the filter to an aquarium air pump (e.g., Silent Giant, from Aquarium Pump Supply Co., Prescott, AZ). Fill the tank with culture solution and start the air pump. As water is displaced by the air entering the bottom of the filter, water is sucked down from the tank through the gravel and filter and will draw with it particulate matter suspended in the water such as egested food waste pellets from the hydra. This detritus will be decomposed by bacteria that will build up in the interstices of the gravel. To remove large amounts of detritus that may

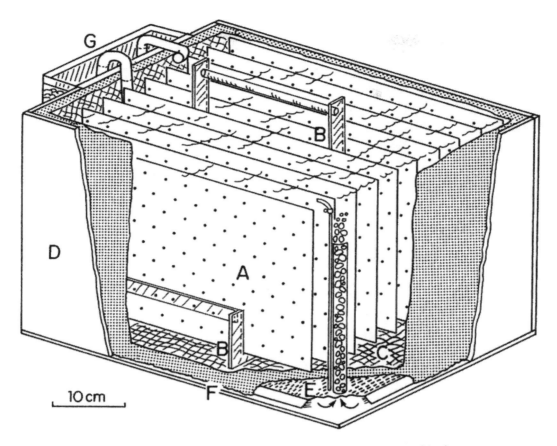

FIGURE 1. Vertical plate apparatus for the mass culture of hydra.

accumulate as you grow large numbers of hydra, you may wish to use an additional outside aquarium motor filter (Fig. 1G) (e.g., Metaframe, Model 410).

To hold the hydra, prepare ten 10 × 14 × 0.06-in. polystyrene plates (Cadillac Plastic and Chemical Co., Anaheim, CA) (Fig. 1A); you may wish to perforate the plates (as seen in Fig. 1) to increase circulation of the fluids, but this step is not absolutely necessary. To hold these plates, construct a rack and holder of 3/16-in. Plexiglas (Fig. 1B) with notches spaced about 1 in apart to hold the plates. Racks constructed in this manner expose as little horizontal surface as possible because such surfaces tend to collect detritus. To trap any detached hydra, you can line the bottom of the tank above the gravel with 38-mesh nylon net, or even line the complete interior of the tank with the net, as illustrated in Fig. 1C.

To seed the hydra onto the plates, construct three tanks 16 × 12 × 3.5 in. of Plexiglas or polystyrene, and six crosses 8 in. long in both directions made of strips of polystyrene (1/8 in. wide and 1/2 in. high).

To seal connections between Plexiglas, use Plexiglas Sealer (e.g., Industrial Polychemical Service, Gardena, CA). To seal connections between polystyrene, use Hot Melt Glue (e.g., Sears Roebuck and Co.). All of these components are not toxic to hydra.

To feed the hydra, use another 18 × 12 × 12-in. tank filled only with M solution (Chapter 4). In order to keep the *Artemia* nauplii in suspension, gently bubble a stream of air through the solution using a pipet attached to an air pump.

TRAY METHOD

PROCEDURES

Feeding

The nauplii collected from one hatching bag (Chapter 6) provide sufficient food for 20–30 densely populated trays (about 5,000–10,000 hydranths per tray) of hydra. After thoroughly rinsing the nauplii free of saline solution, suspend them in hydra culture solution. Using a plastic baster, spread the suspension of nauplii quickly and evenly throughout the tray of hydra. Supply sufficient *Artemia* so that the polyps can feed to repletion within 10–15 min. Do not put so many nauplii in the dish that the water fouls and carcasses of nauplii adhere to the slime in the dish. Do not too heavily feed animals that have been without food for 2 or more days, as they tend to detach from the tray.

First Daily Cleaning

The purpose of this step is to rid the trays of any *Artemia* not ingested. Change the culture solution about 30–45 min after the hydra (e.g., *Hydra attenuata* and *Hydra viridis*) are fed. Because some species, like *Hydra oligactis* and *Hydra pseudoligactis* take longer to release captured but uningested prey, wash these species 60–90 min after feeding the polyps.

Cleaning is relatively simple and rapid. Gently swirl the solution in the tray (to dislodge any nauplii adhering to the bottom) and invert the tray over the sink. Add about 250 ml of clean culture solution, gently swirl, and pour out the contents, making certain to remove all free nauplii. Lastly, add about 1 liter of fresh culture solution to the tray. Pour this solution along the side of the tilted tray and not directly onto the hydra; otherwise the animals may express the contents of their gut or become dislodged. Do not leave the hydra without water for too long because desiccating animals tend to regurgitate.

Such a cleaning procedure is fast. Although a few animals may be lost, it is not economic to take pains to retrieve them. If the dislodged polyps must be recovered, as when starting a new culture, pour the solution from the tray directly into a large casserole dish, not into the sink. If only a few dislodge, retrieve them individually with an eyedropper. If large numbers dislodge, separate them from the nauplii by means of the swirling procedure described below in the section on "total cleaning." Sometimes, however, because of large numbers of free *Artemia*, it may become difficult to retrieve the loose hydra by means of the swirling procedure without carrying along large numbers of nauplii. In such instances, merely allow the casserole dish containing a mixture of hydra and nauplii to sit for an hour or two. By that time many of the hydra will have attached to the dish with their basal disk and simply by inverting it the nauplii can be eliminated. Repeat this process until you retrieve most of the hydra.

Second Daily Cleaning

Once having ingested food, hydra take about 6 hr to regurgitate undigested material, such as exoskeletons of the nauplii. This interval may vary with the species of hydra, with temperature, and with the nutritional state of the animals before they are fed. For example, hydra kept at 22–24°C regurgitate between 4 and 8 hr after feeding, whereas animals kept at 18°C regurgitate within 8–12 hr of the meal. Animals fasted more than 1 day take longer to regurgitate. In all cases it is essential to remove regurgitated pellets from the dishes daily, or they adhere to the dish, the water fouls, and bacterial and fungal contaminants proliferate rapidly. Hydra grown and maintained under conditions in which the regurgitated wastes are not removed daily are unreliable for use in many kinds of experiments unless they are placed in clean culture solution for a day or so before use.

The procedure for the second daily cleaning is much simpler than that for the first cleaning because the solid wastes consist only of about one regurgitated food pellet per hydra, rather than large numbers of nauplii. To remove the regurgitated pellets, gently shake the culture tray and then invert it over the sink. Add about 250 ml culture solution to the tray, swirl the solution to remove any remnants of pellets, pour out this wash solution, and add 1 liter fresh culture solution. The entire procedure takes about 1 min per tray.

Should large numbers of hydra dislodge during the second cleaning, as may occur if the cultures are densely populated, retrieve them by passing the water from the tray through a 125-mesh net. Wash the contents of the net (hydra and pellets) into a casserole dish and separate the animals by the swirling method described under "total cleaning" below. Use a 38-mesh net to separate hydra from some of the excess nauplii during the first cleaning process. The net retains the hydra and allows most of the nauplii to pass through; a disadvantage is that occasionally numerous hydra become enmeshed in the net and are not easily retrieved.

Total Cleaning (Harvesting of Mass Cultures and Cleaning of Culture Trays)

When large numbers of hydra (tens of thousands) are needed for an experiment, or when it is necessary to remove the excess bacterial slime that has accumulated on the bottom of the culture trays, use the following procedures. Pour off about three-fourths of the culture solution from the tray. Dislodge all hydra by gently rubbing your finger tips over the bottom surface of the tray, and pour the solution with hydra into a large casserole dish. (When harvesting 20–40 trays for an experiment, a modified window "squeegee" can be used to dislodge the animals). Usually, the contents of 2–6 trays can comfortably fill a single 2-liter casserole dish. Next, swirl the combined contents, and within a few minutes the hydra will collect in the center of the dish (see Loomis and Lenhoff, 1956, for illustrations). As soon as this happens, transfer the mass of hydra with a baster into a casserole dish containing clean culture solution. If you wait too long, pellets or bits of slime will also collect in the center mass. Repeat the swirling, collecting, and transfer processes two to four times, or until the hydra are free of debris. (Since this cleaning and harvesting process deals with tens of thousands of animals, do not bother to retrieve small numbers of hydra left behind in the dishes.)

The necessity for regular total cleaning depends upon the amount of accumulated slime in the dishes and upon the density of animals. The amount of slime will be substantially reduced by assiduous attention to daily cleaning schedules and by using nauplii hatched fresh from Antiformin-treated cysts (Chapter 6). In our laboratory we totally clean our trays about every 1–2 weeks.

The best time of the day to totally clean, then, is immediately following the second daily cleaning. Hydra cleansed at this time will adhere readily to clean culture trays and can be fed on the following day.

After totally cleaning a densely populated tray of hydra do not place all those animals back into one tray. No matter how clean the tray, crowded animals tend to detach more readily than do animals in sparsely populated trays. Use the animals collected from one dense tray to seed three to six new trays. In this way, large numbers of stock animals can be grown in a few months.

COMMENTS AND PRECAUTIONS

Pyrex trays are ideal for cultivating hydra. They are easily stacked and thereby permit the maintenance of large numbers of animals in a minimum of surface area. Cover the topmost or unstacked tray (1/4-in. Plexiglas cut to 10 × 15 in.) to minimize airborne contamination. The trays may be kept in drawers and cabinets because most hydra apparently have no specific requirements for light. An exception is the symbiotic strain *H. viridis*, which in the absence of light will lose its algal complement (Eakin, 1961).

For convenience in raising 50 large trays of one species of hydra, we have constructed racks into which the trays slide.

The surface on which you observe the hydra in a glass tray or bowl should be of black Formica. The hydra can be most easily seen if a 3- to 4-ft (1 m) fluorescent lamp is placed on the black table top a few inches from the culture tray. In such "dark field" illumination each hydra stands out sharply.

Contamination of cultures of one species of hydra by specimens of another can readily occur unless you take special care. For example, when feeding the hydra cultures, never dip the baster containing the nauplii into the culture medium of any tray, because a floating hydra may adhere to the baster and be transferred to another tray. Likewise, when pouring clean culture solution from a beaker into a tray, do not allow the beaker lip to contact the solution in the tray. Thus, keep separate basters and beakers for each species cultured.

Another possible source of contamination occurs during the total cleaning procedures if casserole bowls are not thoroughly clean. Also, some hydra may adhere to the finger tips while dislodging them from the culture trays, and fall into another tray of animals. To avoid contamination in this manner, it is advisable to wear disposable plastic gloves during the total cleaning process.

TABLE I. Daily Schedule for Rearing Mass Cultures of Hydra (*ca.* 100,000 Hydranths)

Time	Procedure
0830	Start harvesting the nauplii; while the nauplii are settling, seed *Artemia* for the following day
0850–0900	Feed hydra. Between this time and the first daily cleaning period, prepare culture solutions; change the culture solution of those animals being starved
0930–1000	Conduct first daily cleaning to remove uningested shrimps from hydra culture
1630–1700	Conduct second daily cleaning of hydra to remove regurgitated material

A sample daily schedule is given in Table I. By following this schedule (adjusted to the number of hydra), one person can care for 500,000 hydra daily with as little as 2.5 hr of work.

VERTICAL PLATE METHOD

PROCEDURES

Preparing the Culture Tank

Set up the tank as described under Materials and as illustrated in Fig. 1. Before adding the gravel, be certain to boil it in distilled water for about 30 min to remove any contaminants and to kill any bacteria or fungi attached to it. Fill the tank with culture solution, start the air pumps, and check the pH periodically during the next 16–24 hr. If the pH changes significantly, adjust it by adding HCl or NaOH. When the solution has equilibrated to a suitable pH (5–7.5), add the racks with the attached hydra.

Seeding the Plates

Place a polystyrene plate horizontally on two of the "seeding crosses" in a seeding tray containing M solution. Using a pipet, scatter onto the plate about 2000 ± 500 hydra that have been without food for 1 day. Allow them to remain on the plate for 5–15 min. During this time, about two-thirds of the hydra should stick to the plate by their basal disks. Quickly but gently flip the plate over, put it back on the crosses, and seed more hydra on the clean side of the plate. After sufficient hydra have attached to both sides of the plate, put the plate in the Plexiglas rack sitting in the culture tank.

Repeat this process as many times as needed to provide sufficient plates for your tanks. With practice you should be able to seed two to five plates at a time in a single seeding tray as long as you place two crosses between every two plates. Not all the hydra scattered onto the plates will adhere. Therefore, collect the free ones and use them to seed your last plate.

Repeat the seeding process every time the plates become saturated with hydra, or when the plates become covered with bacterial slime and/or with algae. In those cases, remove the hydra from the plates and wash and swirl them just as described in the tray method of this chapter. Be certain to clean the plates before you seed them again, and the racks before they are replaced into the culture tank.

Feeding the Hydra

Lift out the rack with plates having hydra attached to them and place it into another tank filled with M solution and containing *Artemia* nauplii. Gently bubble air through the tank to keep the nauplii suspended evenly. After about 15–30 min, each hydra should have ingested 10 or more nauplii; at that time, lift out the rack and put it back into the culture tank. Use the same suspension of nauplii to feed the hydra attached to the plates of about three to five racks.

Care of the Culture Tank

Unlike the tray method, you do not have to change and discard the culture solution twice daily. To the contrary, it is only necessary to change the solution about once per 2–4 weeks. The frequency with which you change the solution depends upon many factors such as the density of the culture of hydra, the degree to which they feed, the number and kind of microorganisms present, and the efficiency of the filter system.

I recommend that you change the water every 2–3 weeks. Nonetheless, you should observe the hydra cultures as a daily routine. If the animals are not "standing" perpendicular to the vertical plates, and if their tentacles are not outstretched, then change the water. Rather than wait for visible changes to occur in the hydra, you may wish to monitor the solution for sudden changes using a pH meter or ohmmeter. To facilitate emptying of the culture tank, you may wish to install a spigot drain at the bottom of it.

It is not necessary to scrub out the tank every time you replace the culture solution. Occasionally you may wish to wash the gravel free of the debris that collects there. On the other hand, you may wish to leave the gravel undisturbed for a few months at a time, because it is thought that the bacterial colonies thriving in the gravel help break down the water collected there. Accordingly, you will find that the routine you eventually follow will depend upon the special characteristics of your own mass cultures.

COMMENTS AND PRECAUTIONS

This method is sufficiently flexible so that it can be used to grow and maintain either small or large numbers of hydra. We find that using five culture tanks, each containing a rack holding 20 plates, it is possible to raise about 1 kg wet weight of hydra in a month. The animals grow logarithmically on the plates at about half the rate they grow in trays, but by the 14th day, the number of animals falling off the plate is greater than the number of new animals formed per day (R. Erickson and H. Lenhoff, unpublished).

It is even possible to feed and grow hydra in 20-ft-long unpartitioned tanks. These tanks, made of wood and coated with marine paint, can hold around 350 plates. For these tanks, do not use the gravel-type aquarium filters, but instead attach to each tank a heavy-duty filter pump which removes both the uneaten *Artemia* nauplii and the regurgitated food pellets.

The vertical plate method is advantageous in that it provides a simple means for growing large numbers of hydra with relatively little care. A major disadvantage, however, is that the hydra are grown crowded in an environment of unknown composition. Hence, before using animals grown under these conditions in sensitive behavioral and developmental studies, place them uncrowded for a day or so in trays containing solutions of known composition. Another disadvantage of the plate method is that crowded hydra in solutions containing organic wastes tend to become infected more readily than sparse cultures of animals in solutions that are frequently replaced.

REFERENCES

Eakin, R. E. 1961. Quoted in Discussion. In: *The Biology of Hydra and of Some Other Coelenterates* (H. M. Lenhoff and W. F. Loomis, eds.), University of Miami Press, Coral Gables, Fla., p. 266.

Lenhoff, H. M., and Brown, R. D. 1970. Mass culture of hydra: An improved method and its application to other aquatic invertebrates. *Lab. Anim.* 4:139–154.

Loomis, W. F. 1953. The cultivation of *Hydra* under controlled conditions. *Science* 117:565–566.

Loomis, W. F. 1954. Environmental factors controlling growth in hydra. *J. Exp. Zool.* 126:223–234.

Loomis, W. F., and Lenhoff, H. M. 1956. Growth and sexual differentiation of hydra in mass culture. *J. Exp. Zool.* 132:555–574.

Chapter 9

Turbidimetric and Pipetimetric Measurements of Number of Hydra

Howard M. Lenhoff

PURPOSE

To determine rapidly and accurately the number of hydra in dense suspensions by the turbidity of diluted hydra homogenates or by the volume they occupy in a pipet.

INTRODUCTION

Biochemical and physiological research on hydra often demands rapid means for determining numbers of animals and for distributing equal numbers of animals into many reaction vessels. Hydra are too large to measure turbimetrically and are too small to count in large numbers conveniently.

I describe two simple, quick, and accurate methods that overcome these obstacles (Lenhoff and Loomis, 1957). The first is a turbimetric method in which the skeletonless hydra is homogenized and the homogenate is diluted and measured. The second is based on the observation that hydra chilled to 0°C contract into spheres that can be pipetted with much precision.

Howard M. Lenhoff • Department of Developmental and Cell Biology, University of California, Irvine, California.

MATERIALS

Tissue homogenizer; turbidimeter, or colorimeter with blue filter (425 nm); 1-ml-calibrated pipet with its tip removed so that the opening is about 3 mm; Corning utility tray; 0.005 M sodium phosphate buffer, pH 6.

TURBIDIMETRIC METHOD

PROCEDURES

After you are finished using the hydra, such as after measuring their respiration (Chapter 52), concentrate the hydra by either swirling (Chapter 8) or chilling them (see Pipetimetric Assay below). Place them in glass tissue homogenizer containing buffer and prepare a fine suspension of hydra particles by passing the plunger through the sample about eight times. Dilute the suspension with phosphate buffer to give a final volume of 40 ml. Place an aliquot of the dilute suspension in a turbidimeter and measure the turbidity. Compare the measurements to a standard curve made by plotting the turbidity of varying dilutions of a suspension of a homogenate of hydra (ordinate) against the protein content (Chapter 51) of those samples (abscissa). Once you construct standard curves, each assay should take no more than 5 min.

PRECAUTIONS

Be certain to obtain an even suspension of hydra particles in the homogenizing step; thus, depending upon the species of hydra you use and the quality of your tissue homogenizer, you may have to increase the number of plunges in the homogenization step. Turbidity may vary with pH, with the time of the hydra's last feeding, and with the species of hydra used. Thus, carry out suitable controls and preliminary experiments.

PIPETIMETRIC ASSAY

PROCEDURES

Collect about 20,000 hydra by the swirling method (Chapter 8), transfer them into a 10-ml graduated test tube sitting in crushed ice. As the hydra contract into spheres and settle to the bottom of the tube, remove as much of the culture solution as possible using a fine-tipped pipet. After about 30 min, the packed hydra will reach a constant volume. Using a calibrated pipet with an enlarged tip, withdraw aliquots of the spherical animals and pipet the desired amounts into the reaction vessel of your proposed experiment.

Construct a calibration curve by first counting the number of hydranths (Chapter 7) in specified aliquots of the pipetted hydra and next determining the turbidity of a homogenate of those hydra, the protein content of those hydra, or both. To count the hydra in 0.5 ml, for example, spread the chilled hydra over a large glass Corning utility tray which has had a grid of 1-in squares drawn on its bottom with indelible yellow ink.

COMMENTS

Experiments with *Hydra littoralis* gave precise results, duplicate samples of 0.25 and 0.5 ml of chilled hydra giving 688 and 689 hydranths, and 1138 and 1150 hydranths, respectively (Lenhoff and Loomis, 1957).

REFERENCES

Lenhoff, H. M., and Loomis, W. F. 1957. Environmental factors controlling respiration in hydra. *J. Exp. Zool.* **134**:171–182.

Chapter 10

Culturing Hydra of the Same Species but of Different Sizes

Richard D. Campbell and Joann J. Otto

PURPOSE

Size and morphology are controlled by patterning agents such as morphogenetic and positional information fields. In order to study the nature of these fields it is useful to be able to modify them. Controlling hydra size by varying the amounts of food given to them provides an experimental method for manipulating the sizes and properties of patterning fields, and also for obtaining hydra of particular sizes for experiments.

INTRODUCTION

Hydra tissue is continually renewed, with growth balancing cell and tissue loss through budding and tissue atrophy. Under the resultant steady-state condition, the size of hydra can remain constant over a course of months and years (Brien and Reniers-Decoen, 1949) when other environmental conditions (such as temperature) are held constant. Steady-state size can be regulated by the rate of feeding; higher feeding rates produce hydra with larger steady-state size (Otto and Campbell, 1977; Gurkewitz *et al.*, 1980). The steady state of hydra also can be varied by growing them at

Richard D. Campbell ● Department of Developmental and Cell Biology, University of California, Irvine, California.   Joann J. Otto ● Department of Biological Sciences, Purdue University, West Lafayette, Indiana.

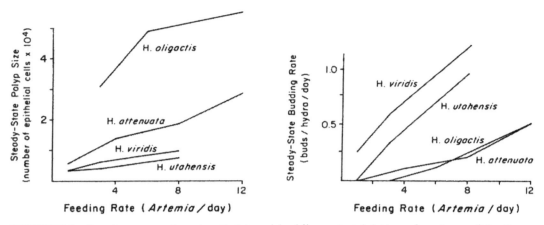

FIGURE 1. Steady-state polyp size (left) and budding rate (right) as functions of feeding rate. The four species included represent the four taxonomic groups of hydra (see Chapter 3). Data from Otto and Campbell (1977) and Gurkewitz *et al.* (1980).

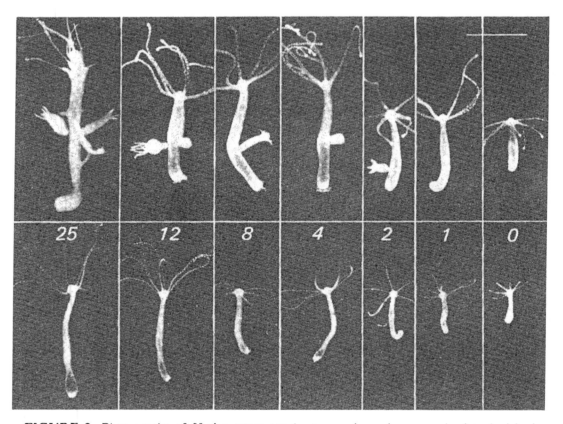

FIGURE 2. Photographs of *Hydra attenuata* (mature polyps above, newly detached buds below) fed 25, 12, 8, 4, 2, 1, and 0 shrimps per day. From Otto and Campbell (1977).

different temperatures, with lower temperatures giving larger hydra (Hecker and Slobodkin, 1976).

MATERIALS

This method requires materials normally used for studies of hydra growth (Chapters 7 and 8).

PROCEDURES

Maintain experimental hydra individually or in small groups. Each day count and discard all detached buds and feed each experimental hydra a counted number of *Artemia* nauplii. Pipet the nauplii onto the tentacles to assure their being caught and ingested. Assess the time at which the hydra in each population achieve steady-state sizes by monitoring the budding rate; a constant rate means the hydra size has stabilized. A more precise method is to determine the number of cells in the hydra (Chapter 20). The budding rates and parent sizes of hydra of four species are shown as a function of feeding rate (Fig. 1). The appearances of steady state hydra, and their buds, are shown in Figure 2.

PRECAUTIONS

Hydra may react adversely to large, sudden increases in feeding rate. Under such conditions, the hydra may go into "depression" or stop feeding after a few days. Therefore, to increase the sizes of animals kept at low feeding rates, increase the feeding rates over the course of a few days.

Hydra may not ingest all the nauplii placed on their tentacles. In these cases check each container for remaining nauplii and feed these hydra the additional nauplii.

REFERENCES

Brien, P., and Reniers-Decoen, M. 1949. La Croissance, la blastogènese, l'ovogenèse chez *Hydra fusca* (Pallas). *Bull. Biol. Fr. Belg.* **83**:293–386.

Gurkewitz, S., Chow, M., and Campbell, R. D. 1980. Hydra size and budding rate: Influence of feeding. *Int. J. Invert. Reprod.* **2**:199–201.

Hecker, B., and Slobodkin, L. B. 1976. Response of *Hydra oligactis* to temperature and feeding rate. In: *Coelenterate Ecology and Behavior* (G. O. Mackie, ed.), Plenum Press, New York, pp. 175–183.

Otto, J. J., and Campbell, R. D. 1977. Tissue economics of *Hydra:* regulation of cell cycle, animal size and development by controlled feeding rates. *J. Cell Sci.* **28**:117–132.

Chapter 11

Culture of Sexually Differentiated Hydra

Charles L. Rutherford, David Hessinger,
and Howard M. Lenhoff

PURPOSE

To induce either the diecious *Hydra littoralis* or the monoecious *Hydra viridis*, to differentiate gonads.

INTRODUCTION

Methods for reliably inducing sexual differentiation in hydra should be useful for the study of factors affecting interstitial cell differentiation as well as for studies of hydra genetics and embryology, dormancy in embryos, and gametogenesis and gonadogenesis in general. Unfortunately, no single method for inducing gonadogenesis works on all species and strains of hydra, and sometimes even "proven" methods show great variability. Perhaps the most reliable method is "calculated neglect." A survey of the literature shows that changes in a number of environmental factors stimulate gonadogenesis: (1) drop in temperature—20 papers on six species (e.g., Burnett and Diehl, 1964; Park *et al.*, 1965); (2) rise in temperature—6 papers on four

Charles L. Rutherford ● Biology Department, Virginia Polytechnic Institute and State University, Blacksburg, Virginia.   David Hessinger ● Department of Physiology and Pharmacology, Loma Linda University, Loma Linda, California.   Howard M. Lenhoff ● Department of Developmental and Cell Biology, University of California, Irvine, California.

71

species (e.g., Brien and Reniers-Decoen, 1950; Itô, 1954); (3) rich feeding (Nussbaum, 1909); (4) starvation (Nussbaum, 1909); (5) intermediate levels of feeding (Rutherford *et al.*, 1965); (6) controlled pCO_2 (Loomis, 1954, 1957); and (7) enriched microenvironment (Loomis, 1964). Because in the current literature the most detailed experimental information is available for only three methods, we present these below.

INCREASING THE TEMPERATURE (PARK ET AL., 1965)

COMMENTS

This method of inducing sexual differentiation by suddenly increasing the incubation temperature is both simple and reliable. The primary disadvantage of the procedure is that temperature itself may not be of significance in a causal sense because other factors, such as nutritional state, will also be affected by temperature. The method is quite useful, however, when a large number of sexual individuals are required for studies of gonadogenesis.

MATERIALS

Controlled temperature incubator; Pyrex glass dishes 6.5 cm in diameter by 3.5 cm deep; dissecting microscope; bulb pipet; BVT culture solution (Chapter 4).

PROCEDURES

In order to obtain temperature-adapted animals, transfer 100 individual *H. littoralis* to 40 ml BVT solution. Maintain the cultures in darkness at four temperatures: $5.0° \pm 0.5°$, $10.0° \pm 0.5°$, $15.0° \pm 1.0°$, and $21.0° \pm 0.5°C$. Transfer the hydra from 21° to 5° in two steps: first to 10° for several days, then to 5°. Maintain the adaptation cultures at their final temperatures for a minimum of 12 weeks (the authors did not determine the minimum period of adaptation required).

Use six hydra for each temperature change or control replicate. Put each animal individually in the Pyrex glass dish containing 10 ml BVT. Keep the temperature of the BVT the same as the temperature at which the hydra had been cultured. Maintain each group of six isolated hydra in a damp chamber for the next 4 weeks at the temperature required by the particular experiment.

Treat stock and experimental hydra as follows. Allow all hydra to feed for 1 hr three times weekly on an excess of *Artemia* nauplii; then rinse the hydra and replace the culture fluid with fresh BVT. On one nonfeeding day each week record the numbers of hydra with and without gonads in the stock cultures, and pick 100 individuals at random from each culture for transfer to clean dishes. On a second nonfeeding day, cleanse each dish of debris with a bulb pipet and replenish the BVT. Discard newly dropped buds from the single hydra experimental and control cultures on each of 5 days every week. Transfer the parent hydra to clean dishes once a week.

Carry out the feeding, cleaning, transferring, and observing as quickly as possible at room temperature. The longest single interval and the longest daily accumulated time that hydra should be kept at this temperature are 20 and 70 min, respectively.

PAST RESULTS

By following this procedure, Park *et al.* (1965) were able to induce sexual differentiation in *H. littoralis*. Groups of six hydra each were subjected to the following temperature increases: 5° to 21°, 10° to 21°, and 15° to 21° for 4 weeks. Hydra began to differentiate sexually within the 1st week after each temperature change. The number of hydra that became sexually mature was essentially stablized by the end of 3 weeks. After each rise in temperature the percentage of hydra that differentiated sexually by the end of 4 weeks was greater than the percentage in the corresponding control group. The most striking effect was observed after a rise from 5° to 21° when 100% of the hydra were sexually developed by the end of 3 weeks. This percentage represents more than a fourfold increase over the control (21°) value of 22%.

CONTROLLING CARBON DIOXIDE TENSION (LOOMIS, 1957)

COMMENTS

This method offers the distinct advantage of highly reproducible results from one experiment to the next. Under the conditions described below, 100% of the individuals treated will be sexually differentiated after only 10–

12 days. Since pH, pO_2, pNH_3, and pCO_2 can be controlled, the causal significance of these feedback variables on sexual differentiation can be investigated. However, if one is interested only in obtaining sexual forms of hydra, the methods of induction by temperature or nutrition are much simpler to perform.

MATERIALS

Several 15-ml beakers; large syringe with No. 18 needle; 100% and 90% oxygen; 10% carbon dioxide; culture solution containing 50 mg $CaCl_2$, 100 mg $NaHCO_3$, and 50 mg EDTA in 1 liter water.

PROCEDURES

Place 10 asexual *H. littoralis* in a 15-ml beaker containing 15 ml culture solution. Feed each culture for 30 min daily with an excess of brine shrimp larvae. Then rinse the beaker with clean culture solution (see below) to remove all uningested brine shrimp. Maintain a constant density of hydra by daily removing all newly detached buds. In addition, rinse the beakers free of regurgitated food wastes about 6 hr after their daily feeding.

To prepare culture solution of known gas mixture, use the following procedures. First, shake the culture solution three times with a large excess of 100% oxygen, yielding a control solution whose pCO_2 is 0.00%. Prepare water with an initial pCO_2 of 8.35% atm twice daily by shaking 20 ml control solution with 100 ml 10% CO_2 and 90% O_2 in a large syringe for 1 min. Inject graded amounts of this pCO_2-rich water twice a day into the experimental cultures. Care must be taken to place the tip of the No. 18 needle as far under water as possible and to inject this pCO_2-rich water with a minimum of bubbling.

PAST RESULTS

Using this method Loomis (1957) found that sexual differentiation may be induced in male *H. littoralis* by artificially increasing the pCO_2 of the water in which they are cultured. Within 9–10 days most of the individuals had initiated sexual differentiation. Reduced oxygen tension was not necessary for sexual differentiation to occur, for oxygen tension in the culture solution was five times higher than that of water saturated with air.

CONTROLLING THE NUTRITIONAL LEVEL
(RUTHERFORD ET AL., 1965)

COMMENTS

By limiting the food intake of *H. viridis*, sexual differentiation can be induced in a short time in virtually all of the treated animals. The procedure, although easy to perform when using a small number of individuals, requires rigid adherence to the feeding schedule. By following the prescribed feeding schedule for an extended period of time, not only are spermaries formed, but ovaries appear and reappear at fairly constant intervals. Modification of the limited feeding procedure can be applied to mass culture of *H. viridis*, but the results are less predictable than those obtained with single individuals.

MATERIALS

Culture dishes, 60×15 mm (Falcon, Oxnard, CA); dissecting microscope; Pasteur pipet drawn to a fine tip; *Artemia* nauplii M solution (Chapter 4).

PROCEDURES

Place single individuals of *H. viridis* (Florida strain, 1961) in culture dishes containing 15 ml of culture solution. Feed each individual three *Artemia* nauplii daily. The number of nauplii consumed can be controlled by placing the nauplii one at a time through the tip of a Pasteur pipet directly into the tentacles of the hydra. Any *Artemia* not captured must be removed from the culture dish and a new one must be fed to the hydra. Feed the control animals excess nauplii (20–25). Excess feeding is accomplished by adding a drop of a dense suspension of nauplii to the tentacles of an individual hydra. Change the culture solution twice daily, at 1 and 7 hr after feeding. Remove all newly detached buds daily from the culture dishes.

PAST RESULTS

By using this method Rutherford *et al.* (1965) found that all 200 animals fed on regimes of from 1 to 13 *Artemia* nauplii daily over extended periods of time developed gonads while 40 control animals fed excess (20–25) nauplii daily did not. Furthermore, the sexual animals reverted to the asexual state when placed on the excess nauplii diet. An additional 60 individuals fed 3 nauplii daily for over 3 months produced ovaries periodically. We quantified this periodicity by recording the number of days between the release of a mature egg and the first appearance of the next ovary. This mean interovary (IO) period was 14 ± 2 days. The first IO period was nearly the same as the second, third, fourth, etc. Hence, it was possible to predict the differentiation of an ovary within a few days. The lengths of the IO periods of hydra fed 1, 2, or 3 nauplii daily were about the same. On the other hand, the number of buds produced by a given individual increased as more food was taken in. As an ovary developed, however, bud production sharply decreased and usually stopped. Immediately after, or at the time the egg was shed, a burst of bud production began.

Although spermary differentiation was also induced by limiting the number of nauplii fed to the hydra daily, spermary development did not appear to exhibit any periodicity. Instead, once induced, spermaries were observed on the hydra for periods ranging up to 80 days. Careful inspection showed, however, that the number of "ripe" spermaries full of active sperm usually peaked as each ovary became fully developed.

PRECAUTIONS FOR ALL METHODS

Because several factors have been shown to induce sexual differentiation in hydra, the effects of a single environmental change can be evaluated only if all others are controlled. Two examples will illustrate this point, the effect of the surface:volume ratio of the culture solution and the pCO_2 level of the diluent water used for preparing culture solutions.

Loomis (1957) showed with *H. littoralis* that altering the surface:volume ratio of the culture solution resulted in sexual differentiation in the absence of any other environmental changes. Presumably changes in surface:volume ratios affect the amount of gases in the culture solution. Thus, culture dishes used must be of sufficient depth to maintain the asexual state throughout the duration of the experiment. Likewise, a constant surface:volume ratio must be maintained in all test cases and in the controls.

The chemistry of the diluent water used in preparing the culture solution also must be rigidly controlled. Loomis (1964) stated that tap water taken from a lake varies in pCO_2 and other factors from one season to the next, "an interesting loophole in an otherwise controlled experiment." Thus, the culture solution should be made from deionized water utilizing a Barnstead "red cap" mixed resin cartridge, or a similar product capable of removing all CO_2 from tap water.

Lastly, regardless of the techniques selected for inducing sexual differentiation, good results will be obtained only if you use a strain of hydra genetically capable of forming mature gonads. Apparently, there are great differences among different strains of the same species (T. Sugiyama, personal communication). Hence, before beginning an extensive study of sexual differentiation, it may be advisable to select a favorable strain from a number of hatched fertilized eggs. But then again, we encounter the proverbial problem: "Which comes first, the hydra or the egg?"

ADDENDUM

Dr. Lynne Littlefield (personal communication) finds that healthy specimens of *H. carnea* and of *H. utohensis* spontaneously differentiate gonads while they are cultured at 18°C. In addition, she finds that *H. oligactis* (*H. fusca*) differentiate ripe gametes if the temperature of the culture solution is lowered to 10° C and the animals are fed at this temperature for about three weeks.

REFERENCES

Brien, P., and Reniers-Decoen, M. 1950. Étude d' *Hydra viridis* (Linnaeus) (La blastogénèse, la spermatogénèse, l'ovogénèse). *Ann. Soc. R. Zool.* 81:33–110.

Burnett, A. L., and Diehl, N. A. 1964. The nervous system of *Hydra*. III. The initiation of sexuality with special reference to the nervous system. *J. Exp. Zool.* 157:237–250.

Itô, T. 1954. Studies on the reproduction of hydras. VI. Induction of the sexual reproduction in *Pelmatohydra robusta* Itô by lowering temperature. *Mem. Ehime Univ. Nat. Sci. Ser. B (Biol.)* 2:51–60.

Loomis, W. F. 1954. Reversible induction of sexual differentiation in *Hydra*. *Science* 120:145–146.

Loomis, W. F. 1957. Sexual differentiation in *Hydra*: Control by carbon dioxide tension. *Science* 126:735–739.

Loomis, W. F. 1964. Microenvironmental control of sexual differentiation in *Hydra*. *J. Exp. Zool.* 156:289–306.

Nussbaum, M. 1909. Uber Geschlechtsbildung bei Polypen. *Arch. Gesamte Physiol. Men. Thiere*, 130:521–629.

Park, H. D., Sharpless, N. E., and Ortmeyer, A. B. 1965. Growth and differentiation in hydra. I. The effect of temperature on sexual differentiation in *Hydra littoralis*. *J. Exp. Zool.* 160:247–254.

Rutherford, C. L., Hessinger, D. H., and Lenhoff, H. M. 1965. Induction of rhythmic differentiation of ovaries in *Clorohydra viridissima*. *Am. Zool.* 5:456.

Chapter 12

Preparing Axenic Hydra

M. Rahat and Vanda Reich

PURPOSE

To prepare axenic ("free of other forms of life") hydra for metabolic, cell, and developmental research.

INTRODUCTION

Hydra are known to be at times infected with bacteria, protozoans, and molds. Some of these infectious agents have been found on the outside surface of the animal, adhering to the mucus produced at the basal disk, inside the gastrodermal cavity, in the mesoglea, and even intracellularly (Margulis *et al.*, 1978). Because the presence of such organisms can interfere with metabolic, cell, and developmental research, we devised a method to rid the hydra of these organisms. This method is based on three basic steps: (1) careful washing of the animals, (2) removal of the usually highly infected basal disk, and (3) treatment with a broad range of antibiotics. We applied this method with success to *Hydra viridis*.

MATERIALS

Antibiotics. Penicillin and streptomycin are available in sterile capped vials for medical use. Neomycin, rifampicin, and chloramphenicol are available commercially (e.g., Sigma or Gibco).

M. Rahat and Vanda Reich ● Department of Zoology, The Hebrew University of Jerusalem, Israel.

Sterile Materials. One 2-ml screw syringe; one 250-ml Erlenmeyer flask; two 5-ml pipets; 20 10-ml screw-capped test tubes; 50 cotton-plugged Pasteur pipets; 500 ml M solution; 0.1 N HCl; 0.1 N NaOH (or KOH); 10 standard 16 $\times$ 220-mm test tubes with 10-ml antibiotic mixture, 10 with 2% proteose peptone solution, and 10 with M solution; three crystallizing dishes or finger bowls.

Nonsterile Labwares. Pasteur pipets with rubber bulbs; three crystallizing dishes or finger bowls; one plastic Petri dish; scalpel with No. 15 blade; test-tube rack; dissection microscope; sterile hood (e.g., with UV light); microbiological incubator; observation stage (see Fig. 1), M solution; 95% ethanol.

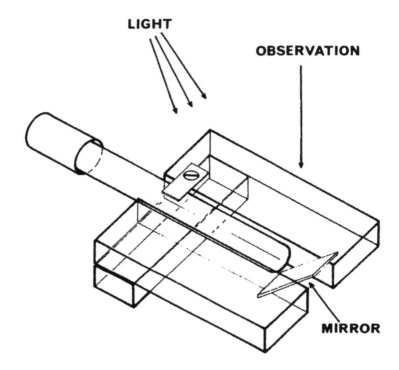

LIGHT

OBSERVATION

MIRROR

FIGURE 1. Observation stage for examination of hydra in test tubes. From a 13-mm Perspex plate cut two pieces measuring 35 $\times$ 90 mm and one piece 22 $\times$ 87 mm. With a few drops of chloroform (which dissolves Perspex), glue the two upper parts onto the lower part as shown. Use laboratory clamps to hold these parts tight for several hours. Between the two upper parts leave about 17 mm for future insertion of standard test tubes. From a mirror glass, cut a piece 30 $\times$ 17.5 mm. Place the stage on a flat surface and insert the mirror at an angle of 45° as shown. You may add a few drops of chloroform to glue the mirror to its place. With a screw, fasten a piece of aluminum 1 $\times$ 15 $\times$ 30 mm to one of the upper parts, as shown in the figure. This holds the test tube in its place while it is examined. To examine any of your test tubes containing hydra, place the observation stage on the stage of your dissection microscope, with the mirror at its center. Use upper oblique lighting. The hydra adhering to the lower part of the test tube are clearly seen in the mirror.

PROCEDURES

Preparing Solutions of Antibiotics

We recommend a final concentration of 100 μg/ml for each of the antibiotics used. We recommend the addition of phenol red to all solutions and media to monitor pH (Chapter 5). Use five antibiotics: penicillin, streptomycin, neomycin, rifampicin, and chloramphenicol. Penicillin and streptomycin are heat labile (Altman and Dittmer, 1964). For these, use the sterile powdered form obtainable in small capped vials to prepare antibiotic stock solutions at 100 times the desired concentration. Following standard sterile practices, remove the protective metal cover from the vial, wipe the rubber stopper with 95% ethanol, and add sterile M solution through the stopper using a sterile hypodermic syringe. The 1,000,000 units of penicillin in a typical vial can be dissolved in about 1–2 ml. To prepare a stock solution of 10,000 units/ml, for example, withdraw the sterile solution with the syringe, transfer it into a 250-ml sterile, covered Erlenmeyer flask and bring up the solution to 100 ml with sterile M solution. With a sterile pipet take out about 29 aliquots of 5 ml and place them into small, screw-capped, sterile test tubes and freeze them.

Follow the same procedure to prepare a stock solution of 10 mg/ml of streptomycin. Add neomycin and chloramphenicol, 100 μg/ml each, directly to M solution and autoclave for 10 min. Note the color of the contained Phenol Red pH indicator while preparing the solutions and after autoclaving them. Adjust the pH if necessary with sterile 0.1 N HCl or NaOH. To prepare rifampicin stock solutions, dissolve 10 mg/ml methanol. We observed no deleterious effect of the added methanol.

To prepare the final antibiotic mixture, aseptically add 1% of each of the penicillin, rifampicin, and streptomycin solutions to the autoclaved M solution containing neomycin and chloramphenicol. To prevent the accumulation of cytotoxic photoproducts of chloramphenicol (Rahat et al., 1979), keep solutions and experimental media containing this antibiotic in dim light (e.g., 500 lux). If rifampicin is used instead of chloramphenicol, no such precautions are necessary.

Cleaning and Transecting Hydra

With a Pasteur pipet, select about 100 hydra from a stock culture that has been starved for 48 hr. Avoid also animals with *Artemia* "eggs" inside their coelenteron. Spores of molds adhere to these eggs, and when they are regurgitated they contaminate the culture. Place the animals into 100 ml M solution, swirl the animals, and transfer them with a Pasteur pipet to another dish with 100 ml M solution. Repeat the washing two more times. Using a dissecting microscope (10–20× magnification), examine the animals before each transfer to ascertain that no observable debris adhere to them.

After the third washing, place animals in sterile M solution at the bottom of a plastic Petri dish. Using a scalpel, transect the hydra immediately below their budding zone and transfer only the upper part of them into a dish containing 100 ml sterile M solution. In this way you get rid of the fauna adhering to the peduncle and to the mucus it secretes. Within 24 hr the hydra regenerate a new basal disk.

Swirl and wash the cut hydra as described above, only this time use three 100-ml portions of sterile M solution and sterile, cotton-plugged Pasteur pipets.

Working in a sterile hood, and with sterile pipets, transfer groups of 10 of the washed hydra into covered sterile test tubes containing 10 ml of the antibiotic mixture. Keep the test tubes in dim light at 20°C for 48 hr.

Sterility Test

Working in a sterile hood and with sterile Pasteur pipette, remove with a minimal amount of fluid one hydra from each test tube containing the animals and the antibiotics and transfer them separately to test tubes containing 10 ml 2% proteose peptone solution. Change pipet for each test tube. Mark these test tubes to match the corresponding tubes from which the hydra were taken. Incubate the test tubes with proteose peptone and the single hydra at 30–32°C for 1 week. Solutions that contain bacteria-free hydra remain clear, while a clouded solution indicates bacterial contamination. Because the hydra decompose rapidly in 2% proteose peptone at 30°C, this sterility test also detects intracellular bacteria.

Maintenance and Examination of Bacteria-Free Hydra

At the same time you transfer the hydra for the sterility test, transfer the rest of the hydra remaining in each test tube (also with as little of the antibiotics as possible) into marked test tubes containing 10 ml sterile M solution. Bacteria-free hydra remain viable in this solution for at least several weeks and can be used for experiments that require bacteria-free animals. To visually examine the hydra closely while they are in test tubes, we recommend using the device depicted in Fig. 1. Such a device facilitates observation of hydra often hidden in the curvature on the bottom of the test tubes.

PRECAUTIONS

Rifampicin has a red color that interferes with that of the Phenol Red pH indicator (see Chapter 5). It does not, however, affect the pH, so add it after final pH adjustment.

COMMENTS

It is now possible to grow cultures of *H. viridis* axenically (Rahat and Dimentman, 1982). Use axenic hydra and axenic *Artemia* nauplii (see Chapter 6) hatched in test tubes containing 3 ml sterile proteose peptone in M solution. Place the tubes with the cysts on a rotating wheel (25 rpm) at 33°C. After 24–48 hr, collect the live nauplii aseptically with a Pasteur pipet, wash them three times in sterile M solution, and offer them to the axenic hydra. Because the uneaten dead larvae will not decay in the bacteria-free medium, you can allow them to remain in the sterile culture. Nonetheless, you may find it convenient to remove routinely (about once a week) and aseptically the accumulated dead larvae and debris.

ACKNOWLEDGMENTS. We thank the United States–Israeli Binational Science Foundation Fund for support (Grant No. 1827).

REFERENCES

Altman, P. L., and Dittmer, D. S., eds. 1964. *Biology Data Book*, 1964. Federation of American Societies for Experimental Biology, Washington, D.C.

Margulis, L., Thorington, G., Berger, B., and Stoltz, J. 1978. Endosymbiotic bacteria associated with the intracellular green algae of *Hydra viridis*. *Curr. Microbiol.* 1:227–232.

Rahat, M. and Dimentman, C.H. 1982. Cultivation of bacteria-free *Hydra viridis*: Missing budding factor in nonsymbiotic hydra. *Science* 216:67–68.

Rahat, M., Zeldes, D., and Reich, Vanda. 1979. Photoproducts of chloramphenicol: Their cytotoxic effects on *Hydra viridis* and its symbiotic algae. *Comp. Biochem. Physiol.* 63C:27–30.

Part II

Histology

Chapter 13

Preparing Hydra for Transmission Electron Microscopy

Richard L. Wood

PURPOSE

The observation of fixed and sectioned material by transmission electron microscopy (TEM) has become a routine extension of light-microscopic methodology. The superior resolution of the electron microscope has obvious advantages for correlative studies of structure and function at the macromolecular level. Modern preparative methods allow the use of a variety of ancillary techniques such as cytochemistry and electron-dense tracers, as well as simply viewing adjacent sections by TEM and light microscopy.

INTRODUCTION

Hydra are prepared for TEM by methods similar to those used for other metazoans. Fixation involves the use of buffered aldehydes and OsO_4, either in sequence or in a combined mixture. The fixed tissues are dehydrated, embedded in epoxy resin, and sectioned with an ultramicrotome. Sections for light microscopy are cut at 0.5–2.0 μm (semithin sections), whereas those for electron microscopy are cut at 0.05—0.1 μm (thin sections). Semithin sections are mounted in immersion oil on glass slides and viewed by phase optics or stained and mounted similarly for examination with regular light

Richard L. Wood ● Department of Anatomy, University of Southern California, School of Medicine, Los Angeles, California.

optics. Thin sections are mounted on copper grids and treated with heavy-metal salts to enhance contrast at the electron microscope. Special procedures useful in preparing hydra for TEM include the following: (1) Anesthetization to keep animals expanded during fixation. (2) Use of low-molarity buffers to reduce osmotic effects of the fixative solution. (3) Use of a dual aldehyde primary fixation (glutaraldehyde and either formaldehyde or acrolein), or a combination of aldehydes and OsO_4 in a single fixative solution. The composition of the fixative influences cellular morphology (Figs. 1 and 2), and more than one type of fixation should be employed if experimental design necessitates interpretation of ultrastructural changes. (4) *En bloc* staining with magnesium uranyl acetate or other procedures such as inclusion of tannic acid (Mitzuhira and Futaesaku, 1972) or H_2O_2 (Peracchia and Mittler, 1972) in the fixatives, to enhance membrane contrast. (5) Use of Araldite embedding for greatest section stability (Luft, 1961). Araldite also provides the best support for nematocyst capsules (Figs. 3 and 4). (6) Use of Spurr's low-viscosity embedding medium to reduce osmotic shrinkage (Spurr, 1969). Low-viscosity resin embedding is of particular value for study of normal cellular relationships in hydra by light microscopy (Fig. 5).

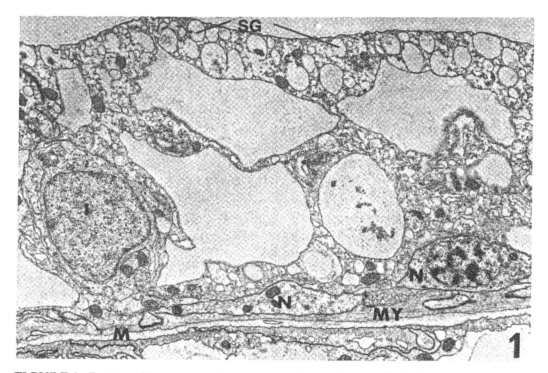

FIGURE 1. Portion of hypostome after combined glutaraldehyde–OsO_4 fixation and Araldite embedding. The general preservation is good, but subsurface granules of epidermal cells (SG) are electron lucent. N, neurons; MY, myonemes; M, mesoglea; and I, I cell, are obvious (4400X, reproduced at 90%).

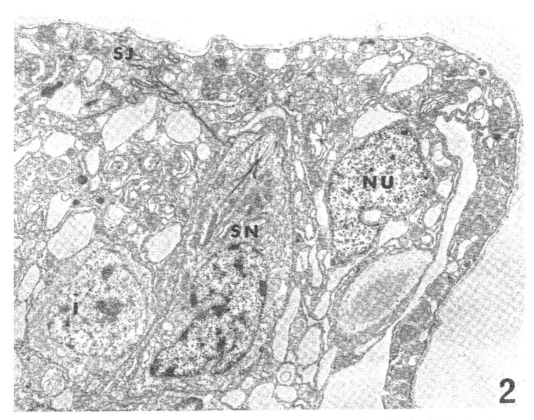

FIGURE 2. Portion of hypostomal ectoderm after sequential aldehyde–OsO$_4$ fixation and Araldite embedding. Subsurface granules (SG) are dense after this fixation. Other preservation appears similar to Fig. 1. I, I cell; SN, sensory neuron; NU, nucleus of epitheliomuscular cell; SJ, septate junctions (5400X, reproduced at 90%).

MATERIALS

All reagents and supplies used for TEM preparation are available from ordinary chemical and electron microscopy supply houses. The reagents and recommended sources are pure glutaraldehyde and embedding resins (Ladd Research Industries, Burlington, VT); paraformaldehyde (Fisher Chemical Company, Pittsburgh, PA); acrolein and magnesium uranyl acetate (K and K Laboratories, Plainview, NY); and sodium cacodylate (Sigma Chemical Company, Saint Louis, MO).

PROCEDURES

1. Anesthetize animals in culture water containing 5–10 mg/ml Nembutal (sodium pentobarbital) for 5–10 min (Wood, 1974).

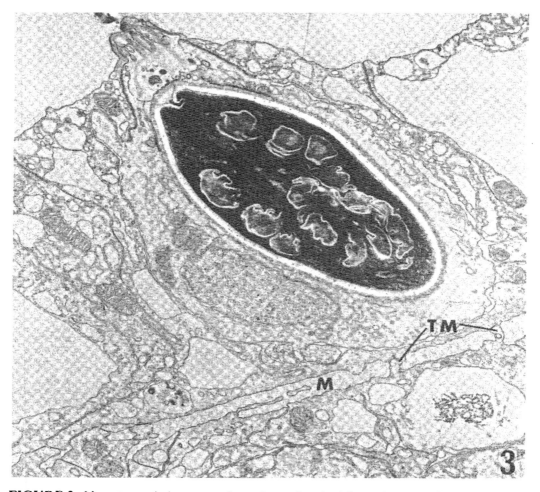

FIGURE 3. Nematocyst in hypostomal ectoderm after Araldite embedding. Glutaraldehyde–OsO₄ fixation. M, mesoglea; TM, transmesogleal contacts (11,500×, reproduced at 90%).

2. Remove excess fluid gently and flood with fixative consisting of (1) 0.75% glutaraldehyde, 0.75% formaldehyde (prepared from paraformaldehyde immediately before use), and 0.05 M sodium phosphate or sodium cacodylate buffer, pH 7.4; or (2) 0.75% glutaraldehyde, 0.5% acrolein, and 0.05 M sodium phosphate or sodium cacodylate buffer, pH 7.4. Fixation in solutions (1) and (2) should be for approximately 30 min at room temperature. After aldehyde fixation the tissues should be washed briefly in 0.05 M buffer and postfixed for 1 hr in similarly buffered ice cold 1% OsO₄. (3) Alternatively, fix for 1 hr in a solution made from equal volumes of double-strength solution (1) mixed with 2% OsO₄ immediately before use. The two solutions should be ice cold before mixing and should be maintained on ice throughout fixation. No postfixation with OsO₄ is required with this method.

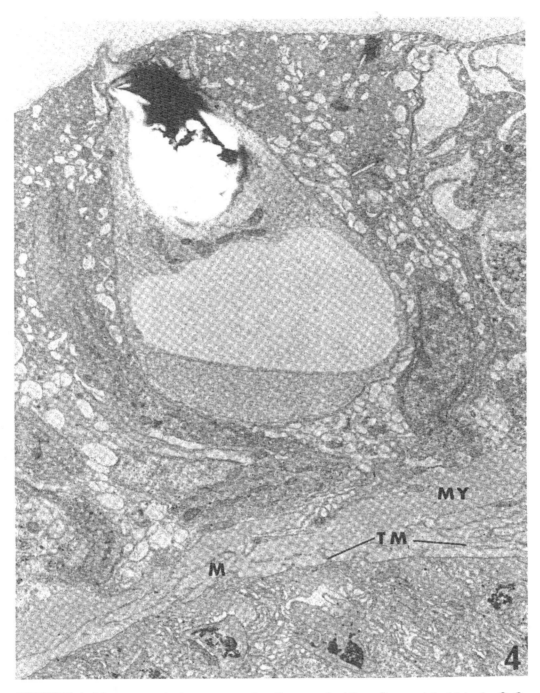

FIGURE 4. Nematocyst in hypostome after Spurr embedding. Sequential aldehyde–OsO₄ fixation. This section was taken from near the mouth and the transmesogleal epithelial contacts (TM) are numerous across the attenuating mesoglea (M); MY, myomeme (5400×, reproduced at 90%).

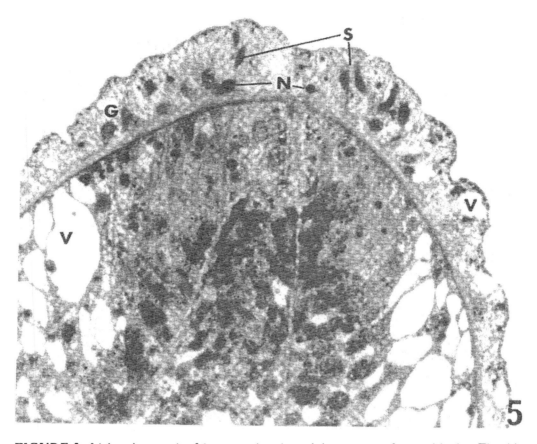

FIGURE 5. Light micrograph of 1-μm section through hypostome of normal hydra. The thin lines in the center (arrows) represent enteric lumen, and the notch in the epidermis represents the edge of the mouth. The large spaces (V) are intracellular vacuoles (both entodermal and epidermal). Note the more condensed arrangement of cells and processes near the mouth and the accumulation of sensory (S) and ganglion (G) cells in this epidermis. Nematoblasts (N) are fixed sequentially in aldehydes and OsO_4 with H_2O_2 added to the aldehydes (Peracchia and Mittler, 1972). Embedded in Spurr's medium. Stained with alkaline Methylene Blue-Azure II (Richardson *et al.*, 1960) (490×, reproduced at 90%).

Variations which employ 1% tannic acid (Mitzuhira and Futaesaku, 1972) or H_2O_2 (Peracchia and Mittler, 1972) should be used with glutaraldehyde alone in the primary fixative and require postfixation with OsO_4.

3. Rinse briefly in 0.05 *M* buffer.

4. Treat for 1–2 hr in magnesium uranyl acetate in 0.3% NaCl at room temperature (optional).

5. Dehydrate in a graded series (30%, 50%, 70%, 95%, and 100%) of ethyl alcohols for a total time of 1 hr.

6. Pass through two 10-min changes of propylene oxide and infilter in epoxy resin (Luft, 1961). For Araldite, it is best to prepare the medium at an

anhydride:epoxy ratio of 3:5. The cutting properties of the cured block are improved by adding 3% Dow Epoxy Resin (DER) 736 to the mixture. Mix aliquots of this stock solution with 1.75% v/v DMP-30 [tri(dimethyl-aminomethyl)phenol)] accelerator immediately before infiltration commences. Infiltration with 1:1 resin and propylene oxide for 1–2 hr and with a 2:1 resin/propylene oxide mixture for 5 hr to overnight is followed by polymerization in an oven sequence of 45–55°C for 8–12 hr each and 68°C for 24 hr. For Spurr's embedding medium, the harder mixture recommended (Spurr, 1969) is most satisfactory. The propylene oxide diluent step is not essential with Spurr's embedding but will speed the replacement of alcohol with resin.

7. Orient tissue as desired and section with a glass knife at 0.5–2 μm for light microscopy. Sections may be transferred to a glass slide by means of a wire loop or a fine camel's hair brush (see Fig. 5).

8. Stain 2–5 min with Methylene Blue-Azure II in borax (Richardson *et al.*, 1960) at 60°C.

9. Cut thin sections approximately 0.1 μm (1000 Å) thick with a glass or diamond knife and collect on carbon-coated copper grids.

10. Stain grids with 2.5% aqueous uranyl acetate for 10 min and lead nitrate (Reynolds, 1963) for 5 min prior to viewing at the electron microscope. After Spurr's embedding, more extended staining time in lead salts is usually required (15–30 min).

PRECAUTIONS

It is particularly important to recognize that morphological features of highly hydrated invertebrate tissue viewed at the ultrastructural level are frequently distorted by the preparative procedures. Although this distortion may not be a serious problem for many types of studies, it can introduce major complications in the interpretation of subtle morphological variations in cells, either normal or experimentally introduced. For example, large vacuolar profiles in hydra epithelia appear to be entirely intracellular in well-fixed and embedded normal animals. After certain experimental manipulations and with some embedding procedures, the vacuoles may appear to be extensions of extracellular space. It is of considerable functional significance to know which situation occurs in the living organism.

REFERENCES

Luft, J. H. 1961. Improvements in epoxy resin embedding methods. *J. Biophys. Biochem. Cytol.* 9:409–414.

Mitzuhira, V., and Futaesaku, Y. 1972. New fixation for biological membranes using tannic acids. *Acta Histochem. Cytochem.* 5:233–234.

Peracchia, C., and Mittler, B. S. 1972. Fixation by means of glutaraldehyde–hydrogen peroxide reaction products. *J. Cell Biol.* 53:234–238.

Reynolds, E. S. 1963. The use of lead citrate at high pH as an electron-opaque stain in electron microscopy. *J. Cell Biol.* 17:208–213.

Richardson, K. C., Jarrett, L., and Finke, E. H. 1960. Embedding in epoxy resins for ultrathin sectioning in electron microscopy. *Stain Technol.* 35:313–323.

Spurr, A. R. 1969. A low-viscosity epoxy resin embedding medium for electron microscopy. *J. Ultrastruct. Res.* 26:31–43.

Wood, R. L. 1974. A closely packed array of membrane intercalated particles at the free surface of *Hydra. J. Cell. Biol.* 62:556–560.

Wood, R. L. 1979. The fine structure of the hypostome and mouth of hydra II. Transmission electron microscopy. *Cell Tissue Res.* 199:319–338.

Chapter 14

Preparing Hydra for Scanning Electron Microscopy

Richard L. Wood

PURPOSE

Scanning electron microscopy (SEM) is used predominantly to study cell surfaces, although slices of tissue or fractured surfaces of fixed or frozen specimens can also reveal some features of internal organelles. Conventional scanning instruments are limited in resolution to approximately 150 Å with most biological material (Everhart and Hayes, 1972). Field emission instruments now coming into more general use are expected to improve this figure significantly (Crewe, 1971). The scanning electron microscope can also be used for x-ray microanalysis. When used with the scanning transmission mode of operation, important information concerning the presence and distribution of specific elements of biological significance can be obtained (Marshall, 1975).

INTRODUCTION

The procedures used to prepare hydra for SEM are similar to those used for other tissues. Techniques especially useful with hydra include (1) anesthetization (Chapter 13) or utilizing OsO_4 in the primary fixative to avoid excessive distortion from agonal myoneme contraction; (2) slicing animals during dehydration, fracturing them in liquid nitrogen, or me-

---

Richard L. Wood ● Department of Anatomy, University of Southern California, School of Medicine, Los Angeles, California.

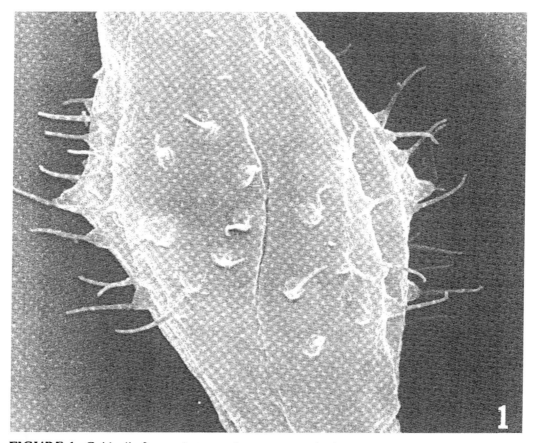

FIGURE 1. Cnidocils from a battery of nematocysts in the tentacle (1900×, reproduced at 85%).

chanically fracturing them after critical point drying in order to expose internal surfaces; (3) embedding in agar and chopping at 100–200 μm with a Sorvall TC-2 tissue chopper to reveal cellular relationships; (4) exposure to thiocarbohydrazide and a second treatment with osmium to enhance tissue contrast (Kelley *et al.*, 1973); (5) stereo viewing and stereophotography to enhance depth perception; and (6) parallel examination of thin sections to aid interpretations.

MATERIALS

Reagents and supplies used in SEM are readily available from ordinary chemical and electron microscopy supply houses. Glutaraldehyde from Ladd Research Industries (Burlington, VT) and paraformaldehyde from Fisher

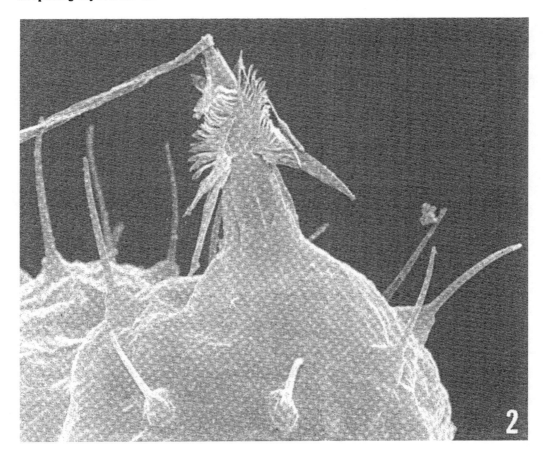

FIGURE 2. Discharged stenotele nematocysts (6400×, reproduced at 85%).

Chemical Co. (Pittsburgh, PA) are recommended.

PROCEDURES (SEE WOOD, 1979)

1. Allow hydra to expand in a small volume of culture water or anesthetize them in culture water containing 5–10 mg/ml sodium pentobarbital.

2. Flood with fixative buffered to pH 7.4–7.5 with 0.05 M sodium cacodylate. If the animals are not anesthetized the fixative should be either 2% OsO_4 or a mixture of aldehydes and OsO_4. Either of these should be kept ice cold. A satisfactory aldehyde–osmium combined fixative consists of 0.75% glutaraldehyde, 0.75% formaldehyde (prepared freshly from paraformaldehyde), and 1% OsO_4 prepared in 0.05 M sodium cacodylate buffer,

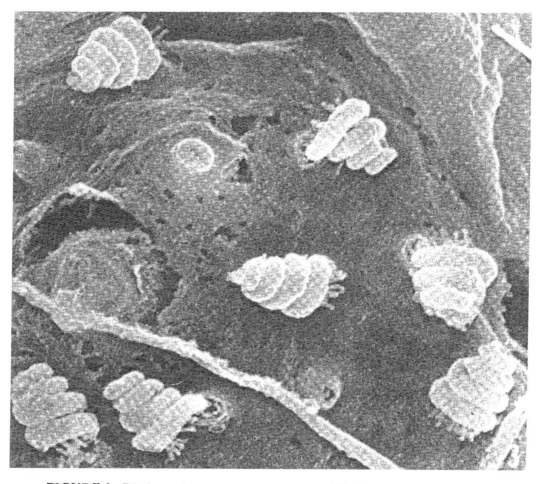

FIGURE 3. Discharged desmoneme nematocysts (4700×. reproduced at 85%).

pH 7.4–7.5. The OsO_4 should be added immediately before use. Anesthetized animals may be fixed sequentially in the aldehyde and osmium mixtures. For sequential fixation the aldehydes should be maintained at room temperature, but treatment with osmium should be done over ice.

3. Dehydrate through an ethanol series (30%, 50%, 70%, 95%, and 100%) and dry by the critical point procedure with either CO_2 or Freon as transition fluids.

4. Alternate methods: (1) Embed individual fixed hydra in 3% agar and slice at 100–200 μm with a Sorvall TC-2 tissue chopper. Recover slices, wash thoroughly in 0.05 M cacodylate buffer, pH 7.4–7.5, and treat with 0.5% thiocarbohydrazide for 15 min. Wash thoroughly and expose to

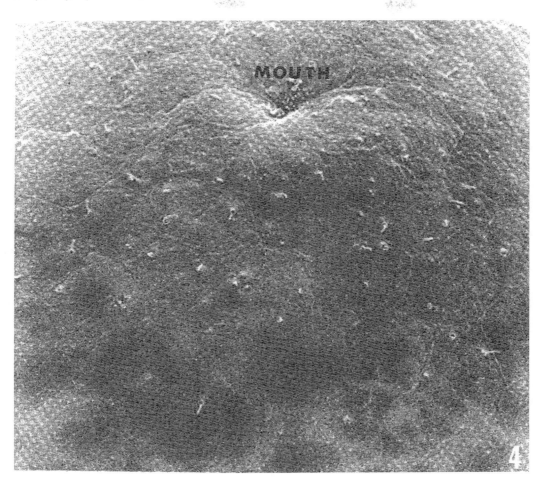

FIGURE 4. Cnidocils (and possibly some sensory cilia) in the ectoderm near the mouth (1050X, reproduced at 85%).

buffered 1% OsO_4 for 1 hr. Wash thoroughly again and proceed with dehydration and critical point drying as indicated above. (2) After ethanol dehydration, freeze in liquid N_2 and fracture with a cold razor blade (Boyde and Wood, 1969). Allow to warm to room temperature in absolute ethanol and proceed with critical point drying.

5. Mount dried specimens on SEM holders with double-stick Scotch tape or in silver conducting paint (Ted Pella, Inc., Tustin, CA).

6. Coat specimens with 50- to 100 Å gold–palladium alloy in a sputter-coater or in a vacuum evaporator.

7. Paint edge of specimen holder with silver conducting paint if specimens are mounted on Scotch tape.

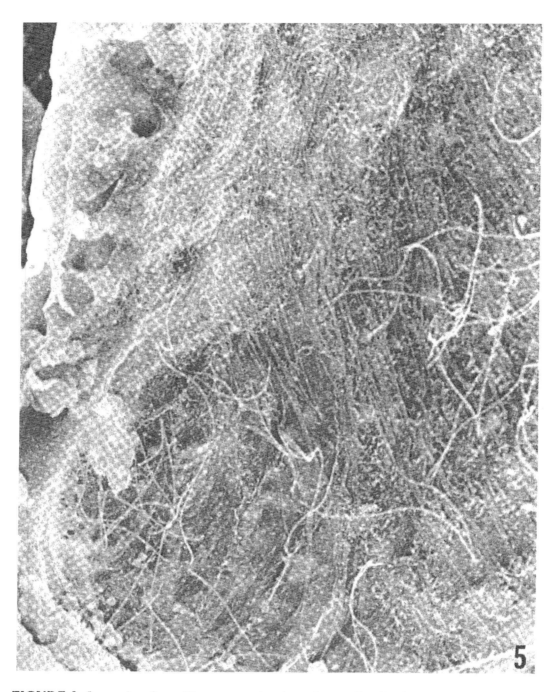

FIGURE 5. Internal surface of hypostome showing adherent flagella (Wood, 1979) (1900×, reproduced at 85%).

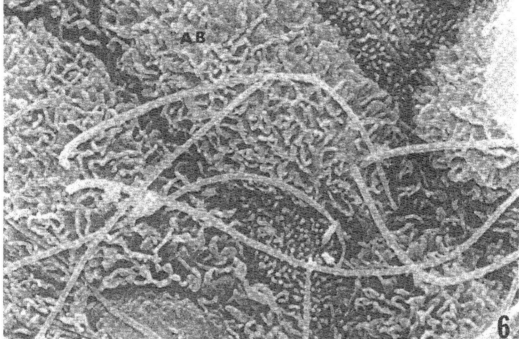

FIGURE 6. Internal surface of enteron showing surface features of absorptive (AB) and glandular cells. Note the differences in microvilli (5550×, reproduced at 85%).

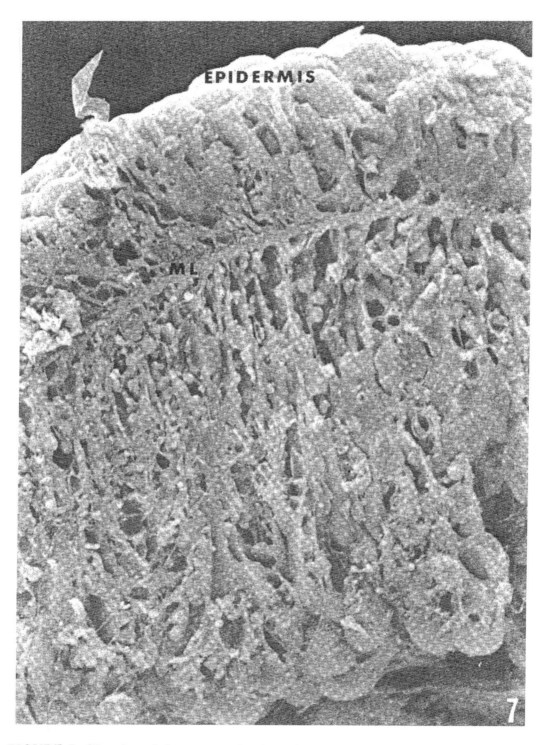

FIGURE 7. Slice through hypostome showing cell boundaries, intracellular vacuoles, the mesolamella, and basally located myonemes (970×, reproduced at 85%).

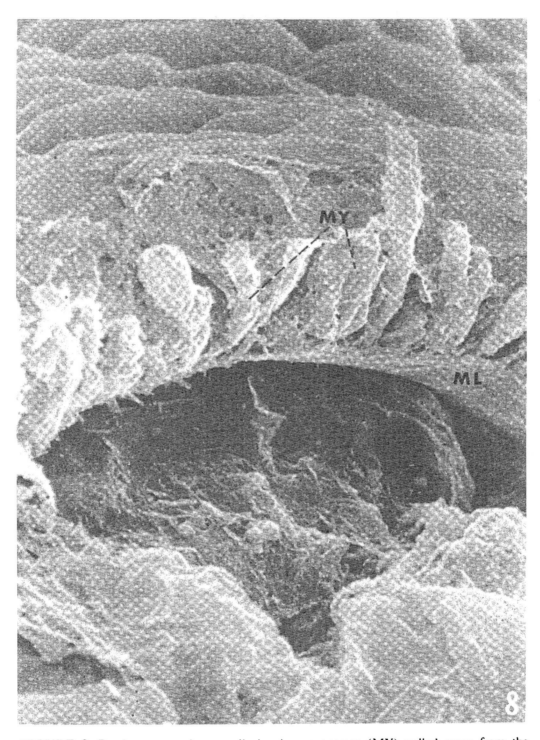

FIGURE 8. Break across column wall showing myonemes (MY) pulled away from the mesolamella (ML) (2600×, reproduced at 90%).

REFERENCES

Boyde, A., and Wood, C. 1969. Preparation of animal tissues for surface scanning electron microscopy. *J. Microsc.* **90**:221–249.

Crewe, A. 1971. A high resolution scanning electron microscope. *Sci. Am.* **224**:26–35.

Everhart, T., and Hayes, T. 1972. The scanning electron microscope. *Sci. Am.* **226**:54–69.

Kelley, R., Dekker, R., and Bluemink, J. 1973. Ligand-mediated osmium binding: Its application in coating biological specimens for scanning electron microscopy. *J. Ultrastruct. Res.* **45**:254–258.

Marshall, A. 1975. Electron probe x-ray microanalysis. In: *Principles and Techniques of Scanning Electron Microscopy: Biological Applications*, vol. 4 (M. Hayat, ed.). Van Nostrand Reinhold, New York, pp. 103–173.

Wood, R. L. 1979. The fine structure of the hypostome and mouth of hydra. I. Scanning electron microscopy. *Cell Tissue Res.* **199**:319–338.

Chapter 15

Preparing Hydra for Freeze-Fracture and Freeze-Etching

Richard L. Wood

PURPOSE

The freeze-fracture technique is particularly advantageous for the study of cell surfaces and intercellular junctions. In general, it involves the rapid freezing of tissues, either with or without partial sublimation of ice (etching). By evaporating a film of pure carbon on the exposed surface, a replica of the cell surface is obtained which reveals its intimate contours. Contrast is obtained by shadowing the exposed surface with evaporated platinum prior to forming the replica. The tissue is removed from the replica by digestion in caustic solutions prior to recovery of the replicas for viewing at the electron microscope (Koehler, 1972). When a fracture occurs along the plane of a biological membrane it tends to split the lipid core and reveal unique surfaces for subsequent replication (Branton, 1966). Junctional regions can be identified by the arrangement of intramembranous particles, which appear to consist predominantly of protein. The distribution of surface components can be localized by combining the freeze-etching procedure with surface probes conjugated with large molecular weight compounds such as ferritin.

Richard L. Wood ● Department of Anatomy, University of Southern California, School of Medicine, Los Angeles, California.

INTRODUCTION

Hydra are prepared for freeze-fracture by procedures similar to those used for other metazoans. Special procedures useful with hydra include the following: (1) Prior to fixation, the animals must be anesthetized to avoid extreme dimensional changes as a result of myoid process contraction during fixation. Such contraction could be prevented by employing direct OsO_4 fixation, but the use of OsO_4 is incompatible with the freeze-fracture technique.(2)There are regional differences in the fine structure of hydra, and interpretation of replica images is greatly aided by knowing beforehand the region being fractured. Therefore, the animals should be dissected or cut into appropriate fragments prior to mounting on specimen holders and freezing. (3) Because of the wide range of cell sizes, the differences in organization of the two epithelia, and the variations in morphology typical of longitudinal and cross sections, the tissues should be mounted so the fracture plane can be reasonably predicted. (4) A briefer than normal aldehyde fixation (10–20 min) makes digestion and removal of the organic material during replica cleaning an easier task. This cleaning is particularly important with hydra because the polysaccharide-rich coatings on cells, and the gastrodermal glandular materials, are not removed readily by standard Clorox treatment. Cleaning of replicas of hydra tissue usually takes longer than for replicas of many tissues of higher organisms. (5) Use of a double replica device that fractures the specimen by means of a free break rather than with a knife blade provides large areas of split membranes, an obvious advantage for studies of membrane specializations.

MATERIALS

Veterinary-grade sodium pentobarbital (50–60 mg/ml) can be obtained through drug suppliers but requires an NDEA permit. Also recommended are high-purity glutaraldehyde from Ladd Research Industries, Burlington, VT; paraformaldehyde from Fisher Chemical Co., Pittsburgh, PA; and sodium cacodylate from Sigma Chemical Co., St. Louis, MO. Freon 22 is available from Virginia Chemical Co. (Portsmouth, VA). Clorox is a commercially available household bleach; the pure active ingredient, sodium hypochlorite, may be obtained from Fisher Chemical Co. but is not necessary.

PROCEDURES (SEE WOOD, 1977, 1979)

1. Place hydra in culture water containing 5–10 mg/ml sodium pentobarbital and allow the animals to relax 5–10 min.

2. Remove excess fluid gently and flood with fixative consisting of 0.75% glutaraldehyde, 0.75% formaldehyde (prepared freshly from para-formaldehyde), and 0.05 M sodium cacodylate buffer, pH 7.4–7.5 Continue fixation for 10–20 min at room temperature.

3. Rinse briefly in 0.05 M cacodylate buffer to remove excess fixative.

4. Glycerinate the specimens for 1.5–2 hr by placing them in a sequence of 10%, 20%, and 30% glycerol diluted with cacodylate buffer (final concentration 0.05 M) for at least 30 min each. Refrigerate the specimens if they are to be stored in glycerol for longer than 2 hr.

5. Mount the specimens on holders and freeze in Freon 22 held close to its freezing point with liquid nitrogen (Koehler, 1972).

6. Transfer to cold specimen stage of the freeze-fracture apparatus.

7. Fracture, shadow with platinum, and replicate with carbon (Koehler, 1972).

8. Transfer replicas with adherent specimens into 100% methanol for 0.5–2 hr.

9. Float replicas onto distilled water and transfer to pure Clorox with a platinum wire loop.

10. Treat with Clorox for 12 hr, changing the solution several times.

11. Transfer replicas to distilled water, then through 25%–50% sulfuric acid and leave for 0.5–2 hr.

12. Transfer replicas to distilled water through 25% sulfuric acid and rinse three times in distilled water.

13. Pick up replicas on 300-mesh uncoated copper grids or larger-mesh coated grids, for viewing at the electron microscope.

COMMENTS

Because of the randomness of the fracture plane through frozen hydra tissues, it is frequently difficult to be certain of their orientation. The presence of nematocysts within an epithelium indicates ectoderm (Fig. 1), and the presence of gland cells or flagellae at a free surface indicates endoderm (Fig. 2). Unfortunately, these features are not always visible in the plane of fracture, but the free epidermal surface has another identifying feature. The plasma membrane contains closely packed aggregates of intramembranous particles on one fracture surface (Fig. 3), or complementary groups of pits on the apposing fracture face (Fig. 4). This arrangement does not occur in the membranes of endodermal cells. An orientation landmark in hydra is the mesolamella. In freeze-fracture replicas the mesolamella can be identified by the appearance of coarse, extracellular fibrils or by its location adjacent to recognizable myonemes (Fig. 5). In the hypostome region indigenous spirochetes are also common in the mesolamella and can be

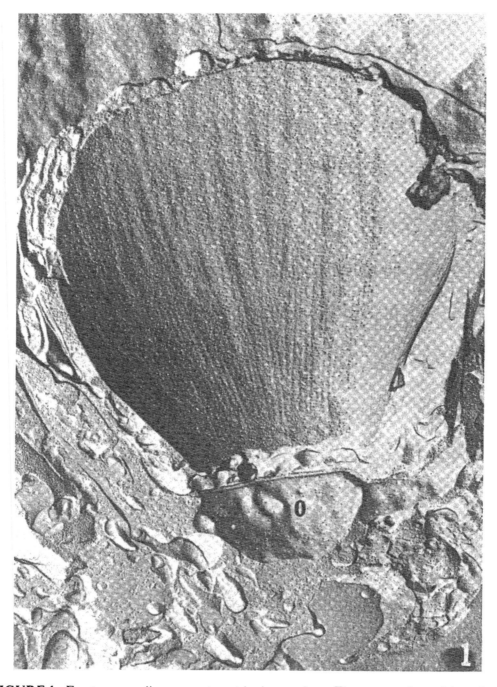

FIGURE 1. Fracture revealing a nematocyst in the ectoderm. The outer surface of the animal is at the lower right. 0, operculum (37,500×, reproduced at 85%).

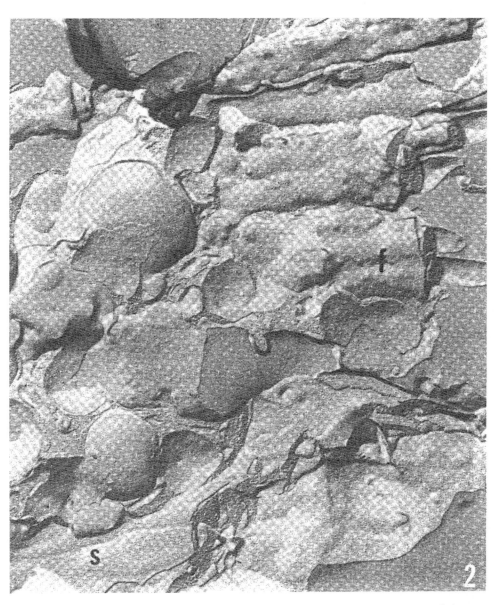

FIGURE 2. Fracture at enteron lumen showing flagellae (f). At the lower left is part of a septate junction (S) (28,700×, reproduced at 85%).

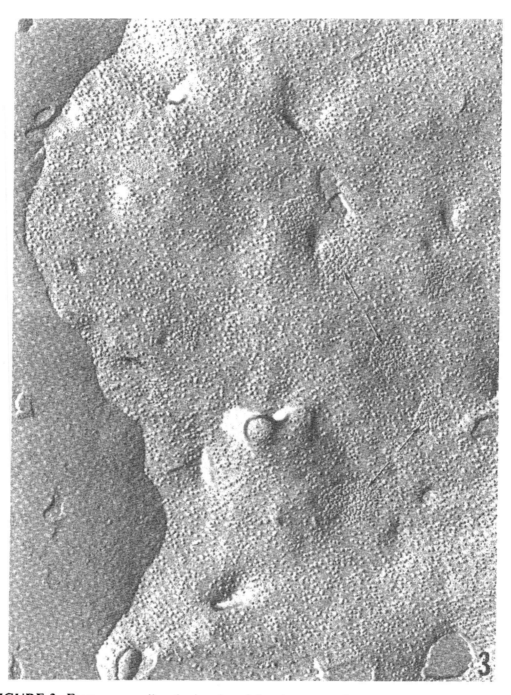

FIGURE 3. Fracture revealing the interior of the plasma membrane, the protoplasmic face. The outside of the animal is to the left. The arrows indicate clusters of intramembranous granules (91,000×, reproduced at 85%).

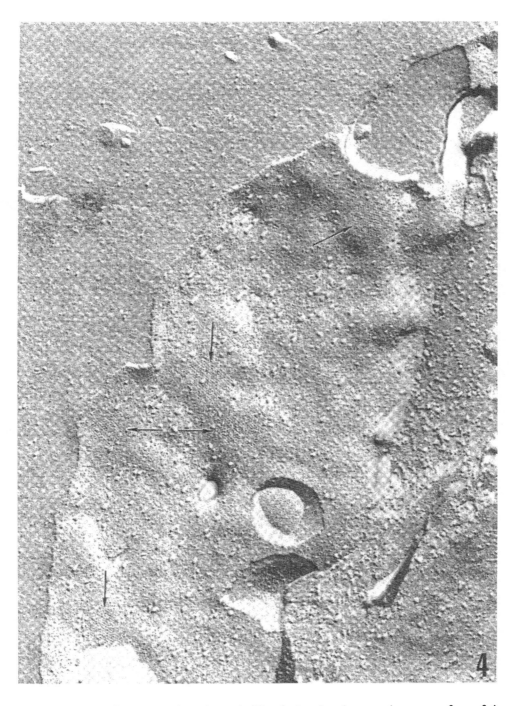

FIGURE 4. Similar fracture to that shown in Fig. 3 showing the complementary face of the membrane interior, the external face. Clusters of pits at the arrows correspond to the clusters of granules in Fig. 3 (91,700×, reproduced at 85%).

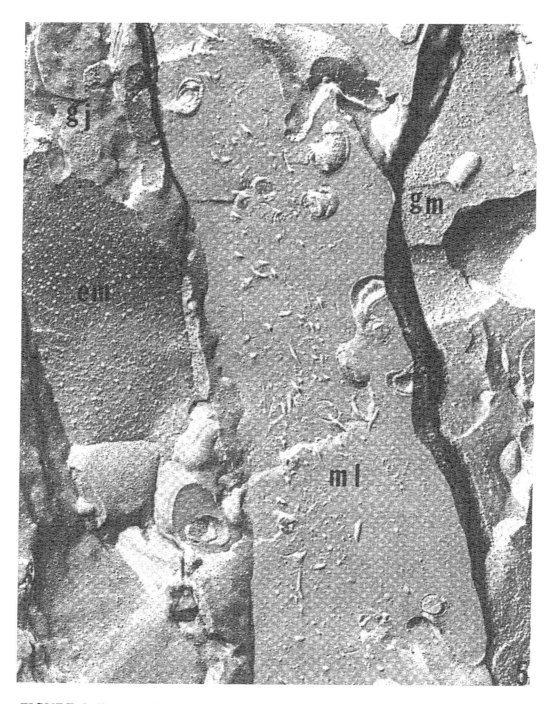

FIGURE 5. Fracture through the hypostome showing the mesolamella (ml) and part of an ectodermal cell myoneme (em). A gap junction appears on the myoneme (g j). The base of an endodermal cell showing myofilaments is at the right (gm) (45,500×, reproduced at 85%).

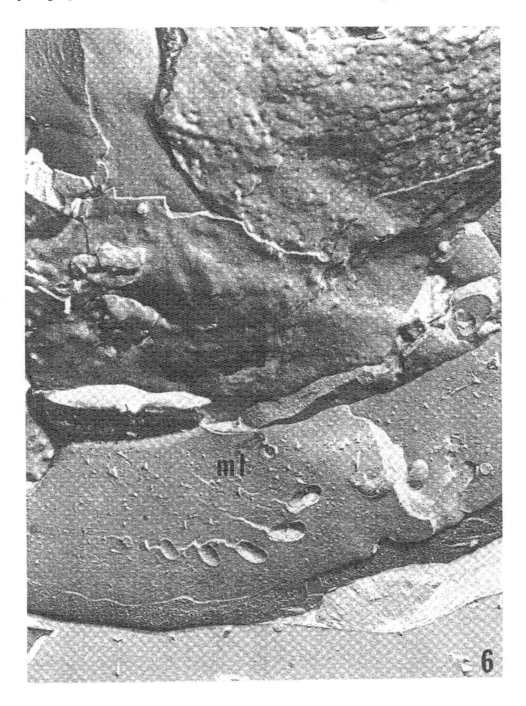

FIGURE 6. Fracture through hypostome showing portions of a spirochete lying in the mesolamella (ml). The ectoderm is at the top, and the endoderm is below (29,000×, reproduced at 85%).

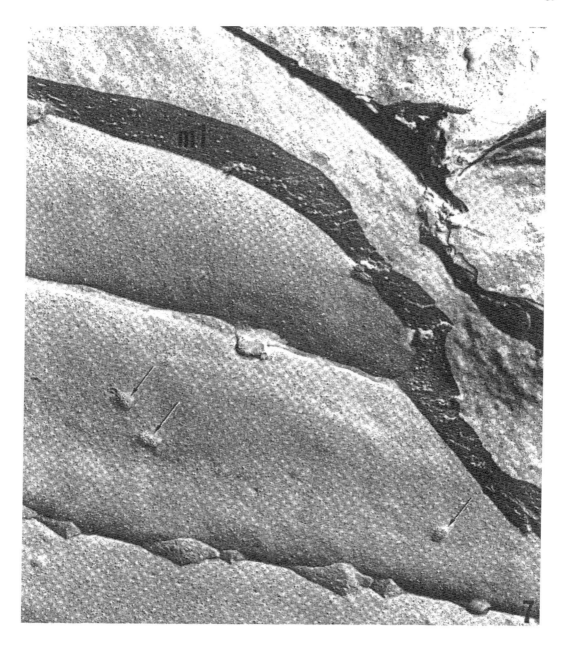

FIGURE 7. Fracture through body wall showing protoplasmic faces of ectodermal cell myonemes at the left. The endoderm is to the upper right with the mesolamella (ml) between the two layers. One myoneme shows focal particle aggregates on small elevations (arrows) (31,000×, reproduced at 85%).

recognized in replicas (Fig. 6). The spirochetes may be eliminated from cultures by treating with antibiotics. When the replica does not display free ectodermal or endodermal surfaces because of fragmentation, it is still possible to recognize ectoderm when fractured membranes show focal particle aggregates located on small elevations (Fig. 7). Again, this particle arrangement is characteristic of the basal region of ectodermal cells and has not been seen in the endoderm.

REFERENCES

Branton, D. 1966. Fracture faces of frozen membranes. *Proc. Natl. Acad. Sci. U.S.A.* **55**:1048–1056.

Koehler, J. 1972. The freeze-etching technique. In: *Principles and Techniques of Electron Microscopy. Biological Applications*, vol. 2 (M. Hayat, ed.), Van Nostrand Reinhold, New York, pp. 53–98.

Wood, R. 1977. The cell junctions of hydra revealed by freeze fracture replication. *J. Ultrastruct. Res.* **58**:299–315.

Wood, R. 1979. The fine structure of the hypostome and mouth of hydra. II. Transmission electron microscopy. *Cell Tissue Res.* **199**:319–338.

Chapter 16

Whole Mounts for Light Microscopy

Richard D. Campbell

PURPOSE

To prepare whole mounts, thereby enabling one to study large areas of hydra in a single microscopic field in which spatial relationships are preserved between cells, and also to preserve experimental animals for future microscopic analyses.

GENERAL METHOD

MATERIALS

Ethanol and xylene for dehydration; mounting medium (e.g.,Permount, Fisher Scientific Co.); small vials; Pasteur pipets; microscope slides; cover slips; No. 1 cover glasses; histological stains.

PROCEDURES

Allow the hydra to elongate, if desired, in 0.25 ml 10% ethanol in a 2- to 5-ml vial (Burnett, 1959). After a few minutes suddenly flood the hydra with several milliliters of fixative, and after 1 min replace with fresh fixative

Richard D. Campbell ● Department of Developmental and Cell Biology, University of California, Irvine, California.

solution. After fixation is complete, draw off the fixative using a Pasteur pipet, and stain the hydra according to the desired processes (see below). Dehydrate them by adding and removing successively 50%, 70%, 95%, and twice 100% ethanol; ethanol xylene (1:1); and twice xylene, all for 5 min each. For particular applications, this schedule can often be shortened as determined by trial.

Pipet the hydra onto a glass microscope slide and draw off most of the xylene puddle using the corner of a sheet of absorbent paper, then promptly cover the specimen with a drop of mounting medium. Slowly lower a cover glass onto the hydra. Adjust the volume of mounting medium so that the cover glass is touching the hydra. It is often advantageous to flatten the hydra somewhat. Absorb mounting medium from around the edge of the cover slip, pressing on the cover glass, if necessary, to flatten the preparation.

SPECIFIC STAINING PROCEDURES

TOLUIDINE BLUE STAINING OF INTERSTITIAL CELLS (BURNETT, 1959; DIEHL AND BURNETT, 1964)

Procedures

Relax a hydra in alcohol for 1 min. Fix in 70% ethanol 5 min, rinse in water and draw off, and add 0.25 ml 0.05% Toluidine Blue (pH 8). Agitate the preparation every 30 sec for 2 min and fill the vial with water. After the hydra settles to the bottom draw off this fluid and add 70% alcohol. Agitate the preparation every minute, changing solutions if necessary to observe the destaining. When the hydra is light blue (about 10 min to 1 hr), transfer it to absolute ethanol and continue as described under General Method.

The ectodermal epithelial cells, after such a staining, should be colorless. The interstitial cells will be deep blue. Nematocytes mounted at the surface of the body column and tentacles will usually be black. Endoderm will be lighter or darker blue depending on the density of food particles in the digestive cells.

Intracellular vital carbon marks (Chapter 24) will remain visible in these preparations.

FEULGEN STAINING FOR LOCATING MITOTIC CELLS

Reagents

Lavdowsky's fixative (ethanol:formatin:acetic acid:water = 50:10: 4:40); 6 N HCl (freshly prepared); "SO_2 water," prepared immediately before use by mixing two stable stock solutions: 5 ml 1 N HCl (stock A) and 5 ml 10% $Na_2S_2O_5$ (stock B) with 90 ml water.

Schiff reagent may be purchased from Fisher Scientific Co. or prepared as follows: cautiously add 1 g Basic Fuchsin to 200 ml boiling water and continue boiling for 5 min. Cool the solution to 50°C and add 2 g $Na_2S_2O_5$ or $K_2S_2O_5$. Shake it well and let stand in a stoppered bottle in the dark overnight. Add 0.5 g neutral activated charcoal (Merck), shake the mixture for exactly 1 min, and filter it rapidly through a double thickness of Whatman #1 paper. Store the reagent in dark at 4°C. The solution may be reused as long as it is clear.

Procedures

Fix hydra at least 4 hr in Lavdowsky's fixative. Hydra may be left in this fixative indefinitely. Wash them twice in water and stain them by the Feulgen procedure: 10 min in 6 N HCl, 1 min in water, 1 hr in Schiff reagent (in dark), three transfers of 2 min each in "SO_2" water, and 10 min of washing in tap water with frequent changes. Dehydrate the specimens and mount them.

After being stained by the Feulgen method, chromosomes should appear magenta. Some endodermal food inclusions will also stain intensely. Interphase nuclei of epithelial and large interstitial cells will stain lightly and uniformly. Interphase nuclei of small cells will stain darkly and irregularly.

OTHER PROCEDURES

The method of preparing whole amounts of hydra can be adapted to many experimental uses. Applications reported in the literature include (1) thiolactic acid Pb^{2+} staining of developing nematoblasts (Chapter 23) David and Challoner, 1974); (2) whole-mount autoradiography of ectoderm (Zumstein and Tardent, 1972); (3) Methylene Blue staining of nematocyst capsules (with specificity for nematocyst type controllable by pH) (Burnett, 1960); (4) interference microscopy of nematocyte orientation (Campbell and Marcum, 1979); and (5) polarization microscopy of muscle processes (Otto, 1977).

REFERENCES

Burnett, A. L. 1959. Histophysiology of growth in hydra. *J. Exp. Zool.* **140**:281–342.

Burnett, A. L. 1960. The nematocyst of hydra. II. The maturation of nematocysts in hydra. *Ann. Soc. R. Zool. Belg.* **90**:269–280.

Campbell, R. D., and Marcum, B. A. 1980. Nematocyte migration in hydra: Evidence for contact guidance *in vivo*. *J. Cell. Sci.* **41**:33–51.

David, C. N., and Challoner, D. 1974. Distribution of interstitial cells and differentiating nematocysts in nests in *Hydra attenuata*. *Am. Zool.* **14**:537–542.

Diehl, F. A., and Burnett, A. L. 1964. The role of interstitial cells in the maintenance of hydra. I. Specific destruction of interstitial cells in normal, asexual, and non-budding animals. *J. Exp. Zool.* **155**:253–260.

Otto, J. J. 1977. Orientation and behavior of epithelial cell muscle processes during hydra budding. *J. Exp. Zool.* **202**:307–322.

Zumstein, A., and Tardent, P. 1972. Autoradiography of whole-mounts of isolated ectoderm of the body column of hydra. A new method. *Experientia* **28**:1124–1125.

Chapter 17

Preparing Histological Sections for Light Microscopy

Richard D. Campbell

PURPOSE

To section hydra that have been embedded in paraffin for histological analysis with the light microscope.

INTRODUCTION

The main stages are fixing, embedding, sectioning, and staining. In general, the methods described in histology books (Gurr, 1958; Pantin, 1962; Humason, 1967; Romeis, 1968) are applicable to hydra. I emphasize certain aspects of these methods that must be observed due to the special characters of hydra.

PROCEDURES

Fixing

The following fixatives have been used most successfully with hydra (references cite reports that may assist you in evaluating the fixative):

Richard D. Campbell ● Department of Developmental and Cell Biology, University of California, Irvine, California.

Heidenhain's Susa (Hadži, 1909); Bouin's (Žnidarić, 1970; Benthin and Davis, 1976); Zenker's (Benthin and Davis, 1976); Lavdowsky's (formalin–acetic–alcohol) (Campbell, 1967). Their compositions are listed in Appendix I. Table I shows the major characteristics of each fixative for use with hydra.

Because tissue sections from contracted hydra are difficult to interpret, fix hydra that are extended and appear relaxed. To prevent hydra from contracting as the fixative is added, consider the following:

1. *Narcosis.* Several agents have been used to relax hydra: (1) Nembutal (see Chapter 13); (2) 10% ethanol (Diehl and Burnett, 1964). Place hydra in this solution for 1 min; then remove as much of the ethanol solution as possible and add fixative; (3) 2% urethan (Macklin, 1976). Add this solution slowly to hydra that are already relaxed in a small quantity of culture solution. After 10 min remove most of the fluid and quickly add fixative.

2. *Choice of fixative.* Certain fixatives induce contraction less than others. The best fixative in this regard is Lavdowsky's.

3. *Rapid flooding of the hydra with the fixative.* Place a single hydra in a vial with the smallest amount of fluid that will allow it to stretch out. An undisturbed hydra will usually elongate within 30 sec when placed in a small drop of water on a clean surface. When it does, flood the hydra with fixative either by pouring a large stream over it or by squirting fixative rapidly from a syringe that has no needle. If you use Bouin's fixative, warm it to 50°C before adding it to the hydra.

To obtain hydra that are straight, allow them to attach to the bottom of a large fixation vessel in a small drop of culture solution and then pour a large volume of fixative over the surface of the vessel as you tilt it. The current should sweep the hydra into a straight condition.

TABLE I. Some Characteristics of Different Fixatives for Hydra Tissue

Characteristics	Fixative			
	Susa	Bouin's	Lavdowsky's	Zenker's
Preserves fine structure	+			
Tissue stains intensely		+		+
Tissue stains uniformly	+		+	
Tissue can be left in fixative indefinitely		+	+	
Highly caustic or dangerous to use	+	+		
Tissue shrinks badly				+
Yields pale staining; suitable for thick sections (>8 μm)			+	

Embedding in Paraffin

Dehydrate the hydra in the series of 50, 70, 80, 95, 100, and 100% ethanol for 30 min each. The 95% solution should contain 0.1% eosin. This dye colors the hydra brilliantly, making it visible after it is embedded in paraffin. Clear the hydra in a 1:1 mixture of methyl salicylate and ethanol for 1 hr, methyl salicylate for 1 hr, and again in methyl salicylate overnight. You can store the tissue for a week in the salicylate. When changing these clearing solutions, first draw off the "old" liquid using a pipet whose tip is immersed just below the surface in order to thoroughly remove the lighter, alcohol-rich fluid; next slowly add the new solution with an immersed pipet tip to the bottom of the vial. Do not agitate the solutions. The alcohol-laden hydra will initially float and then slowly sink into the fresh liquid. Impregnate the animals with paraffin using the following schedule at a temperature 5°C above the melting point of the paraffin: one change of paraffin methyl salicylate (1:1) for 3 hr; three changes of pure paraffin for a total of 24 hr.

To embed in paraffin, first fill a small embedding cup 1 cm deep with melted paraffin; then drop onto the bottom a microscope cover glass that nearly covers the bottom of the cup. The rigid cover glass provides a flat embedding surface. Keep the cup in the incubator so that it remains warm. Use a wide-tipped dropper to transfer one or several hydra into the cup. Examine the hydra using a dissecting microscope to make sure that they are lying flat along the glass bottom; tentacles and buds can hold the hydra off the bottom, in which case you should roll the hydra. If several hydra are to be embedded in the same block, push them close together and into a parallel alignment using a warm needle. Then lift the cup, slowly and without tipping it, and float it on the surface of a beaker filled with water and ice. As soon as the paraffin begins to crystallize around the hydra, thereby holding them in place, agitate the block to cool it quickly. Rapid cooling decreases the crystal size of the paraffin. Do not immerse the blocks.

After about 20 min remove the cups from the water and immediately remove the paraffin block. Lift the coverslip free of the block by slipping a razor blade beneath it. The hydra will be bright orange, lying just under the flat paraffin surface and parallel to it.

Sectioning

The most important special precaution to take in sectioning hydra is to cut the section in the right plane relative to the body column. This plane will be determined by the histological analysis that is to be made. For most purposes, cross sections are the most useful. For example, if the entire hydra is to be analyzed for some aspect of histological structure such as the mitotic index (Chapter 22), then cross sections are suitable. Cross sections cut most cells of the hydra through a plane of symmetry. Any other sectioning plane cuts cells in different planes in different parts of the body column and obscures the bilayered tissue structure. For studies of the basal disk and hypostome, longitudinal sections are often best. Some studies of the longitudinal organization of tissue also require longitudinal sections. In longitudinal sections, only the central few sections show tissue in a plane that can be clearly analyzed. Sections on both sides of the medial region will have the ectoderm and endoderm sectioned obliquely and are difficult to interpret. The extreme lateral sections of a longitudinal series provide grazing (tangential) sections of tissue.

Trim the block precisely to yield perfect cross-sectional (or longitudinally sectioned) planes. Do not alter the flat block face resulting from the cover glass mold; cut the other block faces relative to it. For longitudinal sections, use this flat face as the cutting face, as it will be parallel to the axis of the hydra.

To prepare ribbons of serial sections, trim the block face as closely as possible to the tissue. Do not allow more than a 0.2-mm paraffin margin to lead and trail the sections of the hydra. Otherwise the sections will be too widely spaced on the slide.

Staining

The following are the most useful stains reported in the literature (the references cited may help in selecting and evaluating the stains): Fuelgen method (Campbell, 1967); iron hematoxylin (McConnell, 1932, 1933; Kanajew, 1930); Ehrlich's hematoxylin (Campbell, 1967); Mallory's triple stain (Holmes, 1950; Mueller, 1950; Benthin and Davis, 1976); and Toluidine Blue (Diehl and Burnett, 1964; Davis *et al.*, 1966; Žnidarić, 1970).

Their components and methods for using them are listed in Appendix II. The tissue structures that each stain brings out are shown in Table II. Different stains, or modifications of the way staining is accomplished, may be pursued to obtain particular effects. For such experimentation, general histology books will be useful (Gurr, 1958; Pantin, 1962; Humason, 1967; Romeis, 1968).

When starting a histological analysis with hydra, the most suitable combination of fixing and staining is either Bouin's fixative and Mallory's triple stain, or Lavdowsky's fixative and Ehrlich's hematoxylin. Then, depending on the particular aspects of tissue to be investigated, more specialized methods of preparing the tissue can be chosen using Tables I and II and references to histology books. In some cases, particularly when it is important to delimit cytoplasm and membranes, thin sections of tissue embedded in plastic might be useful (see Chapter 13). These can also be

TABLE II. Some Features of Tissues and Cells of Hydra Brought Out by Different Stains

	Stain				
Features	Iron hematoxylin	Ehrlich's hematoxylin	Mallory's trichrome	Toluidine blue	Feulgen
General tissue					
Detailed structure	+				
Recognition of cell types		+	+		
Specific structures					
I cells		+	+	+	
Nematoblasts		+	+		
Nematocyst structure	+				
Nerve cells	+		+		
Gland cells			+	+	
Muscle processes	+		+		
Mesoglea			+		
Mitotic cells (structure)	+				
Mitotic index		+			+

prepared as ribbons of serial sections (Campbell, 1981). For studies of particular cell types or of some biochemical conditions, histochemical methods may be useful; for these refer to Semal-van Gansen (1954), Gurr (1958), Bouillon (1966), Humason (1967), and Bouillon and Coppois (1977).

APPENDIX I. COMPONENTS AND PROCEDURES FOR USING FIXATIVES LISTED IN TEXT

Heidenhain's Susa Fixative (Humason, 1967, p. 17; Pantin, 1962, p. 8)

Components. 4.5 g $HgCl_2$, 0.5 g NaCl, 2.0 g trichloracetic acid, 4 ml glacial acetic acid, 20 ml formalin (37%), and 80 ml water.

Procedure. Prepare fresh Susa fixative before use. Fix the hydra for 12 hr. Transfer them directly to 70% alcohol for dehydration. Remove the mercuric ions from the tissue either by including iodine in the dehydrating alcohols or by treating sections with Lugol's solution (Humason, 1967, p. 13).

Bouin's Fixative (Humason, 1967, p. 14; Pantin, 1962, p. 9)

Components. 75 ml picric acid (saturated aqueous solution), 25 ml formalin (37%), and 5 ml glacial acetic acid.

Procedure. Fix the hydra 8 hr or longer; you may leave them in this fixative indefinitely. Transfer the hydra directly to 50% alcohol and leave them in this fluid until the yellow color leaches out (6–24 hr). Then continue with the dehydration step.

Lavdowsky's Fixative (Gurr, 1962, p. 230)

Components. 10 ml formalin (37%), 4 ml glacial acetic acid, 50 ml ethanol 95%, and 40 ml water.

Procedure. Fix the hydra for 12 hr or longer; you may leave them in this fixative indefinitely. Transfer the hydra to 50% ethanol and continue with the dehydration step.

Zenker's Fixative (Humason, 1967, p. 17; Pantin, 1962, p. 10)

Components. 5 g $HgCl_2$, 2.5 g $K_2Cr_2O_7$, 1 g Na_2SO_4, and 100 ml water.

Procedure. Fix the hydra 12 hr and then wash them in running water for 12 hr. Remove the mercuric ions from the tissue either by including iodine in the dehydrating alcohols or by treating the sections with Lugol's solution (see Humason, 1967, p. 13).

APPENDIX II. SOLUTIONS AND PROCEDURES FOR USING STAINS LISTED IN TEXT

All stains require practice in use. Always prepare extra sections on which to test stains before using them. Before staining tissue, refer to reports listed in the text and to a general histology book. Most stains can be used in many ways; only a single method for each stain is listed below. Modify the lengths of time suggested in the staining procedures below according to the thickness of the sections, the fixative used, the growth condition and species of the hydra, and the types of observations to be made. Begin all procedures described below with deparaffinized, hydrated sections.

Feulgen Method (Humason, 1967, pp. 309–311; Pantin, 1962, pp. 56–57)

Solutions. 6 N HCl, Schiff's reagent (Fisher Scientific Co.; or may be prepared as described by Humason, 1967, p. 305, or Pantin, 1962, p. 56; keep solution refrigerated in the dark), sulfite water (to 5% aqueous $Na_2S_2O_5$ or $K_2S_2O_5$ add 5% by volume of 1 N HCl just before use), and Fast Green (0.05% Fast Green stain, C.I. 42053, in 95% alcohol).

Procedure. Place sections in 6 N HCl at room temperature for 10 min and rinse them in distilled water. Place the rinsed sections in Schiff's reagent in the dark for 2 hr and rinse them in three changes of bleaching solution for 2 min each. Next, wash them in running tap water for 5 min. Counterstain them in Fast Green for 10 sec while agitating them, and transfer them to 100% ethanol. Finally, mount them on slides.

Special Notes. (1) Counterstain with Fast Green sufficiently lightly to allow the transparent cells to be visualized and to provide contrast with the Schiff reagent's magenta staining. Excess staining will obscure the magenta color. (2) Schiff's reagent is stable for months but is apt to lose its activity unpredictably. Pretest the solution by verifying that it will stain a test slide in 30 min.

Iron Hematoxylin (Humason, 1967, p. 140, 147–148; Pantin, 1962, pp. 39–40)

Solutions. Mordant [4% aqueous ferric alum $(FeNH_4(SO_4)_2 \cdot 12H_2O)$] use within 1 month, and stain (10 ml of a 5% solution of hematoxylin in 95% ethanol mixed with 90 ml distilled water).

Procedure. Place the sections in mordant for 24 hr and rinse them in running tap water for 10 sec. Place the sections in stain for 24 hr and rinse them for 15 sec in tap water. Differentiate (i.e., partially destain) the sections by placing them in fresh mordant solution diluted 1:1 with distilled water.

Check the decreasing intensity of the stain periodically under a microscope. When the sections are sufficiently destained (after 2 min to 2 hr), rinse them for 2 min in running tap water. Counterstain the sections, if desired, and dehydrate and mount them.

Special Notes. (1) The original 5% hematoxylin solution must be "aged" a few weeks before use. To oxidize the solution immediately, add 1 g $NaIO_3$ per gram of hematoxylin. (2) Practice on a series of test sections before staining the experimental sections, in order to gain experience in judging how much differentiation is necessary. (3) This stain gives best results in tissue fixed in Susa fixative and on sections no more than 5 μm thick. (4) Eosin or Biebrich Scarlet serve as suitable counterstains when needed.

Ehrlich's Hematoxylin (Humason, 1967, p. 136; Pantin, 1962, p. 24)

Comments. Numerous one-step hematoxylin staining procedures employ a mordant incorporated in the staining solution. Of these, that of Ehrlich has provided the most satisfactory results with hydra.

Solution. To 30 ml distilled water, add 0.6 g hematoxylin, 1.0 g ammonium alum [$AlNH_4(SO_4)_2 \cdot 12\ H_2O$], 30 ml ethanol, and 30 ml glycerol.

Procedures. Begin with sections maintained in 50% ethanol and stain them for 20 min. Rinse them in distilled water 5 sec while agitating them. To differentiate the stain, dip the sections in acid alcohol (50% ethanol containing 0.2% concentrated HCl) for a few seconds. Then rinse them in tap water a few more seconds. Darken the staining by placing the sections in saturated aqueous $LiCO_3$ for 15 sec and rinse them in tap water for 1 min. Finally, counterstain the sections, if desired, and dehydrate and mount them.

Special Notes. (1) When this stain is applied to specimens fixed in Lavdowsky's solution, the cytoplasm of the epithelial cells stains so faintly that other cells are prominent; all cell types stain. (2) Biebrich Scarlet is the best counterstain to use with hematoxylin. (3) Practice on a series of test sections in order to gain experience in judging how much differentiation is necessary. If the sections become too bleached, as judged after they have been darkened in $LiCO_3$, restain them in the hematoxylin solution.

Mallory's Triple Stain (Humason, 1967, pp. 161–162; Pantin, 1962, pp. 41–43; Benthin and Davis, 1967)

Comments. This staining involves multiple steps (see references). For hydra, better staining can sometimes be achieved by doubling the amount of Orange G normally called for. Cason devised a one-step staining method for accomplishing the Mallory triple stain (Humason, 1967, pp. 165–166). Two disadvantages with this one-step method are that the two principle stains, Basic Fuchsin and Aniline Blue, cannot be separately controlled as they can be in the multistep method, and the heavy-metal mordant cannot be altered. On the other hand, Benthin and Davis (1967) provide a detailed description of excellent results obtained by use of the one-step method on hydra tissue.

Solution (for One-Step Method). To 100 ml distilled water, add 0.5 g phosphotungstic acid, 1 g Orange G, 0.5 g Aniline Blue w.s., and 1.5 g Acid Fuchsin.

Procedure. Stain the sections for 5 min, rinse them for a few seconds in tap water, dehydrate them rapidly, and mount the sections.

Special Notes. (1) Practice on a series of test sections in order to determine the correct staining times and washing rates. (2) To get the best results, fix the hydra in Bouin's fluid.

Toluidine Blue (Humason, 1967, p. 326)

Solution. 0.05% Toluidine Blue in water, buffered at pH 8 with 0.01 M tris or 0.01 M borate buffer.

Procedure. Stain the sections for 2 min, rinse them in distilled water, and differentiate the stain in 70% ethanol for about 0.5–5 min until the stain is light. Finally, finish dehydrating the sections and mount them.

REFERENCES

Benthin, M. G., and Davis, L. E. 1976. The qualitative use of Cason's one-step triple stain on *Hydra. Cytologia* **41**:741–748.

Bouillon, J. 1966. Les cellules glandulaires des hydroides et hydroméduses. Leur structure et la nature de leurs sécrétions. *Cah. Biol. Mar.* **7**:157–205.

Bouillon, J., and Coppois, G. 1977. Étude comparative de la mesoglée des Cnidaires. *Cah. Biol. Mar.* **18**:339–368.

Burnett, A. L. 1959. Histophysiology of growth in hydra. *J. Exp. Zool.* **140**:281–341.

Campbell, R. D. 1967. Tissue dynamics of steady state growth in *Hydra littoralis.* I. Patterns of cell division. *Dev. Biol.* **15**:487–502.

Campbell, R. D. 1981. A method for making ribbons of semithin plastic sections. *Stain Technol.* **56**:247–249.

Davis, L. E., Burnett, A. L., Haynes, J. F., and Mumaw, V. R. 1966. A histological and ultrastructural study of dedifferentiation and redifferentiation of digestive and gland cells in *Hydra viridis. Dev. Biol.* **14**:307–329.

Diehl, F. A., and Burnett, A. L. 1964. The role of interstitial cells in the maintenance of *Hydra.* I. specific destruction of interstitial cells in normal, asexual, non-budding, animals. *J. Exp. Zool.* **155**:253–260.

Gurr, E. 1958. *Methods of Analytical Histology and Histochemistry*, Leonard Hill Ltd., London.

Gurr, E. 1962. *Staining, Practical and Theoretical.* Williams & Wilkins, Baltimore, Md.

Hadži, J. 1909. Ueber das Nervensystem von Hydra. *Arb. Zool. Inst. Univ. Wien* **17**:225–268.

Holmes, W. 1950. The mesoglea and muscle-fibres of *Chlorohydra viridissima. Q. J. Microscop. Sci.* **91**:419–428.

Humason, G. L. 1967. *Animal Tissue Techniques*, 2nd ed, Freeman, San Francisco.

Kanajew, J. 1930. Zur Frage der Bedeutung der Interstitiellen Zellen bei Hydra. *Wilhelm Roux Arch. Entwicklungsmech. Org.* **122**:736–759.

Macklin, M. 1976. The effect of urethan on hydra. *Biol. Bull.* **150**:442–452.

McConnell, C. H. 1932. Zellteilungen bei Hydra. Mitosen in den epithelio-muskulaeren Zellen des Entoderms von Hydra. *Z. Mikrosk. Anat. Forsch.* **28**:578–588.

McConnell, C. H. 1933. Mitosis in hydra: Mitosis of the secretory cells of the endoderm of hydra. *Biol. Bull.* **64**:96–102.

Mueller, J. F. 1950. Some observations on the structure of hydra, with particular reference to the muscular system. *Trans. Am. Microscop. Soc.* **69**:133–1347.

Noda, K. 1968. Migratory cells traversing the mesoglea in hydra. *J. Fac. Sci. Hokkaido Univ. Ser. 6* **16**:353–358.

Pantin, C. F. A. 1962. *Notes on Microscopical Techniques for Zoologists.* Cambridge University Press, Cambridge.

Romeis, B. 1968. *Mikroskopische Technik*, 16th ed., R. Oldenbourg Verlag, Munich.

Semal-van Gansen, P. 1954. L'histophysiologie de l'endoderme de l'hydre d'eau douce. *Ann. Soc. R. Zool. Belg.* **85**:217–278.

Spangenberg, D. B., and Eakin, R. E. 1962. Histological studies of mechanisms involved in hydra regeneration. *J. Exp. Zool.* **151**:85–94.

Žnidarič, D. 1970. Comparison of the regeneration of the hypostome with the budding process in *Hydra littoralis. Arch. Entwicklungsmech. Org.* **166**:45–53.

Chapter 18

Vital Staining: Fluorescent and Immunofluorescent, and Review of Nonfluorescent Dyes

John F. Dunne and C. Lynne Littlefield

PURPOSE

To stain cells and tissues of live hydra with fluorescent dyes or by immunofluorescence. Such methods aid in identifying specific tissues or cells in grafts or in aggregates of cells.

REVIEW OF VITAL STAINING

The techniques of vital staining used to investigate many experimental systems in developmental biology were first developed by Abraham Trembley (1744) with hydra. Trembley stained hydra by feeding them food of different colors.

Since that time a variety of vital stains have been applied to whole hydra. Most acidic dyes were excluded from hydra cells, whereas most basic dyes are readily taken up and at low concentrations will not harm the cells. Hydra have been vitally stained with solutions of neutral red, Methylene Blue, and Nile Blue sulfate (Zoja, 1892; Scholottke, 1932; Rella, 1941). Each dye stains most or all of the cell types to varying degrees. These stains,

---

John F. Dunne and C. Lynne Littlefield ● Developmental Biology Center, University of California, Irvine, California .

however, move as easily out of the tissue as they move in, thereby making them unsuitable for marking cells or tissues to be transplanted or for labeling localized regions along the body column of the hydra.

Weimer (1927) applied particulate Nile Blue sulfate with a needle to a specific region of the body column of hydra and found that the marked tissue remained localized even after it was grafted. More recent techniques devised for labeling specific regions or cell types include the use of colloidal carbon (Chapter 24) to mark epithelial tissue, and radioisotopes, such as tritiated thymidine (Chapter 25), to label cell nuclei. These latter techniques are effective when marking relatively small numbers of animals but can be cumbersome when large numbers of labeled animals are needed.

In an attempt to combine ease of staining and specifity of cells labeled, fluorescent dyes have been recently used with intact hydra tissues or cell suspensions from dissociated hydra. Klimek (1979) applied over 100 fluorescent dyes to cells from dissociated hydra and analyzed some parameters affecting stainability at concentrations which did not adversely affect the viability of the cells. He labeled the cells or tissues directly by soaking them in the dye diluted in hydra culture solution in the presence of dimethylsulfoxide (DMSO). He introduced nonpermeable dyes by feeding whole hydra with shrimp that were labeled with the dye before he dissociated the animals. In this manner, dyes were introduced selectively and permanently into the digestive cells.

INTRODUCTION

We have focused on several fluorescent dyes which we have found to exhibit, to varying degrees, the characteristics necessary for use in research in developmental biology. These characteristics require that the dyes give cells which are viable and intensely stained, and which lose little or no stain to surrounding cells over a minimum of several days. Since most of these dyes fluoresce at different wavelengths, proper combinations of these dyes can be used in double labeling experiments. We gave special attention to Evans Blue, which has been used extensively (Wilby and Webster, 1970; Sugiyama and Fujisawa, 1978; Wanek, 1980) for labeling gastrodermal tissue in intact hydra. Finally we discuss the labeling of specific subsets of cells by indirect immunofluorescence.

MATERIALS

4,6-Diamidino-2-phenylindole-2-HCl (DAPI) (Aldrich, Milwaukee, WI); bis-benzimide trihydrochloride pentahydrate (Hoescht 33258)

(Aldrich); 6-carboxyfluorescein (Molecular Probes, Plano, TX); Evans Blue (Aldrich); fluorescein-isothiocyanate-conjugated (FITC-conjugated) goat anti-mouse Ig (Antibodies Inc., Davis, CA).

FLUORESCENT MICROSCOPY

The descriptions of various dyes in this chapter are based on observations made on a Zeiss photomicroscope equipped for epifluorescence with a 100-W high-pressure mercury lamp. Signals for Hoescht 33258 and DAPI were filtered with the Zeiss combination filter 48 77 02, which is a broad-excitation filter with a peak transmission at 365 nm, and a barrier filter transmitting wavelengths above 420 nm. Carboxyfluorescein and FITC-conjugated goat anti-mouse Ig were visualized through Zeiss filter 48 77 17, an excitation filter transmitting from 475 to 495 nm, and a barrier filter transmitting from about 520 to 560 nm. The fluorescent signal from material stained with Evans Blue was seen through Zeiss filter 48 77 12, which has an excitation filter with a peak transmission of 546 nm and a barrier filter transmitting above 590 nm.

METHOD I. HOESCHT 33258

COMMENTS

Hoescht 33258 binds to A–T-rich regions of DNA (Mueller and Gautier, 1975) and becomes brightly fluorescent with an excitation maximum at 343 nm and an emission peak around 460 nm. Hydra nuclei are easily visualized *in situ*. The nuclear morphology is distinct, and various cell types are recognizable. Clusters of very bright nematocyte nuclei are embedded in a regular matrix of large and more diffuse epithelial nuclei. Internal morphology is particularly clear in these large nuclei.

PROCEDURES

Prepare a solution of 50 μg Hoescht 33258 per milliliter of culture solution. This solution may be stored cold and in the dark for many months and may be reused many times. Place from 1 to 100 hydra into 20 ml staining solution for 1 hr. Wash them carefully with several changes of culture solution before observing them.

Alternatively, you can examine the tissue while it sits in dilute, 1-μg/ml staining solution. Since the Hoescht dye fluoresces only when it is intercalated, there is no background fluorescence of the dye even in concentrated solutions.

Fix the tissue by flooding it with 100% ethanol. This treatment increases tissue autofluorescence (see below) and also greatly enhances the nuclear signal of stained tissue. Thus, even after the stain appears to fade out of living tissue, ethanol fixation selectively increases the fluorescent signal from nuclei stained with Hoescht 33258.

PRECAUTIONS

Like any DNA dye, Hoescht is almost certainly a potent carcinogen. Because it is rapidly absorbed through the skin, great care is advised even when handling dilute solutions.

Wash stained tissue thoroughly to avoid contaminating unstained tissue.

OBSERVATIONS

In many respects tissues stained with Hoescht 33258 have an image similar to that shown by tissue stained with DAPI (see below). Two distinctions are noteworthy. (1) Hoescht stain fades much more rapidly than DAPI, remaining easily detectable in epithelial nuclei for only 4 or 5 days after staining. Nematocyte nuclei, on the other hand, remain bright much longer, up to 2 weeks in the tentacles, presumably owing to their highly condensed state and/or lowered mitotic activity. (2) Our stock of *Hydra attenuata* shows a distinct chartreuse signal after Hoescht staining, which is not seen in animals stained with DAPI. This chartreuse image is apparently extracellular in origin and is on the ectodermal surface; it appears as a "latticework" whose density is correlated with the clefts between the domed apical surfaces of ectodermal cells. The signal rigidly respects graft junctions between stained and unstained tissues for about 1 week, after which a faint signal begins to appear across the junction, probably the result of dye diffusion and secondary uptake. In spite of this faint spreading of dye, the graft junction remains distinct for several weeks. This signal remains bright much longer than the nuclear signal in live animals, but is completely obliterated following ethanol fixation.

Unfortunately, unstained hydra tissue autofluoresces weakly when seen through filter combinations suitable for observing tissue stained with DAPI and Hoescht dyes. This autofluorescence is not restricted to the nuclei of hydra cells and is therefore easily distinguished from the nuclear specific

DAPI and Hoescht signals. Nonetheless, this autofluorescence defines a lower limit below which DAPI and Hoescht signals are not discernable.

METHOD II. DAPI

COMMENTS

DAPI fluoresces blue with an emission peak at about 450 nm and a excitation frequency of 365 nm (Russell *et al.*, 1975). DAPI is intercalated into DNA, localizing the fluorescence to the nucleus of the cells. All cell types stain intensely with DAPI, and the level of photobleaching is negligible after prolonged periods of observation.

PROCEDURES

Whole Animals. Soak whole hydra in 0.05 μg/ml DAPI in hydra culture solution for approximately 30 min (T. Honegger, personal communication). Wash the animals several times in culture solution and place them in a dish of fresh culture solution. Keep these animals in a light-tight container. After 24 hr you can use these stained hydra for grafting experiments, or you can dissociate the tissue and reaggregate the cells.

Dissociated Cells. Stain cells from dissociated hydra by incubating them in 0.05 μg/ml DAPI in reaggregation solution (Chapter 32) for 15 min. Wash the cells several times and resuspend them in fresh reaggregation solution. You may make aggregates with various ratios of stained and unstained cells.

PRECAUTIONS

DAPI intercalates into DNA and may be carcinogenic. Handle it with extreme care.

OBSERVATIONS

Animals stained with DAPI remain as viable and healthy as unstained control animals. Fluorescing nuclei remain bright in unfed animals for at least 1 month. In grafts, DAPI remains in the cells originally stained ("cell autonomous") for at least up to 5 days. DAPI also appears to remain cell autonomous in aggregates (R. Stidwill, 1981; personal observations). The development of aggregates composed of stained cells is slightly slower than that of unstained controls. In both grafts and aggregates it appears that the migration of interstitial cells, nematocytes, and nematoblasts may be somewhat hindered. Because fixed hydra cells are seen to autofluoresce intensely under the filter combinations used to visualize the DAPI and Hoescht stains, cells stained with DAPI are difficult to distinguish from unstained cells in preparations from macerated hydra (Chapter 20) or fixed whole mounts.

METHOD III. EVANS BLUE DYE

COMMENTS

Evans blue is a blue-colored dye when observed under transmitted light. When observed with fluorescent microscopy, it fluoresces red with an excitation maximum at 611 nm, although fluorescence was readily observed using Zeiss filter combination 48 77 12, which has a peak excitation of 546 nm (also see van der Kooy, 1979). Evans blue has been used primarily to stain digestive cells of the endoderm (Wilby and Webster, 1970; Sugiyama and Fujisawa, 1978; Wanek, 1980) by feeding *Artemia* nauplii stained with Evans Blue to intact hydra. The stain appears to localize in the cytoplasm of both endodermal epithelial cells and gland cells.

PROCEDURES

Two methods are available for staining hydra tissue with Evans blue. In the first, add 1 ml 1% w/v Evans blue solution made up in culture solution to 50 ml *Artemia* nauplii in sea water. Leave the nauplii in this solution approximately 24 h or until they are dark blue. When the nauplii appear thoroughly stained, feed them to hydra. Repeat this entire procedure two to three times to ensure intensive staining of the hydra's gastrodermal tissue.

In the second method, feed hydra lightly with unstained *Artemia* nauplii. Fifteen to 30 min after feeding inject a 1% solution of Evans Blue directly into the gut of the hydra through a drawn glass needle (see Chapter 25). The hydra should appear deep blue immediately and can be used for experiments 1 day after they are stained.

PRECAUTIONS

Evans Blue is reported to be a "cancer suspect agent." Do not breathe in the powder or allow the solution to contact your skin.

OBSERVATIONS

No harmful effects to the hydra have been observed using the dye administered by either of these two methods. The second method offers the advantage of being able to label a few animals quickly, whereas with the first method, many animals can be labeled with little effort. In grafts Evans Blue remains cell autonomous for several days when observed with transmitted light. Under fluorescence microscopy, however, some turnover of the dye is observed in 1–2 days, becoming extensive after 3 days.

METHOD IV. CARBOXYFLUORESCEIN

COMMENTS

The carboxylic acid derivatives of fluorescein can be useful vital dyes since their permeability to membranes can be controlled by varying extracellular pH. Below pH 5.5 the molecule is neutral and can cross membranes readily, but in more alkaline solutions the carboxylic acid is charged and membrane passage is blocked. A 1-hr incubation of hydra in dilute carboxyfluorescein in mild acid results in some labeling of all endoderm cells and bright labeling of hundreds of cells in the ectoderm.

PROCEDURES

Dissolve 50 mg 6-carboxyfluorescein in 10 ml hydra culture solution (0.5%) and adjust the pH to 5.4 with 1 N HCl (some dye precipitation may occur, but the solution will retain its ability to stain). Transfer the hydra in a small volume of hydra culture solution to the staining solution and readjust the pH to 5.4. After they incubate for 1 hr at room temperature, carry the hydra through repeated washes until you observe no dye in the culture solution. Longer incubation times give more thoroughly stained hydra but may impair the general health of the animals. A 24-hr incubation leaves animals contracted and ragged, but they generally recover.

OBSERVATIONS

The washed animals usually maintain a high concentration of stain in their gut until their first feeding. The bright light generated by excitation of this stain results in a dark field image of the ectoderm, making nuclei and nematocytes clearly visible.

After the first feeding, the gut is cleared and intracellular labeling is apparent. Sparse, very bright areas represent stained cells in the ectoderm, while the fluorescence from the endoderm is more continuous and muted. View the horizon of the cylindrical body wall to unambiguously characterize the tissue layer containing a fluorescent spot. On the horizon you should see a generally dark ectoderm overlying a smooth boundary of green light adjacent to the mesoglea.

Ectoderm labeling is discrete. Cells are either brightly labeled or not labeled at all. The frequency of ectodermal cell labeling is grossly correlated with incubation time in 6-carboxyfluorescein.

Labeling of the endoderm by this stain is complete but not homogeneous. All cells appear fluorescent, and adjacent cells are generally not similar in intensity; thus endodermal cell boundaries can be easily defined.

Graft junctions between labeled and unlabeled animals remain visible for many days, or even several weeks in unfed animals. Though some secondary uptake is seen in originally unlabeled endoderm, an abrupt change in intensity is easily seen at the graft junction.

METHOD V: INDIRECT IMMUNOFLUORESCENCE

COMMENTS

We find that live hydra cells are highly immunogenic and readily bind antibody from immune serum. The binding of hydra-specific mouse antibodies can be visualized by subsequent incubation of antibody-bound cells in fluorescein-conjugated goat antibodies purified against mouse immunoglobulins. The lability of this staining technique makes it unsuitable for long-term labeling studies. The power of this technique lies in the potential for labeling antigenically defined subsets of cells. This potential is probably only dependent on the specificity of the mouse antibody.

PROCEDURES

Inject 1 million hydra cells dissociated in aggregation solution (Chapter 32) intraperitoneally into a mouse on day 0. Inject 1 million to 2 million more dissociated cells intravenously on days 7–10, and on days 10–15 isolate serum from whole blood. This serum can typically be diluted as much as 200-fold and be used as a source of antibodies which bind to hydra cell surfaces as described below.

Incubate dissociated hydra cells in immune serum diluted in aggregation solution for 15–30 min. Wash cells three times by centrifuging them and resuspending them in serum-free aggregation solution. After the third wash resuspend the cells in a dilute solution of FITC-conjugated goat anti-mouse Ig in aggregation solution ($\sim$20 μg/ml) and incubate them for 15–30 min. Wash cells as before and examine them with fluorescence microscopy.

PRECAUTIONS

Fluorescein, either as FITC or as carboxyfluorescein, is sensitive to photobleaching. Thus, in preparations that are sparsely labeled, the signal can rapidly diminish at a rate proportional to the intensity of the excitation. In some cases, weak signals can be lost in seconds.

OBSERVATIONS

The fluorescence seen after treatment is proportional to the concentration of immune serum over a broad range (typically up to 200-fold), and far above preimmune control serum treatments, which in turn are brighter than hydra cell autofluorescence.

In live hydra cells, capping of some antibodies occurs at temperature-dependent rates. At room temperature, the fluorescent signal is easily visible and restricted to the cell surface for at least 1 hr, after which it can be localized on part of the surface, internalized, or lost at various rates.

ACKNOWLEDGMENTS. This research was supported by the USPHS Training Grant HD-07029 and postoctoral fellowship HD-05637.

REFERENCES

Gierer, A., Berking, S., Bode, H., David, C. N., Flick, K., Hansmann, G., Schaller, H., and Trenkner, E. 1972. Regeneration of hydra from reaggregated cells. *Nature (London)* **239**:98–101.

Klimek, F. 1979. Untersuchung zur Separation und Aggregation von Hydrazellen. Ph.D. thesis, Eberhard-Karls University, Tubingen.

Mueller, W., and Gautier, F. 1975. Intercalation of heteroaromatic compounds with nucleic acids; A-T specific nonintercalating DNA ligands. *Eur. J. Biochem.* **54**:385.

Rella, M. 1941. Vitalfarbungsuntersuchungen an Süsswasserhydrozoen. *Protoplasma* **35**:298–317.

Russell, W. C., Newman, C., and Williamson, D. H. (1975). A simple cytochemical technique for demonstration of DNA in cells infected with mycoplasmas and viruses. *Nature (London)* **253**:461–462.

Schlottke, E. 1932. Zellstudien an Hydra. III. Versuche mit Vitalfarben. *Z. Mikrosk. Anat. Forsch.* **28**:298–336.

Stidwill, R. 1981. Interspezifische Inkompätibilitaten zwischen Arten der Gattung *Hydra (Hydrozoa, Cnidaria)*, Ph.D. thesis, University of Zürich.

Sugiyama, T., and Fujisawa, T. 1978. Genetic analysis of developmental mechanisms in hydra. II. Isolation and characterization of an interstitial cell-deficient strain. *J. Cell Sci.* **29**:35–52.

Trembley, A. 1744. Mémoires pour servir à l'histoire naturelle d'un genre de polype d'eau douce à bras en forme de cornes, Leyden.

van der Kooy, D., and Kuypers, H. G. J. M. 1979. Fluorescent retrograde double labeling: Axonal branching in the ascending raphe and nigral projections. Science **204**:873–875.

Wanek, N. L. 1980. Roles of ectodermal and endodermal epithelial cells in hydra morphogenesis. Ph.D. thesis, University of California, Irvine.

Weimer, B. R. 1927. The use of Nile Blue sulfate as a vital stain on *Hydra*. *Biol. Bull.* **52**:219–222.

Wilby, O. K., and Webster, G. 1970. Experimental studies on axial polarity in *Hydra*. *J. Embryol. Exp. Morphol.* **24**:595–613.

Zoja, R. 1892. Die vitale Methylenblaufarbung bei Hydra. *Zool. Anz.* **15**:241–242.

Part III

Macrophotography

Chapter 19

Macrophotography

Richard D. Campbell

PURPOSE

Photography permits recording and storing of data concerning the distribution, morphology, and histology of hydra, and is useful in illustrating studies on hydra.

INTRODUCTION

I present a method for photographing hydra at magnifications of 1–5×. Macrophotography is useful in recording and illustrating the appearances of whole polyps. More extensive information on macrophotography and other types of photography useful in hydra research can be found in three Kodak publications (Eastman Kodak Company, 1970, 1974, 1975) and Blaker (1965, 1976).

The following are general rules for successful hydra macrophotography: (1) The subject should fill the entire film field. (2) The subject should be reasonably oriented in the field, and in grouped photographs the subjects should be aligned and photographed similarly. (3) The culture solution and optical components must be clean.

Richard D. Campbell ● Department of Developmental and Cell Biology, University of California, Irvine, California.

143

MATERIALS

Thirty-five-millimeter reflex camera body; lens with focal length of about 50 mm; bellows attachment with excursion of three to five times the focal length of the lens (if all photographs are to be taken at the same magnification, extension tubes are satisfactory; the appropriate length of the tubes can be determined from Fig. 1); adapter to mount lens on the bellows attachment with the lens in an inverted orientation (so that the back of the lens faces the specimen); flash illuminator coupled electrically to camera but not mounted on camera; camera stand; stand for the flash illuminator (e.g., ringstand); clean glass or plastic dish with an unscratched bottom; two alternate stands for specimen: (1) a ringstand with a ring support to hold the culture dish, and (2) a box (~5-in. sides such as a lantern slide plate box) lined with a black interior, with a hole cut in the top which is slightly smaller than the culture dish; plastic needle to position the hydra; small fluorescent lamp (8 W).

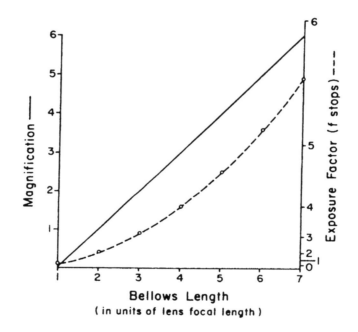

FIGURE 1. Use of bellows length to calculate magnification and exposure factor. Bellows length refers to total distance between film and center of the lens and expressed in units of lens focal length. Total bellows length should be graduated on the bellows track. To calculate magnification (ratio of image size to object size) for a particular bellows length, read the solid line on the left hand ordinate. The relative exposure factor in going from one bellows length to another (dotted line) is on the right-hand ordinate. Exposure factor is expressed as the number of *f* stop increases needed when changing from one bellows length to another. To change from a bellows length of three to four, approximately one *f* stop change is required.

It is preferable to have this equipment permanently set up; it requires only about 2 ft² of solid bench space (Fig. 2).

PROCEDURES

Taking the Photograph

Pipet the hydra into the photographic chamber and wait until it elongates. Then reposition it to the center of the photographic field using a

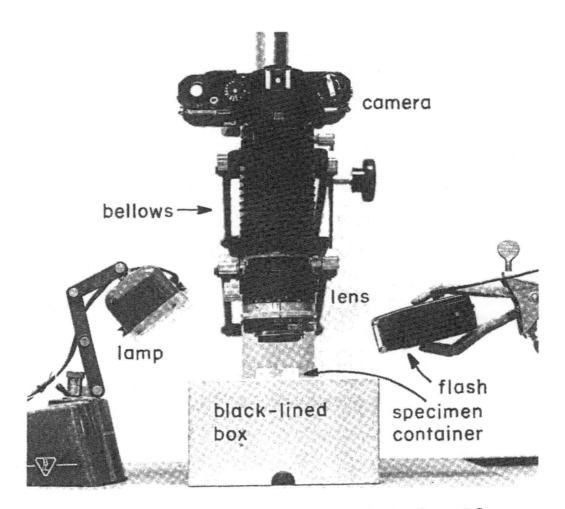

FIGURE 2. Photographic apparatus for macrophotography of hydra. The small fluorescent lamp at left is for providing illumination during focusing. It is so dim that it does not contribute to the exposure illuminated by a flash unit at right. The lens is attached upside down to the end of a bellows extension. The specimen is in a culture dish centered over a hole in the box lined with black. The hole is not visible in the photograph.

probe made of plastic so it will not scratch the dish. Photograph the hydra in a position which best illustrates the point under discussion. Focus with the lens aperture fully opened using the fluorescent light for illumination. Close the lens aperture to a predetermined setting (see below) and take the photograph.

Exposure Control

Control exposure by varying the distance separating the flash illuminator from the specimen. The other parameters affecting exposure are not easy to vary. For example, lens–subject distance must be held constant so that magnification does not change, and effective exposure time is constant and determined by the flash duration. Calibrate a scale on the desk top to position the flash at predetermined distances.

Do not use the lens aperture to control exposure, because the lens aperture also affects resolution and depth of field. A lens aperture of $f\,11$ or $f\,16$ will usually provide the best combination of resolution and depth of field. Under the conditions described, the best resolution will be approximately equal to micrometers to the f-stop setting ($11\ \mu m$ at $f\,11$), and the depth of field will be about $40\ \mu m \times f$ stop.

To calibrate exposure for each magnification to be used, photograph one specimen at several different flash–specimen distances. Select the best distances and post these above the camera.

Place the flash illuminator slightly above the specimen plane and aimed toward the specimen. Do not directly illuminate the camera lens with the flash illuminator or else glare or reflections will result.

Vary exposure with the thickness and density of a specimen when using side illumination as described above. For example, a small, starved hydra requires twice the exposure needed for a hydra of average size, whereas a large, well-fed hydra requires only one-half the exposure of a normal hydra.

Vary exposure for films of different sensitivity. To use a film whose ASA exposure index is twice that of the film used in the calibration, increase the flash illumination distance by a factor of 1.4 for an ASA index one-half that of the calibrated film, decrease the distance by a factor of 0.7.

As a general starting value for Kodachrome II (ASA 25) at $f\,11$, magnification 3:1 and a 50-mm lens, with a flash guide number of 30, use a flash–subject distance of 3 in.

Background of Photograph

The color and darkness of the background should suit the purpose of the photograph. For showing the general form of a hydra, a black background is satisfactory. For the best black background, use the method in which the specimen is placed over a hole in a box lined with black.

To indicate dark markings on a hydra, a gray background must be produced by placing a gray card below the specimen. On the other hand, too light a background will make the hydra itself difficult to see. For a background in color photographs, use black or a color which is complementary to the color of the marking. To prevent the background material from imparting a texture to the photograph, maintain it several inches away from the specimen.

Film

Ordinarily it is not important to use a highly sensitive film since the flash–illuminator is intense. Slow films such as Kodak Panatomic-X or Kodachrome 25 are preferable to fast ones since they yield better images.

Magnification

Control magnification by varying the length of the bellows extension. The approximate magnification can be computed using Fig. 1. Calibrate the bellows attachment by photographing a ruler as the first or last photograph of each film.

Exposure varies with magnification. For higher magnification admit more light. Either use a larger lens aperture, in which case the required change can be estimated from Fig. 1, or move the flash illuminator closer to the specimen.

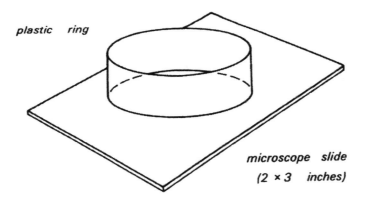

FIGURE 3. Specimen chamber. See text.

Photographic Chamber

Use a chamber having a clean, flat, transparent bottom of uniform thickness. Any such dish is suitable, for example, a Petri dish made of glass or plastic. Most dishes, however, are too irregular, and plastic dishes are easily scratched. To make an excellent photographic chamber (Fig. 3), saw off the bottom of a 35-mm-diameter Petri dish, glue the remaining plastic ring to a 2 × 3-in. glass microscope slide or cover glass. Use silicone stopcock grease for making temporary chambers, and silicone glue for permanent chambers.

PROBLEMS

Unsharp Photographs. Either the camera was not focused properly, or the negative was overly enlarged.

Uneven Illumination. This problem may arise from the refraction of light by the curvature of the dish or from shadows. Make certain that the specimen is in the center of the dish with nothing blocking light on the background.

Background Texture in Focus. To eliminate such texture, increase the distance between the specimen chamber and the background.

Bright Specks in Photograph. These arise from dirt particles and scratches on the bottom of the dish and particles in the culture fluid. Therefore, use a clean, unscratched dish with clean water.

Ghost Image of Hydra Next to the Main Image. This ghost image is the reflection of the hydra in the bottom of the specimen chamber. It arises if the camera is not aimed perpendicular to the bottom of the chamber. Therfore, be certain that the camera is exactly vertical and the chamber is horizontal.

REFERENCES

Blaker, Alfred A. 1965. *Photography for Scientific Publications*, Freeman, San Francisco.
Blaker, Alfred A. 1976. *Field Photography*, Freeman, San Francisco.
Eastman Kodak Company. 1970. *Basic Scientific Photography*, Kodak Scientific Data Book N-5.

Eastman Kodak Company. 1974. *Photography through the Microscope*, Kodak Scientific Data
    Book P-2.
Eastman Kodak Company. 1975. *Close-up Photography and Photomacrography*. Kodak
    Scientific Data Book N-16.

Part IV

Quantitative Cytology

Dissociating Hydra Tissue into Single Cells by the Maceration Technique

Charles N. David

PURPOSE

To rapidly and completely dissociate hydra tissue into its individual cells and to fix them for identification and counting.

INTRODUCTION

Quantitative data on the abundance and distribution of each cell type in hydra is essential to investigating a variety of problems concerning the cell biology and morphology of hydra. Obtaining such data in histological sections is difficult and time-consuming. We have, therefore, developed a maceration technique for rapidly and completely dissociating hydra tissue into individual cells (David, 1973). Each cell type is readily distinguishable under phase microscopy in such macerations, and its abundance can be determined by counting.

MATERIALS

The maceration solution is glycerin/glacial acetic acid/water (1:1:13). As a fixative, use formaldehyde (8%) or osmium tetroxide (1%). "Subbed"

Charles N. David ● Department of Molecular Biology, Albert Einstein College of Medicine, Bronx, New York.

microscope slides are prepared by dipping washed slides in a solution of 5% (w/v) gelatin and 0.5% (w/v) chrome alum. Dry the slides before use. Other materials are 1% Tween 80 detergent (Sigma), small disposable polyethylene tubes (4 ml), Falcon Microtest dish (96 0.4-ml wells), and hemoctyometer.

PROCEDURES

Dissociating Tissue

Place pieces of hydra or whole hydra in disposable polyethylene tubes, draw off excess medium with a Pasteur pipet and add about 0.1 ml maceration solution per hydra. Let the tissue soak for 2–3 min and then dissociate it by gently shaking the tube (tapping it on fingernail or table works well). It is best to carry out the procedure under a dissecting microscope in order to monitor the extent of the dissociation.

Tissue from the gastric region gives a homogeneous turbid cell suspension without noticeable clumps with very little shaking. Samples which include hypostome, basal disk, or tentacles require longer soaking and more vigorous shaking to dissociate; even vigorous shaking may not yield a suspension free of clumps. However, the cells in small clumps can usually be identified and counted when the preparations are examined in a microscope.

There are differences between species in the susceptibility to maceration. *Hydra attenuata* macerates easily; *Hydra viridis*, by comparison, requires more vigorous dissociation to yield good cell suspensions.

Fixing Cells and Preparing Cell Spreads for Counting

When dissociation is complete, add fixative. To examine cells and determine cell counts, transfer an aliquot of the suspension to a hemocytometer or to a subbed microscope slide on which a small drop of detergent has been placed. Spread the drop over an area of 1–3 cm^2 on the slide, depending on the concentration of cells in the suspension; the more cells, the greater the area. For example, if five hydra (about 250,000 total cells) are macerated in a final volume of 1.0 ml maceration solution plus fixative, spread 0.1 ml of the suspension containing 25,000 cells over an area of 200 mm^2 on the slide to yield a density of 125 cells/mm^2. This density corresponds to about 40 cells per field when viewed with a 25-power objective lens. For most purposes this density of cells on a slide is convenient for counting. With lower densities, one has to scan large areas to find enough cells when minor cell types such as nerves are being scored. (For illustrations of individual cells, see Chapter 1).

Microtechnique for Individual Pieces of Tissue

To dissociate individual small pieces of tissue, use the wells in Microtest dishes (volume 0.4 ml) for maceration in place of tubes. While observing the whole process under a dissecting microscope, transfer a piece of tissue to the well, draw off excess medium with a pipet, and add one or two drops of maceration solution. To shake the microtiter dish, slide it back and forth on the bench top, banging it against an object like a bottle cap. This sort of vigorous motion is required to stir the small volume in the well. After dissociation is complete, add one drop of fixative and transfer the entire contents of the well with a Pasteur pipet to a slide and spread it over about 1 cm^2. To rinse the last few cells out of the well, add another drop of fixative, shake the well, and transfer the rinse to the slide.

After spreading, place slides on a level surface so that the solution dries evenly; otherwise cells which settle out of the suspension slowly will accumulate on the last part of the suspension to dry on a tilted slide. Such assymmetric drying can seriously distort cell counts.

Counting Cells

After drying on slides, macerations can be examined in several ways. To count cell types, place a drop of 10% glycerin and a coverslip on the slide and examine the preparation using a 25- or 40-power objective lens in a phase contrast microscope. All cell types can be easily recognized with phase optics, and no cells are lost from the slide. To preserve the preparation for a period of months, ring it with a coat of lacquer (nail polish).

To count cells on slides, determine the boundaries of the cell spread using a stage micrometer. Then count all the cells in several complete passes across the spread. From the width of the field and the dimensions of the spread, calculate the total cells on the slide. If a known volume of cell suspension was dried on the slide, calculate the cell concentration in the original suspension. This technique is particularly useful for counting minor cell types such as nerves since large areas of the spread of cells can be easily scanned.

Autoradiography

Macerations on subbed slides are suitable for autoradiography using stripping film or dipping film. Before covering the slides with film, rinse them for 5–10 min in water in order to remove the glycerin and formaldehyde, which cause chemical "exposure" of the film and make scoring labeled cells difficult to carry out. To score labeled cells in autoradiographs, develop the film and dry the slides. Then place a drop of water and a coverslip over the film and examine the preparation by phase contrast microscopy.

Staining

Macerations are suitable for staining by a variety of standard histological techniques. For example, Feulgen-stained preparations can be used for counting mitotic cells and determining the DNA content of individual nuclei by microspectrophotometry (David and Campbell, 1972). Although cells in macerations stick to subbed slides fairly well, the frequent dipping and washing procedures involved in staining may cause some loss of cells from the slides.

REFERENCES

David, C. N. 1973. A quantitative method for maceration of *Hydra* tissue. *Wilhelm Roux Arch. Entwicklungsmech. Org.* 171:259–268.
David, C. N., and Campbell, R. D. 1972. Cell cycle kinetics and development of *Hydra attenuata*. I. Epithelial cells. *J. Cell Sci. 11*:557–568.

Chapter 21

Cell Cycle Analysis of Hydra Cells

Charles N. David

PURPOSE

To measure kinetics of cell cycle and differentiation kinetics, and nuclear DNA content.

INTRODUCTION

Knowledge of the cell cycle kinetics and differentiation kinetics of all hydra cell types is essential to understanding the contribution of each cell type to tissue level development. Obtaining such information has been greatly facilitated in recent years by techniques for labeling hydra with [^{3}H]thymidine (Chapter 25), analysis of cells by maceration (Chapter 20), and microfluorometric techniques for determination of nuclear DNA content. Using these techniques it has been possible to determine the cell cycle kinetics of epithelial cells, interstitial stem cells, and proliferating nematoblasts (David and Campbell, 1972; Campbell and David, 1974) and the differentiation kinetics of nerve cells and stenotele, desmoneme, and isorhiza nematocytes (David and Gierer, 1974).

Charles N. David ● Department of Molecular Biology, Albert Einstein College of Medicine, Bronx, New York.

MATERIALS

[^{3}H]Thymidine (20–100 μCi/ml; 30 mCi/mM); 2,5-bis(4'-amino-phenyl-1')-1,3,4-oxdiazole (BAO) (Fluka, A.G., Buchs, Switzerland); $K_2S_2O_5$; Kodak AR10 Stripping Film or Kodak NTB Autoradiographic Liquid emulsion.

PROCEDURES

Doubling Time of Populations of Cells

Basic information about the doubling time of a cell population is obtained from growth curves of hydra cultures by analyzing the increase in number of the various cell types. Prepare replicate dishes with 10 hydra each and feed all of them daily being careful not to lose any animals or detached buds. On various days, macerate (Chapter 20) the entire contents of a dish and count the number of cells of a given cell type. Cell numbers of hydra fed daily should increase exponentially; the doubling time of the cell population can be read directly from a semilog plot of cell number versus time. If the entire cell population is dividing mitotically (proliferative fraction = 1.0), then the population doubling time equals the average cell cycle time. If the proliferative fraction is less than 1.0, then the population doubling time will be longer than the cell cycle time.

Cell Cycle Time and Proliferative Fraction

Estimate both cell cycle time and proliferative fraction from the kinetics with which a cell population becomes labeled when continuously exposed to [^{3}H]thymidine. To label hydra continuously with [^{3}H]thymidine, inject animals with 0.1 μl of isotope (20–100 μCi/ml) every 8–12 hr. (Each injection results in a pulse label. However, since the S phase of hydra cells is about 12 hr, repeated pulsing with [^{3}H]thymidine at intervals shorter than 12 hr assures that every cycling cell picks up the label at some point in its S phase). Macerate samples of labeled hydra at various times during the course of the labeling experiment and determine by autoradiography the labeling index (labeled cells/total cells) of the cell type being investigated. Expose auto-radiograms of hydra labeled with [^{3}H]thymidine at a concentration of 20–100 μCi/ml for 2 weeks.

An example of a continuous labeling experiment for epithelial cells is shown in Fig. 1. The initial [^{3}H]thymidine pulse labels about 20% of epithelial cells, and the labeling index increased monotonically to 95% by 3 days. The results indicate that 95% of epithelial cells cycled through S phase

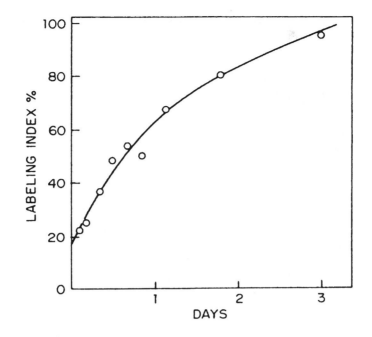

FIGURE 1. Increase in the labeling index of epithelial cells in hydra "continuously" exposed to [³H]thymidine.

in 3 days, and thus the proliferative fraction is at least 0.95. The length of time required to label the entire proliferative fraction of a population is equal to the length of the cell cycle minus the S phase. From the data in Fig. 1, the total epithelial cell cycle is estimated to be 72 hr + S phase, or 84 hr assuming an S phase of 12 hr (see below).

S Phase

Estimate the duration of S phase by using a double labeling technique in which a population of cells in S phase is first labeled with [³H]thymidine and then, after an interval, relabeled with [¹⁴C]thymidine (Wimber and Quastler, 1963). Pulse labeling with [³H]thymidine identifies a population of cells in S phase. With time this population proceeds through S phase and enters G2. The fraction of S-phase cells which have moved into G2 after a given interval can be determined by relabeling with ¹⁴C; cells in G2 do not take up the [¹⁴C]thymidine. The time required for all ³H-labeled cells to move into G2 and therefore not to be labeled by a second ¹⁴C pulse is a measure of the length of S phase.

To determine S phase by this procedure, label several groups of 5–10 hydra with [³H]thymidine. Immediately relabel one group with [¹⁴C] thymidine; relabel the other groups with [¹⁴C]thymidine after 5, 10, 15, and

20 hr, respectively. Macerate each group about 30 min after the $[^{14}C]$ thymidine pulse. Count the percentage of cells labeled only with ^3H in autoradiograms prepared with Kodak stripping film. (Cells labeled with ^3H and ^{14}C can be distinguished from each other in autoradiograms because ^{14}C decays are more energetic and penetrate the film whereas ^3H decays are less energetic and only expose the film immediately above the nucleus of a labeled cell).

A simpler version of the double labeling procedure can be carried out by using only one interval between ^3H and ^{14}C. Cells which leave the S phase between the two isotope pulses will be labeled with only $[^3H]$thymidine. The ratio of cells labeled solely with ^3H to all cells labeled with ^{14}C increases as the interval between pulses increases. For any given interval between pulses (t) the following relationship holds:

$$^3H/^{14}C = t/S$$

where S is the length of S phase, ^3H is the fraction of cells labeled solely with ^3H, and ^{14}C is the fraction of cells labeled with ^{14}C alone or with ^{14}C and ^3H.

G2 Phase

Estimate the duration of G2 by the method of labeled mitoses (Quastler and Sherman, 1959). In most cases mitotic figures in epithelial cells, gland cells, and interstitial cells can be identified in macerations of hydra tissue. However, to obtain data on nests of mitotic interstitial cells (nematoblasts) it is necessary to use histological sections since nests of mitotic interstitial cells are fragile and break up into single cells upon maceration.

To analyze labeled mitoses, pulse label several groups of 5–10 hydra with $[^3H]$thymidine. Macerate (or fix and section) one group of hydra at various times after the pulse. The choice of the time to take those samples depends on the cell type being analyzed: epithelial and gland cells have G2 periods of from 24 to 72 hr and samples can be taken every 8 hr; interstitial stem cells and nests of nematoblasts have G2 periods of from 4 to 24 hr and samples must be taken every 2–3 hr. Mitotic figures can be identified in maceration preparations using phase optics. Staining those cells with Feulgen reagent, however, makes mitotic figures more conspicuous and facilitates scoring. Map mitotic figures on the slides and then cover them with autoradiography film. Expose the slides for 2 weeks, develop them, and determine which mitotic figures are labeled. Plot the fraction of labeled mitoses versus time.

Examples of labeled mitoses curves for nests of two and four interstitial cells are shown in Fig. 2. for synchronous cell populations, the labeling index

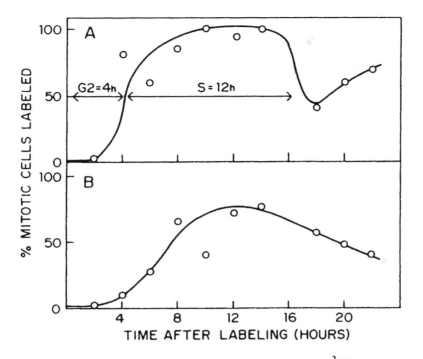

FIGURE 2. Percentage of mitotic figures labeled following pulse of [^{3}H]thymidine. (A) Nests of four interstitial cells: (B) nests of two interstitial cells.

for mitoses rises rapidly from 0 to 100% at a time when the block of cells labeled in S phase has progressed through G2 and entered mitosis. The labeling index remains 100% for a period corresponding to the duration of S and then decreases to 0%. When the block of labeled cells again moves through mitosis, the index again rises to 100%. Natural cell populations are not normally so synchronous because of variations in the speed with which individual cells progress through the cycle. Nevertheless, nests of four interstitial cells yield a fairly square wave of labeled mitoses from which it is possible to estimate G2 = 4 hr and S = 12 hr (Fig. 2A). By comparison, nests of two interstitial cells yield a broad curve which never reaches 100% labeled mitoses (Fig. 2B). Such behavior indicates *variability* in the length of G2 that is significantly greater than the length of S phase (12 hr). Such variability in G2 is a characteristic feature of hydra cells.

Duration of Mitosis

Estimate the duration of mitosis (t_m) in exponentially growing population from the relationship: $t_m = (MI \times T)/2$, where MI is the mitotic index and T the population doubling time (Cleaver, 1967).

Nuclear DNA Content

Measurements of nuclear DNA content on individual cells provide useful additional information about the distribution of cells in various phases of the cell cycle. Cells in G1 have 2C, cells in S have 2C–4C, and cells in G2 have 4C nuclear DNA content, respectively. Measurements of nuclear DNA content are made by staining macerations with a fluorescent Feulgen reagent (Ruch, 1966) and determing the fluorescence intensity of individual nuclei. From the frequency distribution of cells with DNA contents between 2C and 4C, it is possible to estimate the proportion of cells in G1, S, and G2. Proliferating epithelial cells, interstitial stem cells, and nematoblasts have S or G2 DNA contents; virtually none of these cells have G1 DNA contents. By comparison, differentiating nerve cells and nematocytes have G1 DNA contents.

To determine nuclear DNA contents, prepare macerations as described in Chapter 20. Wash the slides briefly and dip them in 1 N HCl at 60°C for 10 minutes. Rinse slides in water and stain them for 2 hr with a solution containing 0.01% BAO and 0.5% $K_2S_2O_5$ in 0.05 M HCl. Wash slides three times in freshly prepared solution of 0.5% $K_2S_2O_5$ in 0.05 M HCl. Determine the fluorescence intensity of individual nuclei using a fluorescence microscope equipped with a photomultiplier.

Differentiation Kinetics and Turnover of Time of Nonproliferating Differentiated Cell Populations

Nerves and nematocytes are nonproliferating differentiated cells derived from stem cells and have G1 nuclear DNA content, indicating they differentiate following a terminal mitosis. To determine the time course of their differentiation and the rate (cells per hydra per day) at which these cells are being produced by hydra tissue, pulse label several groups of hydra with [3H]thymidine and sample macerations of the animals at various times after labeling. Following autoradiography, score the labeling index of nerve cells or nematocytes. The lag time between [3H]thymidine labeling and the first appearance of labeled nerve cells or nematocytes is a measure of the time from the end of the last S phase of the precursor to the appearance of the differentiated cells. For nerve cells it is commonly 12–24 hr; for stenotele nematocytes, 72 hr; for desmoneme and isorhiza nematocytes, 50 hr.

To determine the rate of differentiation of nerve cells and nematocytes, label groups of hydra continuously with [3H]thymidine and sample animals at various times after the start of labeling. The continuous labeling procedure labels the entire precursor cell population and thus after a period of time all newly differentiated nerves and nematocytes will be labeled. From the increase in labeled cells per unit time, estimate the rate of differentiation in cells per hydra per day.

REFERENCES

Campbell, R. D., and David, C. N. 1974. Cell cycle kinetics and development in *Hydra attenuata*. II. Interstitial cells. *J. Cell Sci.* **16**:349–358.

Cleaver, J. R. 1967. *Thymidine Metabolism and Cell Kinetics*, North-Holland, Amsterdam.

David, C. N., and Campbell, R. D. 1972. Cell cycle kinetics and development in *Hydra attentuata*. I. Epithelial cells. *J. Cell. Sci.* **11**:557–568.

David, C. N., and Gierer, A. 1974. Cell cycle kinetics and development in *Hydra attenuata*. III. Nerve and nematocyte differentiation. *J. Cell Sci.* **16**:359–375.

Quastler, H., and Sherman, F. G. 1959. Cell population kinetics in the intestinal epithelium of the mouse. *Exp. Cell Res.* **17**:420–438.

Ruch, F. 1966. Determination of DNA content by microfluorometry. In: *Introduction of Quantitative Cytochemistry*, Academic Press, New York, pp. 281–294.

Wimber, D. E., and Quastler, H. 1963. [14]C- and ^{3}H-thymidine double labeling technique in the study of cell proliferation in *Tradescantia* root tips. *Exp. Cell Res.* **30**:8–22.

Chapter 22

Mitotic Index

Richard D. Campbell

PURPOSE

The mitotic index (percentage of cells in mitosis at any time) provides a measure of the capacity of cells to divide and of the rate of cell division. It is used to identify the sites of growth within a tissue and to determine which cell types are dividing.

INTRODUCTION

Mitotic indexing is superior to isotopic labeling methods for estimating growth in that (1) it can be carried out with cell and tissue preparations of much higher histological quality, (2) the tissue preparations can be used for other purposes, and (3) the special methodology and precautions of isotope use are not required. It is inferior to isotopic methods in that it alone cannot provide information on absolute rates of cell turnover or cell cycle duration.

MATERIALS

Supplies for histological techniques (Chapter 17) and for the maceration technique (Chapter 20) are needed, depending on the method used.

Richard D. Campbell ● Department of Developmental and Cell Biology, University of California, Irvine, California.

PROCEDURES

Tissue Sections of Hydra Fixed with Lavdowsky's Fluid (Campbell, 1967)

Allow each hydra to elongate in a small volume of culture solution, and then flood them suddenly with Lavdowsky's fixative (alcohol : formalin: acetic acid: water ratio = 50 : 10 : 4 : 36). Fix more hydra than will be finally needed so that individuals can be selected which are well extended and straight. Fix the hydra for 24 hr, embed them in paraffin, and section the animals transversely to the body column (Chapter 17). Stain tissue by the Feulgen method (Chapter 17); if this staining does not sufficiently discriminate between cell types, use hematoxylin (Chapter 17) or some other staining method.

Examine all sections or representative sections through the region of interest. Analyze every cell in each selected section. Count and record each nucleus and mitotic figure. Score any stage of mitosis as long as it is consistently recognizable. Calculate the percentage of nuclei in mitosis. Make separate counts and calculations for each cell type of interest. When presenting the data, include a statement as to which stages of mitosis were recognized.

Stained Macerated Preparations

Stain preparations of cells separated by the maceration procedure (Chapter 20) by the same methods as used with tissue sections cited above. Determine the mitotic index by systematically scanning the slide and counting all nonmitotic and mitotic cells of a given type.

Macerated Preparations Viewed with Phase Contrast Microscopy (Schaller, 1976)

Carry out the counting as above, but using phase contrast microscopy to view the cells; the cells need not be stained. Cells in mitosis are not as easily distinguished under phase contrast microscopy, but the method is simpler and faster than procedures involving staining.

Stained Whole Mounts (Park et al., 1970)

Stain whole mounts (Chapter 16), either flattened or opened longi-tudinally, with hematoxylin or by the Feulgen method; count the mitotic figures. Whole mounts preserve the relations between the mitotic cell and the hydra's morphology and are easier to prepare. The disadvantages are that cells are rather difficult to identify in whole mounts and that it is difficult to scan the tissue systematically.

PRECAUTIONS

Prepare histological sections in a plane of section which allows identification of the cells (Chapter 17). Section cells parallel to their axes of symmetry. The best tissue plane of section is transverse to the polyp axis. In a series of longitudinal sections, only the medial sections allow identification of cells. For cells in the hypostome, however, longitudinal section may be preferable although not all sections will be usable.

Cell division in hydra is partially synchronized and is affected by the degree to which animals are fed and by probably other environmental variables. Hydra grown on a daily culture cycle have a pronounced daily rhythm in the mitotic index (Campbell, 1967; David and Campbell, 1972). Fasted hydra have a low mitotic index (Campbell, 1967, Park *et al.*, 1970). Possibly the distribution of dividing cells along the body varies with nutritional level.

In determining mitotic index, systematically scan the preparation and count every cell; otherwise, you will miss cells and not see those in mitosis. Failure to count every cell may account for the inability of some workers to find mitotic activity in epithelial cells.

Do not use colchicine to make mitotic cells accumulate. Some workers claim that colchicine is effective for mitotic analysis (Sturtevant *et al.*, 1951; Corff, 1973). I do not because colchicine has various effects on hydra tissue, one of which is to damage interstitial cells (Campbell, 1976). Damaged interstitial cells may acquire pycnotic nuclei which resemble "c figures."

REFERENCES

Campbell, R. D. 1967. Tissue dynamics of steady state growth in *Hydra littoralis*. I. Patterns of cell division. *Dev. Biol.* 15:487–502.

Campbell, R. D. 1976. Elimination of *Hydra* interstitial and nerve cells by means of colchicine. *J. Cell Sci.* 21:1–13.

Campbell, R. D., and David, C. N. 1974. Cell cycle kinetics and development of *Hydra attenuata*. II. Interstitial cells. *J. Cell Sci.* 16:349–358.

Corff, S. 1973. Organismal growth and the contribution of cell proliferation to the net growth and maintenance of form. In: *Biology of Hydra* (A. L. Burnett, ed.), Academic Press, New York, pp. 345–389.

David, C. N., and Campbell, R. D. 1972. Cell cycle kinetics and development of *Hydra attenuata*. I. Epithelial cells. *J. Cell Sci.* 11:557–568.

Park, H. D., Ortmeyer, A. B., and Blankenbaker, D. P. 1970. Cell division during regeneration in hydra. *Nature (London)* **227**:617–619.

Schaller, H. C. 1976. Action of the head activator as a growth hormone in hydra. *Cell Differ.* **5**:1–11.

Sturtevant, F. M., Sturtevant, R. P., and Turner, C. L. 1951. Effect of colchicine on regeneration in *Pelmatohydra oligactis*. *Science* **114**:241–242.

Chapter 23

Measurement of the Numbers of Nematoblasts, Nematocytes, and Nematocysts

Hans R. Bode, G. Scott Smith, and Patricia M. Bode

PURPOSE

To quantitate the numbers of nematocytes, nematoblasts, and nematocysts in different body regions and in different stages of development.

GENERAL INTRODUCTION

The ability to measure the number of nematocytes of each of the four types in the whole animal or in a particular body region rests on the distinctive morphology of the nematocyst capsule of each type. Using phase microscopy (160–400×), the capsule types are easily distinguishable from one another when isolated free of tissue (Fig. 1), in single-cell suspensions of macerated animals, or in whole mounts. The same clear-cut differences can be used to quantitate the nematoblasts of each type at a late stage in their differentiation where capsule morphology becomes recognizable. Four methods exploiting these differences are described.

Hans R. Bode, G. Scott Smith, and Patricia M. Bode ● Developmental Biology Center and Department of Developmental and Cell Biology, University of California, Irvine, California.

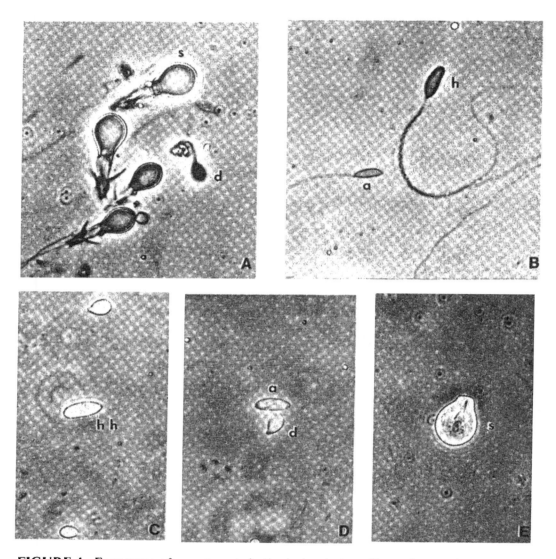

FIGURE 1. Four types of nematocysts in the isolated state. Photomicrographs were taken with phase optics. (A) Discharged desmoneme (d) and stenotele nematocysts (s). (B) Discharged holotrichous isorhiza (h) and atrichous isorhiza (a) nematocysts. (C) Intact holotrichous isorhiza nematocyst (h). (D) Intact desmoneme (d) and atrichous isorhiza (a) nematocysts. (E) Intact stenotele nematocyst (s) (640×, reproduced at 85%).

METHOD I. NEMATOBLASTS IN LATE STAGE OF DEVELOPMENT: LEAD NITRATE–THIOACETIC ACID STAIN

INTRODUCTION

Developing nematoblasts are found in the body column, but not the extremities, and always occur in the syncytial clusters or nests of cells usually numbering 8, 16, or 32 (Lehn, 1951; Slautterback and Fawcett, 1959; Rich and Tardent, 1969). All members of a nest are of the same type. Tardent (1954) and Tardent *et al.* (1969) developed a method in which the hydra was fixed and the ectoderm removed, displayed on glass, and then stained, rendering the nests of nematoblasts clearly visible and identifiable by type. More recently, David and Challoner (1974) described a simpler procedure for specifically staining the nematocyst capsules of late-stage nematoblasts in whole mounts with lead nitrate–thioacetic acid. These capsules stain dark brown, whereas the stain is not taken up by earlier stages of nematoblasts in which the capsule has not acquired a definitive shape and by capsules of mature nematocytes. No other cell type or organelle stains by this reagent. Several nests of nematoblasts with stained developing nematocysts are shown in Figs. 2 and 3.

MATERIALS

Reagents: 0.15 *M* sodium cacodylate (K & K Laboratories) buffer, pH 6.0; 0.1 *M* lead nitrate (reagent grade); thioacetic acid (Matheson, Coleman & Bell, practical grade); 1 *N* NaOH; and 1 *N* HCl.

Hood; disposable gloves; glass filter paper (Whatman 6 P/A, 12.5 cm, or Whatman No. 1 filter paper); ethyl alcohol; xylene; plastic and glass Petri dishes; mounting medium; ocular micrometer; Linde Molecular Sieve (Type SA, 1/16-in. pellets, Allied Chemicals, Morristown, NJ).

Be careful to note that the staining characteristics of different batches of thioacetic acid vary. Newly opened bottles of the acid often give poor stains. To overcome this problem, add a small volume of thioacetic acid from a new bottle to the remaining volume of an old bottle and mix. Warming new thioacetic acid at 37°C with magnetic stirring followed by stirring at room temperature also enhances its staining properties. To prevent a general darkening of the stained tissue, do not heat at too high a temperture or for too long, and do not stir too long.

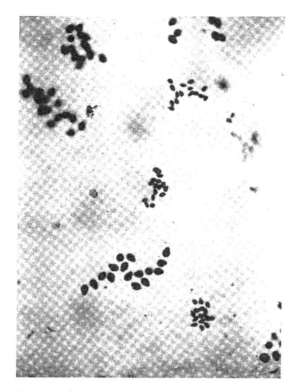

FIGURE 2. Several nests of stenoteles and desmonemes in the body column of a whole mount stained with lead nitrate–thioacetic acid (240×, reproduced at 85%).

PROCEDURES

Preparing Thioacetic Acid–Lead Nitrate Stain

Because the odor of thioacetic acid is highly unpleasant, prepare and use the stain in a fume hood. As the odor is difficult to remove, keep a special set of glassware either in the hood or in a container away from working areas. Carry out all steps connected with the stain wearing a lab coat and disposable gloves. (Dry cleaning removes the odor from clothes. Ethanol reduces it considerably from glassware and other materials.) Keep stock reagent solutions in the hood. Make up the stain just prior to use.

Add 2.35 ml 1 N NaOH to 50 ml distilled water in a glass beaker. Using a calibrated Pasteur pipet, add 0.42 ml thioacetic acid to the alkaline solution. Mix well by pipeting up and down with the Pasteur pipet for 3 min. The solution will become cloudy. Adjust the pH with 1 N NaOH to between 5.5 and 6.0 using a broad-range pH paper (e.g., Panpeha). With a graduated cylinder measure 18 ml of this thioacetic solution and place it in a glass

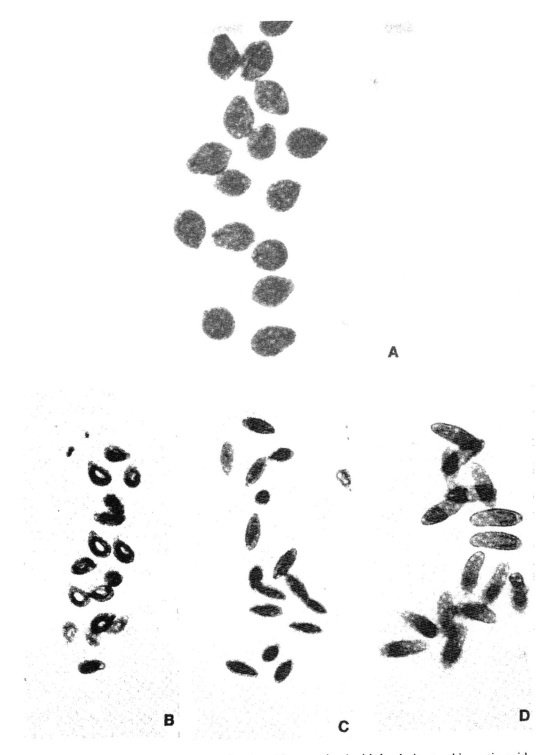

FIGURE 3. Nests of the four types of nematoblasts stained with lead nitrate–thioacetic acid. (A) Nest of 16 stenoteles. (B) Nest of 16 desmonemes. (C). Nest of 16 atrichous isorhizas. (D) Nest of 16 holotrichous isorhizas (1040×. reproduced at 85%).

beaker. Add, in order, 2 ml cacodylate buffer and 1 ml lead nitrate buffer. Mix and allow the solution to stand 25 min. It will turn brown and later black due to precipitation. Then, filter solution through glass fiber paper (Whatman 6 P/A, 12.5 cm; Whatman No. 1 filter paper will probably work as well). Let filtered solution sit 30–40 min. At this point it is convenient to fix the animals prior to staining.

Fixing Animals

Fix the animals when they are extended to ensure fewer nematoblasts per unit area, thus rendering the counting easier and errors fewer. Place an individual animal in 2% urethane solution in distilled water in a 35-mm plastic Petri dish. The animal will stretch out. Then remove the urethane solution and rapidly add 100% ETOH. Allow 1–2 min for fixation.

Collect all fixed animals in a 60-mm Petri dish and remove the alcohol from the tissue by successive rinses in 95% ETOH, 70% ETOH, 35% ETOH, and three changes of distilled water. Allow 2 min for the ethanol steps and 0.5–1 min for each water change. When animals are completely hydrated, they will sink instead of float. Place the dish in the fume hood and start staining as soon as possible because the animals tend to disintegrate in water.

Staining Tissue

Before applying the stain, filter it once more through glass fiber paper. Remove the distilled water from around the animals, immediately add the stain solution, and expose them to the stain for 20–25 min. Exposure for more than 30 min results in heavy black precipitates forming in the tissue which obliterates the stained nematocysts. Thereafter remove the stain solution and wash the animals twice by flooding the dish with distilled water. Rinse twice with 70% ETOH. The animals may then be removed from the hood.

Preparing Whole Mounts

Once the hydra are in 70% ETOH, the stain is stable for many hours. Dehydrate the tissue with the following schedule (1 min each): 95% ETOH, 95% ETOH, 100% ETOH, 100% ETOH, 100 ETOH–xylene at 1:1, and xylene. Carry out the steps up to and including the last 100% ETOH in plastic Petri dishes, and the last two steps in glass dishes because xylene dissolves plastic. Transfer animals from solution to solution using a Pasteur pipet with a large orifice. Once the animals are in the 1:1 ETOH–xylene mixture, transfer them by gently grasping the tentacles with watchmaker's forceps. The animals become sticky in xylene and are lost when they adhere to the inside glass walls of the Pasteur pipet.

If at the end of the dehydration the tissue appears white or milky instead of translucent, it contains water. Therefore, rehydrate by tracing the steps back to 95% ethanol and repeat the dehydration procedure. To prevent this problem, fill the bottle containing the 100% ethanol one-fourth full of Linde Molecular Sieve granules. Transfer the dehydrated animals to a glass slide. Once they are on the slide, push tentacles and buds aside to prevent them from obscuring the body column. Add a drop of mounting medium (e.g., Histoclad or Permount) to the animals and apply a cover glass. Slight pressure to the slide will flatten the animal a little to aid in visualizing the nest in one plane. In some mounting media, but not the two mentioned, the stain fades and vanishes after 2–3 days.

Quantitation

To observe and count all the nematoblast nests on both sides of the animal and along the edges use bright field optics at 160–400×. An ocular micrometer with cross hairs or a net helps in delineating areas to be counted, thereby reducing the errors due to missed or repeated counts. Determine axial distribution of nests by locating each nest with respect to the head and foot. A simple method consists of dividing the body column into a number of units, each unit being defined by the area covered by a net of lines on an ocular reticule. Assign every nest to a unit which then defines its axial location. A more precise, but far more tedious method, is to determine the coordinates of each nest, the head, the foot and other prominent features of the whole mount in terms of the horizontal and vertical vernier scales of the microscope stage. The relative location of each nest can then be calculated.

COMMENTS

These methods have been used to quantitate the numbers and axial distributions of late-stage nematoblasts in steady-state *Hydra attenuata* (David and Challoner, 1974; Bode and Flick, 1976; Bode and Smith, 1977). It is worth noting that the number of nests of each nematocyte type reflects the numbers of interstitial cells committed to the differentiation of each type. Thus, the technique can be used to study aspects of interstitial cell behavior. Finally, the size (length) of the stenotele capsule depends on the axial position of the nest where the capsule develops (Lehn, 1951; Rich and Tardent, 1969; Bode and Smith, 1977). The length of the capsule decreases monotonically as the distance of the stenotele from the head increases. The length of a capsule is easily measured in these preparations with an ocular micrometer with a scale using phase optics under oil at 1000×.

METHOD II. NEMATOCYTES IN THE TENTACLES: NEMATOCYST SUSPENSIONS

INTRODUCTION

This procedure, based on the resistance of the nematocyst capsule to reagents that dissolve most tissue, yields suspensions of nematocyst capsules that can be easily counted (Bode and Flick, 1976). We describe methods for preparing nematocyst suspensions from tentacles both of groups of animals and of single animals.

MATERIALS

Construct scalpels by mounting a ~ 3-mm sliver of razor blade at a 45° angle in a slot at the end of a wood application stick, and cemented with glue, prepare the sliver by using tin snips to cut a double-edged razor blade perpendicular to the edge into 15–30 pieces.

One-tenth of one percent sodium dodecyl sulfate (SDS); 10% formaldehyde; 0.5 N NaOH–7% glycerol solution; syringe with a 18- to 21-gauge needle; Neubauer cell-counting chamber; polyethylene tubing (Intramedic tubing, PE 60, Clay-Adams); 50 μl Hamilton syringe; tungsten needle.

PROCEDURES

Groups of Animals

Isolate tentacles of 5–10 animals by first severing the heads (hypostome and tentacles) from the body columns followed by cutting the tentacles from the hypostomes with a scalpel. Plastic Petri dishes offer a good soft surface for cutting.

Place the tentacles in a plastic test tube which has a hydrophobic surface so as not to lose any volume. Dissolve the tentacles in a known volume (0.1 ml) of 0.1% SDS in distilled H_2O. (Use distilled water since 0.1% SDS forms precipitates and/or crystals with potassium ions, and these tend to obscure the nematocysts.) Within 10–15 min the tentacles should have dissolved, leaving only nematocyst capsules visible, most of which will be undischarged. If left in SDS, however, they all eventually discharge. To prevent discharge, add 1/10 volume of 10% formaldehyde after the tissue is dissolved. Stenotele and desmoneme nematocysts can be easily recognized when discharged or undischarged, whereas the atrichous and holotrichous isorhizas are less distinct when discharged (Fig. 1).

Suspensions of nematocysts can also be obtained by dissolving the tentacles in 0.5 N NaOH–7% glycerol (T. Fujisawa and T. Sugiyama, personal communication) A third method is based on disrupting the tentacles and releasing the nematocysts by forcefully expelling a suspension of tentacles a number of times through a syringe with a small-gauge (18–21) needle. This procedure is as effective as the use of dissolving reagents, but has the disadvantage that some of the solution (and suspension) may be lost in the syringe.

Individual Animals

The same procedure can be used for single animals by modifying the method to deal with small volumes. A convenient volume is 20 μl, as it is just sufficient to fill both fields of a Neubauer cell-counting chamber with a depth of 0.1 mm. Draw the severed tentacles into a piece of polyethylene tubing (Intramedic tubing, PE 60, Clay-Adams) from the Petri dish with a 50-μl Hamilton syringe attached to the tubing. With a tungsten needle, tamp down the tentacles to one end of the fluid column and expel the excess fluid. Draw 1/10 volume of 1% SDS into the tubing and mix it with the tentacles by stirring with the tungsten needle and moving the fluid column up and down with the plunger of the attached syringe. After the tissue dissolves, draw in 1/10 volume of formaldehyde and mix it with the nematocyst suspension. For storage, seal the two ends of the tubing by heating them over a Bunsen burner and store the sample at room temperature. Samples can be stored at least 4 weeks without loss of material (A. Kobrin and H. R. Bode, unpublished results). When the sample is to be counted, cut off the ends of the tube, mix the suspension as before, and expel into a cell-counting chamber.

Quantitation

To determine the total number of nematocytes in the cell suspension, measure the volume of the sample and the number of nematocytes per unit volume. Measure the volume for samples of several animals by weighing. For samples of single animals, measure the length of the fluid column in the polyethylene tube and convert it to a volume using a previously established calibration curve. Determine the number of nematocytes per unit volume with a Neubauer cell-counting chamber specially designed for use with a phase microscope (0.1-mm depth) at 250 or 400×. Obtain differential capsule counts of the four types of nematocysts by counting 500–1000 capsules in the cell-counting chamber. Samples to be analyzed for differential counts at a later time can be preserved for a period of days to weeks by placing a drop of the suspension on a glass slide, covering it with a cover slip, and sealing the edges with nail polish or mounting medium (e.g., Permount).

METHOD III. STENOTELES ON THE TENTACLES: DIRECT OBSERVATION IN SITU

INTRODUCTION

With phase microscopy the nematocysts of nematocytes mounted in the battery cells of the tentacles are recognizable (Fig. 1). The large stenoteles are particularly recognizable. Simply place a live animal in a large drop of culture solution on a glass slide and gently flatten it with a cover slip. It should become immobile, but intact. With phase microscopy (250 or 400×) first examine for all the stenoteles on the surface of a tentacle facing the objective. Next count the stenoteles on the visible half of three to six tentacles; their number can vary from tentacle to tentacle.

After counting, carefully remove the cover slip and return the animal to a culture dish. One hour later such animals appear normal and are capable of feeding. Work fairly rapidly so that the animal is not in the flattened state for too long. The procedure can be repeated on the same animal every 2–3 days for extended periods of time without detectable damage to it.

COMMENTS AND PRECAUTIONS

This method was used to examine changes in the population size of stenoteles in the tentacles over a period of 4 months (Bode and Flick, 1976). In principle the method can be applied to the other nematocyte types, but not readily in practice. The desmonemes are simply too numerous to count without error and tedium, while the two types of isorhizas are not readily distinguishable by this method.

METHOD IV. NEMATOCYTES ON THE SURFACE OF THE BODY COLUMN BY TOLUIDINE BLUE STAIN

INTRODUCTION

The nematocysts of nematocytes mounted on the surface of the body column (and tentacles) can be selectively stained in whole mounts with Toluidine Blue (Figs. 4 and 5), (Diehl and Burnett, 1967). The procedure is a little tricky as the length of time the tissue is stained is critical. If too short, staining is incomplete, and if too long, late stage nematoblasts and mature migrating nematocytes as well as mounted nematocytes also will be stained.

MATERIALS

Fixatives (see Method I); ethanol; 0.05% Toluidine Blue in 0.01 M tris, pH 7–8.

PROCEDURE

For ease of counting, fix individual animals while they are extended as described for staining for nematoblasts (see Method I). Allow 1 min for

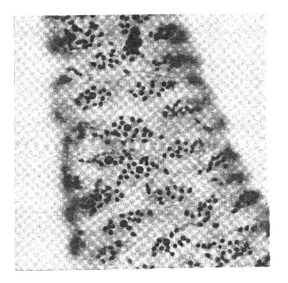

FIGURE 4. Toluidine Blue-stained nematocysts within nematocytes mounted in battery cells of a tentacle (280×, reproduced at 85%).

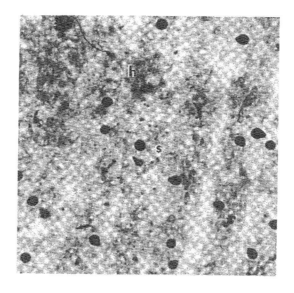

FIGURE 5. Toluidine Blue-stained nematocyst capsules of stenoteles (*s*) and holotrichous isorhizas (*h*) within nematocytes mounted in the ectoderm of the body (280×, reproduced at 85%).

fixation, and pool the animals into one dish. Hydrate them through the following solutions, each for 1 min: 70% ETOH, distilled water, distilled water. This process is readily performed by exchanging the 2 ml of each solution in the Petri dish. Transfer the animals to a smaller container such as a 10-ml beaker or 10-ml screw cap vial. Remove the water and add 0.5 ml 0.05% Toluidine Blue in 0.01 M tris, pH 7–8. Stain for 60 sec only, agitating the solution constantly to ensure uniform staining of the animals. To stop the staining, immediately and rapidly dilute the stain either by pouring water into the beaker or vial or by pouring stain and animals into a beaker filled with water. Transfer the animals with a wide-bore Pasteur pipet to a dish of distilled water for 2 min. Use the same dehydration schedule and mounting procedure as described for whole mounts stained for late-stage nematoblasts in Method I.

COMMENTS AND PRECAUTIONS

During the staining period, the side of an animal in contact with the container will be stained either very lightly or not at all. Staining time is critical. Determine the optimal staining time for each species of hydra and each fresh stain solution. With practice you will recognize the characteristic intensity of the blue color of the animal when the nematocytes are appropriately stained.

Quantitation

To determine the number of nematocytes on the body column, count, using bright-field microscopy (250×), all stained nematocysts on the half of the hydra facing the objective and on one edge (tentacles, hypostome, and buds excluded). Multiply this number by two because the nematocytes on the side of the animal away from the objective are hard to count. If necessary, however, you can turn the slide over and count the nematocytes.

Since the long axis of the mounted nematocysts is perpendicular to the surface of the body column, you will see the capsules in cross section. Distinguishing among the desmonemes and the two isorhizas is quite difficult, but can be achieved by examining the capsules at several focal planes. In *H. attenuata* that problem does not arise since only stenoteles and holotrichous isorhizas, which are easily distinguishable, are mounted on the body column. Hence, it is advisable to cursorily examine of the surface of other hydra species before staining them to identify the types of nematocysts present.

In principle this procedure is not useful for counting nematocysts in tentacles because it is difficult to keep them from becoming twisted and looped around one another during the dehydration procedure.

REFERENCES

Bode, H. R., and Flick, K. M. 1976. Distribution and dynamics of nematocyte populations in *Hydra attenuata*. *J. Cell Sci.* 21:15–34.

Bode, H. R., and Smith, G. S. 1977. Regulation of interstitial cell differentiation in *Hydra attenuata*. II. Correlation of the axial position of the interstitial cell with nematocyte differentiation. *Wilhelm Roux Arch. Entwicklungsmech. Org.* 181:203–213.

David, C. N., and Challoner, D. 1974. Distribution of interstitial cells and differentiating nematocytes in nests in *Hydra attenuata*. *Am. Zool.* 14:537–542.

David, C. N., and Gierer, A. 1974. Cell cycle kinetics and development of *Hydra attenuata*. III. Nerve and nematocyte differentiation. *J. Cell Sci.* 16:359–375.

Diehl, F. A., and Burnett, A. L. 1964. The role of interstitial cells in the maintenance of hydra. I. Specific destruction of interstitial cells in normal, asexual and non-budding animals. *J. Exp. Zool.* 155:253–259.

Lehn, H. 1951. Teilungsfolgen and Determination von I-Zellen für die Cnidenbilding bei Hydra. *Z. Naturforsch.* B6:388–391.

Rich, F., and Tardent, P. 1969. Untersuchungen zur Nematocyten-Differenzierung bei *Hydra attenuata* Pall. *Rev. Suisse Zool.* 76:779–787.

Slautterback, D. B., and Fawcett, D. W. 1959. The development of the cnidoblasts of hydra. An electron microscope study of cell differentiation. *J. Biophys. Biochem. Cytol.* 5:441–452.

Tardent, P. 1954. Axiale Verteilungs-Gradienten der interstitiellen Zellen bei *Hydra* und
    Tubularia and ihre bedeutung für die Regeneration. *Wilhelm Roux Arch.
    Entwicklungsmech. Org.* **146**:5932–649.
Tardent, P., Rich, F., and Schneider, V. 1971. The polarity of stenotele differentiation in *Hydra
    attenuata* Pall. *Dev. Biol.* **24**:596–608.

Chapter 24

Marking Epithelial Cells in Living Hydra with India Ink

Joann J. Otto and Richard D. Campbell

PURPOSE

To vitally mark epitheliomuscular cells with carbon particles so that those cells can be used to follow the displacement of small groups of cells or to demarcate the boundary of a tissue graft.

INTRODUCTION

Carbon particles injected into the ectodermal tissue layer are taken up by the epithelial cells through phagocytosis and are sequestered in terminal lysosomes (Campbell, 1973). When a cell marked in this way divides, the carbon is retained in the daughter cells. Thus, the carbon serves as a permanent marker for a cell and some of its descendants. The marks are visible with a dissecting microscope for days or weeks although in time the marked area becomes diffuse due to tissue growth and to a slow loss of marks from cells.

Joann J. Otto ● Department of Biological Sciences, Purdue University, West Lafayette, Indiana.   Richard D. Campbell ● Department of Developmental and Cell Biology, University of California, Irvine, California.

MATERIALS

India ink (Pelikan 11/1431a); Pasteur pipet to use as mouth pipet; plastic Petri dish; flexible Tygon tubing (outer diameter 1/8 in., inner diameter 1/16 in.) which will fit tightly on tip of Pasteur pipet; glass thin-walled capillary tubing (outer diameter 2 mm) for micropipets (should fit tightly inside the flexible tubing); watchmaker's forceps; dissecting micro-scope with white background; to hold needles, a plastic foam block which fits under jar or beaker.

Also needed is a small Bunsen burner for making micropipets. This burner can conveniently be made by placing a No. 20-gauge syringe needle, attached to a gas outlet, into the edge of a large rubber stopper.

PROCEDURES

Preparing and Caring for Micropipets

Make the tips of the micropipets relatively short (about 5 mm), since longer needles tend to break easily, and with a tip diameter of about 5 μm. To make a micropipet by hand, heat the capillary tube with the smallest possible Bunsen microburner flame ($\sim$5 mm) and pull hard and constantly on the ends of the tube as the glass melts. The glass should produce a dull snapping noise as it breaks. If the tip is too long, you overheated the glass. Store the needles, with their tips projecting upward, in slits made in the side of a foam pad. Cover the foam and needles with a beaker or jar to prevent damage to the tips and injury to people.

Marking the Hydra (Fig. 1)

Place the hydra in a Petri dish on a white background under a dissecting microscope. When first trying this procedure, use large hydra. With practice, you should also be able to mark small hydra. Insert a micropipet into the end of the polyvinyl tubing of the mouth pipet. Holding the immersed needle with one hand and forceps with the other and while looking at the tip under the microscope, determine if the tip diameter is the proper size. Fluid should move slowly ($<$0.5 mm/sec) up the open tip when you apply suction. If it moves more rapidly, the tip is too large and you must make a new one. If it moves too slowly, the tip is too small and you should break it by very gently touching it to the forceps. Place a small drop of ink on a clean hydrophobic surface such as a small, inverted plastic Petri dish. Fill the micropipet with ink by placing the tip horizontally into the drop of ink and applying a great

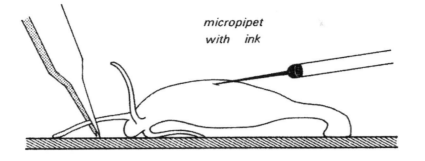

FIGURE I. Positioning of hydra while injecting it with India ink.

deal of suction to the mouthpiece. Do not apply suction when the pipet is in the air, because a bubble will ruin the micropipet.

Move the micropipet to the dish of hydra and immediately insert the tip into the medium in order to keep it wet. From this time on keep the tip wet to prevent the ink from drying and clogging the tip.

Find an attached and extended hydra to mark, and hold it horizontally by grasping a tentacle lightly with the forceps. Blow hard into the pipet to remove the medium from its tip and to bring the ink back to the extreme tip. Continue blowing ink out while carefully inserting the pipet into the ectoderm until you get the impression of the tip of the micropipet contacting the thin collagenous mesoglea. Withdraw the pipet from the hydra. Ink will pour out of the wound for a few moments. After the wound heals, gently brush away with the forceps the ink which accumulates around the hydra and examine the mark.

The size and extent of a mark can be somewhat controlled by the angle the pipet penetrates, tip size, the force of ink injection, and the state of contraction of the hydra. When a small tip is inserted at an acute angle, the marks tend to be small. When a larger tip is inserted at right angles to the hydra, the marks are more extensive. Smaller marks can be made in an extended hydra than in a contracted one. To mark an entire hydra or large portion of the body, press a fairly large tip at right angles against the surface of a contracted hydra and apply much force through the mouth pipet.

To clear a needle that clogs with ink or tissue debris, try (1) blowing very hard with the tip suspended in the medium, (2) gently touching the tip to the forceps to rebreak the tip, or (3) drawing up more ink into the needle.

ALTERNATE MATERIALS AND TECHNIQUES

1. Colloids other than India ink and particle suspensions can be used to produce different types or colors of marking. Small glass or latex beads (1–

$20\mu m$ in diameter) are suitable. Beads greater than 10 mm in diameter can be held individually by suction at the tip of a small micropipet and inserted into the ectoderm individually to produce single, point marks.

2. To mark the endoderm in spots, press the micropipet tip through the ectoderm and mesolamella before expelling ink. In this case, expel the ink with a very light pressure or else ink will flow into the gastric cavity and label the entire endoderm.

3. To mark the entire endoderm with ink, inject the ink directly into the gastric cavity. Insert the micropipet either through the mouth or through the column tissue. Endodermal marking fades more rapidly than ectodermal marking, presumably due to the expulsion of the particles from the digestive cells.

4. To mark the mesolamella in spots, drive the micropipet through it while expelling ink. This procedure also marks the overlying ectoderm and endoderm. However, after several hours the intracellular carbon moves away from the basal surfaces of the cells, so that mesolamella marks can be recognized by their central position between the ectoderm and endoderm.

REFERENCES

Campbell, R. D. 1973. Vital marking of single cells in developing tissues: India ink injection to trace tissue movements in hydra. *J. Cell Sci.* 13:651–661.

Part V

Techniques Using Isotopes

Chapter 25

Incorporating [³H]Thymidine into Hydra by Microinjection

Charles N. David

PURPOSE

To label hydra by injecting [³H]thymidine into the gastric cavity (Campbell, 1965; David and Campbell, 1972).

INTRODUCTION

Hydra, because of their low permeability, cannot be effectively labeled with radioactive materials by the usual method of soaking animals in a solution containing the isotope. Injection of [³H]thymidine into the gastric cavity offers several advantages over soaking hydra in medium containing isotope. (1) [³H]Thymidine is taken up 10 to 20 times more effectively from the gastric cavity than from the external medium, and only small amounts of isotope are required for injection. (2) The injected [³H]thymidine labels primarily hydra cells and not bacteria, which exist in large numbers on the outside of hydra. By comparison, >95% of the label is incorporated into bacterial DNA when hydra are soaked in [³H]thymidine. (3) Injection of [³H]thymidine yields a natural pulse label. A single injection is taken up within 45 min in unfed animals and within 90 min in fed animals.

Charles N. David • Department of Molecular Biology, Albert Einstein College of Medicine, Bronx, New York.

MATERIALS

Hamilton syringe (10 or 25 μl; Hamilton Co., Reno, NV), polyethylene tubing (Intramedic PE 50; Clay-Adams, Parsippany, NJ).

PROCEDURES

Preparing Polyethylene Needles

Polyethylene needles are superior to glass needles for injecting hydra because they are slightly flexible. Prepare the needles by warming polyethylene tubing (PE 50) near a small flame such as the pilot light of a Bunsen burner. When the tubing starts to melt, remove it from the flame and draw it out. The short melted section pulls out into a thin tube which hardens almost immediately. Cut the tubing with a razor blade on an angle at the point where its diameter is about 0.1 mm. Attach the needle to the end of a Hamilton syringe.

Filling the Needle

Remove an appropriate small amount (20–100 μl) of isotope from the stock solution and place it on the bottom of a 20-mm plastic Petri dish. The solution forms a round drop since the plastic surface is hydrophobic. Keep the dish covered to avoid evaporation. Draw up the isotope solution into the polyethylene needle but not into the syringe itself. Discard the needle at the end of the experiment.

Injection Procedure

Place 5–10 hydra in 10 ml medium in a 50-mm plastic Petri dish. Move the hydra to the center of the dish, loosen them from the bottom, and wait for them to stretch out a bit. During injection, view the hydra under low power in a dissecting microscope. With tweezers in one hand, position a hydra and hold it lightly behind the tentacles. With the other hand bring the Hamilton syringe into position and insert the needle into the mouth of the animal. The insertion is generally easy to do with thin needles and does not normally cause the animal to contract much or to open its mouth. Once the needle is inserted, gently press the plunger of the syringe to expel a small volume of solution into the hydra's gastric cavity. Estimate the amount injected by watching the movement of the meniscus of the solution in the needle; usually 0.25 μl occupies a length of 1 mm.

After the hydra swells up, wait a few second before withdrawing the needle. The mouth usually closes tightly as the needle is withdrawn and the hydra remain somewhat swollen. If individual animals contract immediately upon withdrawal of the needle, reinject them a minute or two later. With practice one can inject two to three hydra per minute.

For individuals with unsteady hand, the Hamilton syringe may be mounted in a motor-driven syringe pump activated with a foot pedal. If the injection volume does not need to be controlled, the injection needle may be connected directly to a mouth pipet and the isotope expelled by blowing gently.

REFERENCES

Campbell, R. D. 1965. Cell proliferation in *Hydra*: An autoradiographic approach. *Science* **148**:1231–1232.

David, C. N., and Campbell, R. D. 1972. Cell cycle kinetics and development of *Hydra attenuata*. I. Epithelial cells. *J. Cell Sci.* **11**:557–568.

Chapter 26

Labeling with Gaseous $^{14}CO_2$ or by Feeding on Radioactive Tissues

Howard M. Lenhoff

PURPOSE

To label hydra directly by feeding them on tissues that have been previously made radioactive or by exposing them to $^{14}CO_2$. The ingested radioactive tissue labels the endoderm first and, within a day, most of the hydra's cells (Lenhoff, 1961). The labeled $^{14}CO_2$ passes directly into hydra and labels most intensely the interstitial cells and their derivative cells (Lenhoff, 1959); in the case of green hydra, the $^{14}CO_2$ labels the endosymbiotic algae most intensely (Muscatine and Lenhoff, 1965).

INTRODUCTION

Hydra, like most freshwater organisms, are relatively impermeable to ionic compounds. Thus, it is not possible to label them as is commonly done with microorganisms, i.e., by simply bathing them in a nutrient medium containing the desired label. Furthermore, in the bathing experiments a significant portion of radioactive compounds are usually taken up by the bacteria and molds frequently adhering to hydra, especially those living in the sticky secretions of the basal disk.

Thus, hydra can be conveniently and efficiently labeled by one of three methods: (1) by the injection technique (Chapter 25); (2) by feeding them on

---

Howard M. Lenhoff ● Department of Developmental and Cell Biology, University of California, Irvine, California.

radioactive tissues; or (3) by exposing them to $^{14}CO_2$, a gas that permeates hydra's cell membranes.

MATERIALS

For Feeding Radioactive Tissue

Yeast protein or whole yeast cells made radioactive with ^{35}S may be either purchased (e.g., from Schwartz-Mann Co.) or prepared economically by growing yeast on $^{35}SO_4^{2-}$ (Cowie *et al.*, 1952). Other materials needed are physiological saline solution, $\sim 0.1\%$ NaCl; a young mouse in a cage; small syringe; scalpels with No. 15 blades; a razor blade; fine forceps (No. 5); scissors; plastic test tubes; Petri dishes; ether; 500-ml beaker; cotton; $10^{-4} M$ reduced glutathione made up in culture medium.

For Supplying $^{14}CO_2$

Prepare an apparatus consisting of a structure identical to the side arm of a Warburg respirometer flask and attach it to the upper third of 50- or 100-ml pyrex beaker that previously had its top rim sawed off. The side arm should have a separate opening closed by a ground glass stopper. Prepare flat glass plates that will cover these modified beakers. I recommend these modified beakers rather than commercially available Warburg vessels because the wide opening of the beaker makes it easier to manipulate the hydra. Other materials needed are $NaH^{14}CO_3$, concentrated phosphoric acid, and stopcock grease.

LABELING BY FEEDING HYDRA

PROCEDURES

Prepare the labeled tissue. This example is for ^{35}S-labeled tissue; therefore, most of the isotope is found in the cysteine, cystine, and methionine of tissue proteins. Similar procedures can be followed using other isotopes. For example, tissue labeled with ^{32}P will have its nucleic acid fractions heavily labeled.

To prepare ^{35}S-labeled tissue, hydrolyze commercially available ^{35}S yeast or protein in 1 ml 6 N HCl in a sealed test tube at $100°C$ for 10–16 hr.

Dry the hydrolysate in an evaporating dish over a steam bath, or in a test tube under vacuum. To remove the residual HCl, add a few drops of distilled water to the residue and dry again. Dissolve the dry radioactive residue in 2–3 ml physiological saline.

Inject about 0.5 ml of the solution into the peritoneal cavity of a young, growing mouse and leave it alone for about 16–24 hr. Make certain that the mouse has food and water. Kill the mouse; a simple way is to put it into a covered beaker containing cotton slightly soaked with ether. When the mouse is inert, remove it from the beaker, place it on a small pad of newspapers, cut it open and remove the liver, kidney, lungs, and other organs of interest. Put each organ in a separate plastic test tube, mark it accordingly, and freeze it for future use. Dispose of the mouse carcass and of the litter in the cage according to standard practices for handling radioactive wastes.

Hydra that are affixed by their basal disks are much easier to feed labeled tissues. Therefore, in the late afternoon before labeling the hydra, place about 10–12 large ones in a Petri dish three-fourths full of culture solution. By morning when you should label the hydra, their basal disks should be affixed securely to the bottom of the dishes.

Using a razor blade, cut off a small piece (~ 1 cm^3) of radioactive mouse tissue (e.g., liver) and place it in 1 ml $10^{-4} M$ glutathione. While observing the tissue under the dissecting microscope, cut it into 10–15 smaller bits and allow them to remain in the glutathione for an additional 5 min. Pick up a small bit of radioactive tissue with the forceps and place it in the center of a hydra's ringlet of tentacles as close to the mouth as possible. Then immediately add a drop of fresh glutathione near the mouth of the same hydra.

Once you feed one hydra in a Petri dish in this manner, continue immediately to feed the rest of the animals starting with the ones closest to the first animal fed. If you do not, the glutathione will diffuse throughout the dish and will cause the animals to contract their tentacles prematurely, making it difficult to feed them the labeled tissue.

COMMENTS

By following these procedures, you should be able to feed over 50 hydra in a half-hour. You may find it worthwhile to practice the feeding process using unlabeled liver.

Once a hydra has ingested such radioactive tissue, it will proceed to process it by a combination of extracellular and intracellular digestion. After 6 hr it will regurgitate any undigestible wastes. Experiments feeding hydra on ^{35}S-labeled mouse liver show that hydra retain 80% of the ingested radioactivity (Lenhoff, 1961).

LABELING WITH GASEOUS $^{14}CO_2$

PROCEDURE

Place from 10 to 1000 hydra (depending upon the experiment) in a modified beaker one-fifth full of culture solution. Before covering the beaker with glass plates, apply a thin film of stopcock grease to its rim. Carry out all subsequent operations with your materials in a fume hood. Using a fine-tipped micropipet, place 100 μl of a $NaH^{14}CO_3$ (200 μCi/ml) solution into the side arm of the modified beaker. Holding the greased glass stopper of the side arm in the left hand, carefully and quickly add 200 μl concentrated phosphoric acid to the side arm to evolve the $^{14}CO_2$ and immediately put the stopper into place. (Phosphoric acid is used because it is not volatile.) Keep the beaker in the hood for the duration of the experiment.

After various periods of incubation, remove the individual hydra with an eye dropper, removing as little fluid as possible with the hydra. Wash the hydra by three serial rinses in pH 7.6 medium (Chapter 4). At some stage while you are processing the animals for analysis [(e.g., whole-animal radioautography (Chapter 28) or fractionation (Chapter 27)], be certain to add a drop or two of 0.1 N HCl to them to evolve $^{14}CO_2$, from any $H^{14}CO_3^-$, $^{14}CO_3^{2-}$, or labeled amino acid carbamates.

PRECAUTIONS

For all experiments with isotopes use standard procedures of caution and of waste disposal. All experiments with $^{14}CO_2$ should be done in a fume hood approved for use with radioactive materials. At the end of the experiments with $^{14}CO_2$, add 0.5 N NaOH to the reaction beakers to sequester free $^{14}CO_2$ before you dispose of the radioactive wastes. Speed is essential when working with radioactive gases.

REFERENCES

Cowie, D. B., Bolton, E. T., and Sands, M. K. 1952. The labeling of bacterial cells with S^{35} for the production of high specific activity compounds. *Arch. Biochem. Biophys.* 35:140–145.
Lenhoff, H. M. 1959. Migration of ^{14}C-labeled cnidoblasts. *Exp. Cell Res.* 17:570–573.
Lenhoff, H. M. 1961. Digestion of protein in hydra as studied using radioautography and fractionation by differential solubilities. *Exp. Cell Res.* 23:335–353.
Muscatine, L., and Lenhoff, H. M. 1963. Symbiosis: On the role of algae symbiotic with hydra. *Science* 142:956–958.

Chapter 27

Fractionating Small Amounts of Radioactive Tissue

Howard M. Lenhoff

PURPOSE

Following the administration of a labeled substance to hydra, it may be necessary to determine the metabolic fate of that substance kinetically. I describe here two methods which make use of microfilters to fractionate labeled hydra. One uses a combination of centrifugation and microfilters to fractionate as few as 5–10 hydra. The second uses only microfilters during the separation procedures. I place particular emphasis on methods fractionating for proteins, nucleic acids, or carbohydrates.

INTRODUCTION

The first method uses Millipore filters primarily to eliminate a major source of error that usually occurs when working with small amounts of tissue. When separating soluble from insoluble components by centrifuging small volumes of a mixture, some particles of the precipitate often dislodge from the tube and contaminate the soluble fraction. Although the actual amount of precipitate that dislodges may be minute, its radioactivity may significantly alter the results. Hence, before being counted, all solutions should first be passed through a Millipore filter. The filters are also used to

Howard M. Lenhoff ● Department of Developmental and Cell Biology, University of California, Irvine, California.

197

eliminate the last centrifugation step in the fractionation procedure in which soluble material is separated from insoluble material. This method is particularly useful when fractionating for proteins or for nucleic acids, and it can be used with as few as two to three labeled hydra.

The second method, rather than separating soluble from insoluble material mostly by centrifuging, separates them entirely through use of Millipore filters. This method is particularly useful for separating polysaccharides from monosaccharides in the TCA-soluble fraction. Although more rapid than the first method, it requires a larger initial sample of tissue. Depending upon the amount of radioactivity in the sample, usually 50–200 hydra homogenized in a 3-ml volume are required for a fractionation.

MATERIALS

Trichloroacetic acid (TCA), 5 and 10% solutions; 80% ethanol; ether; 0.1 N HCl; micropipets, 100 μl and 200 μl; Millipore filter (HA 0.45 μm, 13mm); microanalysis filter holder (Millipore Filter Corp., xx 10 000 00); constant-temperature water baths; heat lamp and warm air source (hair dryer) for drying samples; small glass tissue grinder marked at the 1-ml level; Buchner flask; vacuum source; equipment for counting radioactivity, preferably liquid scintilation.

METHOD I. (LENHOFF, 1961)

PROCEDURES

Ten labeled animals usually suffice. Before fractionating, wash the animals in clean culture solution. Place them with about 0.3 ml solution in a chilled glass homogenizer, gently homogenize, and bring the suspension up to the 1-ml mark while carefully rinsing the glass plunger into the tube of the homogenizer.

Fraction 1. From a 1-ml suspension of homogenized tissue, remove 0.1 ml for counting.

Fraction 2. To the remaining 0.9 ml homogenate, add 0.9 ml 10% TCA let the mixture stand at room temperature for 15 min, and centrifuge at about 10,000g for 15 min. Pass all the supernatant through a Millipore filter set on a filter holder sitting in a Buchner flask connected to a vacuum pump. Collect the TCA-soluble material in a clean test tube set at the bottom of the buchner flash near the opening of the filter holder (see Precautions). Extract the TCA from this solution by shaking it with three 2-ml portions of ether.

Fraction 3. Wash the "TCA particles" remaining on the filter disk three times with 10-ml portions of 5% TCA.

Fraction 4. To the TCA-insoluble precipitate remaining in the centrifuge tube, add 4 ml 80% ethanol and one drop 0.1 N HCl; in this step, first add a few drops of the ethanol and, using a glass rod, carefully break up the precipitate into a fine suspension before adding the rest of the ethanol. Heat the tube in a 45°C water bath for 30–40 min, and stir the contents occasionally. Centrifuge the tube and its contents at 10,000g for 15 min. Pour the supernatant through a Millipore filter into a clean test tube (as described under Fraction 2) to get the TCA-insoluble, alcohol-soluble material. [Depending upon the label used and the amount of lipid material labeled, the remaining precipitate can be extracted again with a 1:1 ratio of 80% ethanol/ether (see Roberts *et al.*, 1955).]

Fraction 5. Wash the "alcohol particles" remaining on the filter three times with 10-ml portions of 80% ethanol.

Fraction 6. To the alcohol-insoluble precipitate remaining in the centrifuge tube, add 4 ml 5% TCA and heat the resultant suspension in a boiling water bath for 30 min. Cool the tube and pass 1 ml of the suspension through a Millipore filter and collect the "TCA- and alcohol-insoluble, hot TCA-soluble" material in a clean tube. Extract the TCA as in fraction 2.

Fraction 7. With three 10-ml portions of 5% TCA, wash the filter pad containing the TCA-, alcohol-, and hot TCA-insoluble material.

Assay for Radioactivity

Count the filter pads with radioactive material from fractions 3, 5, and 7 directly. The volume of the soluble material counted depends upon the type of label and its distribution among the fractions. Usually 200-μl portions from fraction 2, 1 ml from Fraction 4, and 0.4 ml from fraction 6 suffice to give reliable counts.

Calculations

Calculations of the total radioactivity in a particular chemical fraction appear complicated because they not only have to take into account the obvious dilution and size of sample factors (discussed more fully with examples under Method II), but they also have to account for the radioactivity in the dislodged particles that were salvaged in fractions 3 and 5. Fraction 5, for example, contains both material which is soluble and material which is insoluble in hot TCA (i.e., materials that belong in fractions 6 and 7), whereas fraction 3 contains not only these, but in addition, some alcohol-soluble materials (as in fraction 4). Thus, once you determine the percent distribution of radioactivity for fractions 2, 4, 6, and 7 you can calculate the relative amounts of fractions 4, 6, and 7 in fraction 3 and the amounts of fractions 6 and 7 in fraction 5. Then add these values to those of the proper major fraction.

An example of the above is illustrated as follows. Let x = the counts in fraction 5, y = those in 6, and z = those in 7. Thus the counts of fraction 6 represented in the counts of the particles of fraction 5 would be $[y/(y+z)] \cdot x$. Then add this value to the counts of fraction 6 that were originally counted. After you do the same kind of calculation for the particles of fraction 3, and correct for the dilution factors, you can compute the final percentage distribution of radioactivity present in the four major fractions.

You can express the final distribution of label as four major fractions: (1) TCA-soluble, containing mostly small molecules and sugars; (2) TCA-insoluble, alcohol-soluble, containing lipids, lipid-soluble materials, and small proteins; (3) TCA- and alcohol-insoluble, hot TCA-soluble, containing nucleic acid components; and (4) TCA-, alcohol-, and hot TCA-insoluble, containing mostly protein.

Modification for Fractionating ^{35}S-Labeled Tissue

Hydra fed on ^{35}S-labeled tissue (Chapter 26) distributes most of the label into amino acids (cold TCA-soluble), peptides (cold TCA-insoluble, alcohol-soluble) or proteins (cold TCA-insoluble, alcohol-insoluble). Because no label will go into the nucleic acid (cold TCA-insoluble, alcohol-insoluble, hot TCA-soluble), most of the steps in Method I involved in obtaining fractions 6 and 7 can be eliminated. Therefore, for ^{35}S-labeled hydra, carry out the steps necessary to obtain fractions 1, 2, 3, and 4. After the 45°C incubation step, do not centrifuge your sample but simply pass the entire suspension through a Millipore filter. The filtrate will be the TCA-insoluble, alcohol-soluble fraction (i.e., fraction 4), and the material on the filter will contain all the labeled protein (i.e., fraction 7). Before counting the labeled protein in the filter, however, rinse it three times with 10-ml portions of 80% ethanol.

PRECAUTIONS

For all filtrations in which the filtrates are to be saved and counted, rather than use separate Buchner flasks, simply place a test tube inside the flask so its lip will cover the tip of the filter holder and will receive all of the filtrate.

In the steps under Fraction 4, after you pass the hot ethanol extract through the filter, turn off the vacuum immediately; otherwise, some of the warm ethanol will evaporate, the alcohol soluble material will be concentrated, and the calculations will be off. Likewise, when heating the tubes in a boiling bath (step described under Fraction 6), cover each tube with a glass marble to prevent evaporation.

You may wish to have a number of filter apparatuses set up so that you can go from one filtration to the next quickly without taking time to wash the filter holders between steps to prevent contamination.

METHOD II. (LENHOFF AND ROFFMAN, 1971)

PROCEDURES

Fraction 1. Because this method requires more hydra than Method I (use 50–200 animals), begin with the hydra homogenized in a total volume of 3 ml. Remove 0.4 ml for counting.

Fractions 2 and 3. To 1 ml of suspension, add 1 ml 10% TCA and allow the mixture to stand at room temperature for about 15 min. Filter 1.5 ml of the now 5% TCA mixture and collect the filtrate in a clean test tube. Mark the TCA-soluble material fraction 2, and the TCA-insoluble material on the filter as fraction 3. Wash fraction 3 on the filter pad with three 10-ml portions of 5% TCA. (See next steps for obtaining fractions 8 and 9.)

Fractions 4 and 5. Repeat the above step, only this time heat the mixture for 30 min in a boiling water bath after adding the 10% TCA.

Separate through the filter into the hot TCA-soluble (4) and hot TCA-insoluble (5) fractions. Wash fraction 5 as above.

Fractions 6 and 7. To 0.6 ml of the suspension, add 3.2 ml of 95% ethanol and incubate at 45°C for 45 min. Remove 3 ml of the stirred suspension and pass it through the Millipore filter. An alcohol-soluble (6) and an alcohol-insoluble (7) fraction result. Wash fraction 7 with three portions of 80% ethanol.

Fractions 8 and 9. To 0.6 ml of the TCA-soluble material from fraction 2, add 3.2 ml of 95% ethanol and heat at 45°C for 45 min. Remove 3 ml of the stirred suspension and filter into the TCA-soluble alcohol-soluble fraction (8) and the TCA-soluble, alcohol-insoluble fraction (9). Wash fraction 9 with three portions of 80% ethanol.

Assay for Radioactivity

Count the filter pads with radioactive material from fractions 3, 5, 7, and 9 directly. The volume of the soluble material to be counted depends upon the distribution and type of label. For example, if you are investigating distribution of $^{14}CO_2$ in green hydra, use 0.4 ml from fractions 1, 2, and 4, and 1 ml from fractions 6 and 8.

Calculations

Calculations for the total radioactivity in a particular sample have to take into account the dilution of the sample in each procedure and the size of the sample counted. For example, to determine the amount of activity in the original homogenate represented by fraction 4, three adjustments must be made: only one-third of the original homogenate is used, only 1.5 ml of the 2-ml extraction mixture is filtered, and only 0.4 ml of a 1.5-ml portion of the filtrate is assayed for radioactivity. Thus the factor used to correct for these three steps is derived from the reciprocals of the dilution factors: i.e., $3/1 \times 2/1.5 \times 1.5/0.4 = 15$. Dilution factors are calculated for all fractions in this manner.

The percentage of radioactivity in the major biochemical fractions of the original radioactive tissue analyzed can be easily calculated from the radioactivity found in each of the filter fractions. Table I lists the major fractions, the possible components of each, and the corresponding filter fractions from which the radioactivity in the major fraction was derived.

TABLE I. Composition of Major Classes of Chemical Components

Major fraction	Probable components	Corresponding fraction of Method I	Corresponding fraction of Method II
A (TCA-soluble, ethanol-soluble)	Small molecules, such as amino acids and mono-saccharides	2	8
B (TCA-soluble, ethanol-insoluble)	Oligosaccharides, oligonucleotides	2	9
C (TCA-insoluble, ethanol-soluble)	Lipids and lipid-soluble compounds; small proteins	4[a]	6–8
D (TCA- and ethanol-insoluble, hot TCA-soluble)	Nucleic acids	6[a]	4–2
E (TCA-, ethanol-, and hot TCA-insoluble)	Proteins	7[a]	5–(6–8)

[a] Must be corrected for the materials in fractions 3 and 5.

PRECAUTIONS

When using larger numbers of hydra, take care not to clog the filters. On the other hand, if only two to three hydra have sufficient radioactivity to count, add seven to eight unlabeled hydra to the radioactive animals so you will at least be able to see the precipitates as you fractionate the homogenate.

REFERENCES

Lenhoff, H. M. 1961. Digestion of protein in hydra as studied using radioautography and fractionation by differential solubilities. *Exp. Cell Res.* 2:335–353.

Lenhoff, H. M., and Roffman, B. 1971. Two methods for fractionating small amounts of radioactive tissue. In: *Experimental Coelenterate Biology* (H. M. Lenhoff, L. Muscatine, and L. V. Davis, eds.), University of Hawaii Press, Honolulu, pp. 265–271.

Roberts, R., Abelson, P., Cowie, D., Bolton, E., and Britten, R. 1957. *Studies of Biosynthesis in Escherichia Coli*, Carnegie Institute of Washington Publication 607, Washington, D. C.

Chapter 28

Rapid Whole-Mount Radioautography

Howard M. Lenhoff

PURPOSE

To prepare labeled live hydra as intact extended specimens for whole-mount radioautographs.

INTRODUCTION

Hydra are one of the few animals used in research from which it is possible to make whole-mount radioautographs. They have neither a hard exoskeleton nor an endoskeleton and can be dried while they are outstretched to yield a specimen thin enough for use in radioautography.

MATERIALS

Millipore membrane filter disk, 1-in. diameter; microanalysis sintered glass filter holder for the disk (Millipore xx 10 100 00); Buchner flask and rubber stopper for sintered glass holder; vacuum source; infrared heat lamp; 1 × 3-in. glass slides; fine forceps; rubber cement; either NTB_3 Eastman Kodak nuclear track plates (Eastman Kodak Co.) or stripping film; strong binder clips; aluminum foil.

Howard M. Lenhoff • Department of Developmental and Cell Biology, University of California, Irvine, California.

PROCEDURES

Place a moist Millipore filter disk on the sintered glass holder set on the Buchner flask. Attach the Buchner flask to a vacuum source by means of an on–off stopcock. Have the vacuum on, but set the stopcock at the off position position. Put a few drops of culture solution on the disk, and then place one or two hydra in that solution. When the animals appear completely relaxed with their tentacles outstretched and their body tube extended, quickly turn the stopcock to the on position (i.e. vacuum on) without jarring the Buchner flask and hydra. As soon as the culture solution is drawn through and the hydra are flattened onto the disk (about 5 sec), turn on the heat lamp placed 6 in. from the disk. Using a wash bottle, and while the vacuum is still on, gently wash the flattened hydra and the disk a few times to free them of any soluble radioactive contaminants that might have been transferred in the medium surrounding the hydra. Turn off the vacuum. Using forceps, remove the disk with the hydra from the sintered glass holder and attach it to the center of a 1×3-in. glass slide onto a smear of fresh rubber cement. Dry the preparation for about 5 min under the infrared lamp, and with a scalpel trim away any excess glue.

These slides with disks are now ready for radioautography. You may use standard stripping film or dipping methods (David and Campbell, 1972). I find the use of 1×3-in. NTB$_3$ nuclear track plates sufficiently sensitive for whole mounts and simple to use. While in the dark, simply place the emulsion side of the NTB$_3$ plate against the glass slide with the filter paper disk, hold them together by strong clips, make them light-tight by wrapping them with aluminum foil, and place them in a dark place until the plate is ready for developing. Develop the plates per directions accompanying the NTB$_3$ plates, superimpose each developed plate on the slide with disk, examine them under the dissecting microscope, and note any special correlation of the developed silver grains with particular portions of the dried hydra specimens.

COMMENTS

The length of time the plates with hydra are to remain in the dark will vary depending upon the radioactivity of the hydra specimen. Clear radio-autographs can be obtained after 12 hr exposure of the plates if the hydra are made radioactive by feeding them heavily labeled radioactive tissue (Lenhoff, 1961) or after 2–3 weeks if they were labeled weakly with $^{14}CO_2$ gas (Lenhoff, 1959) (both in Chapter 27).

REFERENCES

Lenhoff, H. M. 1959. Migration of 14C-labeled cnidoblasts. *Exp. Cell Res.* 17:570–573.

Lenhoff, H. M. 1961. Digestion of protein in hydra as studied using radioautography and fractionation by differential solubilities. *Exp. Cell Res.* 23:335–353.

David, C. N., and Campbell, R. D. 1972. Cell cycle kinetics and development of *Hydra attenuata*. I. Epithelial cells. *J. Cell Sci.* 11:557–568.

Part VI

Isolating Hydra Mutants by Sexual Inbreeding

Chapter 29

Isolating Hydra Mutants by Sexual Inbreeding

Tsutomu Sugiyama

PURPOSE

To isolate mutant hydra by sexual inbreeding.

INTRODUCTION

The genetic approach for the study of hydra development promises to be a powerful one. This approach, however, has been attempted only in a few cases (Lenhoff, 1965; Moore and Campbell, 1973; Sugiyama and Fujisawa, 1977a), presumably because (1) hydra's sexual reproduction is sporadic, slow, and difficult to control; and (2) the design of efficient screening procedures for mutants appears at present not practical.

To isolate mutants, we use inbred strains of hydra obtained from the field rather than attempting to induce mutagenesis in cultures of animals grown in the laboratory for long periods. The field animals that are heterozygous recessive for mutant genes are made homozygous recessive by reproducing sexually in the laboratory. The resultant inbred mutants are propagated by asexual breeding as clones.

In screening for mutants, we restricted ourselves to searching for developmental mutants that can be discovered by simply examining many animals visually. The procedure is designed for *Hydra magnipapillata*, a

Tsutomu Sugiyama  National Institute of Genetics, Mishima, Shizuoka-ken , Japan.

dioecious species commonly found in Japan. We describe representative types of mutants that appear to be useful for research in developmental biology. Detailed studies on these mutants are reported elsewhere (Sugiyama and Fujisawa, 1977a,b, 1978a,b; Fujisawa and Sugiyama, 1978).

MATERIALS

When preparing culture solutions, such as M (Chapter 4), use the best-grade chemicals available and high-purity water because sexually differentiated animals, unfertilized eggs, and newly hatched hydra appear to be much more sensitive to the quality of the culture water than hydra reproducing solely asexually. Use the same culture solution in all procedures.

Other reagents required are the antibiotic rifampicin (Boehringer-Mannheim) at 50 μg/ml of culture solution; Penicillin-G and Mycostatin (Grand Island Biological Co.) at 40 and 50 units, respectively, per milliliter of culture solution; and 0.3% (w/v) NaCl in culture solution.

PROCEDURES

Collecting Strains from Natural Environment

Collect wild strains, preferably from small and well-isolated ponds because animals from such ponds are more highly inbred (Sugiyama and Fujisawa, 1977a). Do not put freshly collected animals from the field near stock cultures of hydra maintained in the laboratory, because animals from the field frequently carry parasites (see below). Once the new hydra are in the laboratory, allow them to adapt to the defined culture solution. Because sudden changes of the culture water occasionally harm the animals, use varying mixtures of the original pond water and the defined culture solution at first. During this transition period parasites, usually small protozoans, may appear in large numbers. Remove them by washing the hydra in the 0.3% NaCl solution for several minutes. If heavy fungal growth appears, or if hydra appear "depressed," treat them with the antibiotic solutions for about 7 days.

As soon as the animals appear healthy in the laboratory culture solution, treat them in such a way as to induce them to differentiate gonads (see below and Chapter 11). Select two male and two female animals from the group of animals collected from the same ponds, and allow them to multiply in separate Petri dishes asexually by budding in order to start two male and two female clones to be used later for crossing.

Induction of Sexual Differentiation

Different hydra species apparently require different stimuli for sexual differentiation (Chapter 11). For *H. magnipapillata*, we suggest you use the modified procedure of reduced feeding described for *Hydra viridis*.

Prior to inducing sexual differentiation, feed animals heavily on *Artemia* nauplii every day for 2–3 weeks. Place 10–15 animals each of a male and a female strain in a 600-ml beaker containing 400 ml of culture solution; gently aerate the culture at 18°C. Provide small amounts of food (one to two *Artemia* nauplii per animal) daily, but do not change the culture water for a week or sometimes longer unless it becomes turbid.

This procedure usually induces gonad development within 2–3 weeks. It is not always successful, however; with some strains, repeated trials may be necessary in some cases. Shifting temperature from 18 to 23°C is successful with some strains (Chapter 11).

Hatching of New Animals

Fertilized hydra eggs form a clearly visible theca when examined under a dissecting microscope. Collect the fertilized eggs and place them in groups of 5–10 in a 50-mm plastic Petri dish containing culture solution. Keep the eggs at 18°C, examine them once a week, and change the culture water once every 2–3 weeks. When newly hatched small polyps emerge, transfer them individually to new Petri dishes and hand feed them (see Chapter 37) freshly crushed and immobilized *Artemia* nauplii. It is important to place the immobilized food directly on the tentacles of the young animals for the first few feedings because they frequently have difficulty in capturing prey. After you give them a few meals during a 2- to 4-day period, they should be able to feed normally, grow, and bud to start new clonal lines.

The hatching period varies greatly both within embryos from the same cross and between embryos from different crosses (Fig. 1). The hatching rate is generally low, and many eggs remain unhatched for more than 6 months; others may decompose during this period. We find, for example, a hatching rate of 21% with eggs from crosses between strains from the same pond, and 41% with eggs from crosses between strains from different ponds. Also, some young animals die soon after hatching in spite of the special care given them. The low hatching rate of embryos from hydra of the same pond may be due to "inbreeding depression" (Sugiyama and Fujisawa, 1977a).

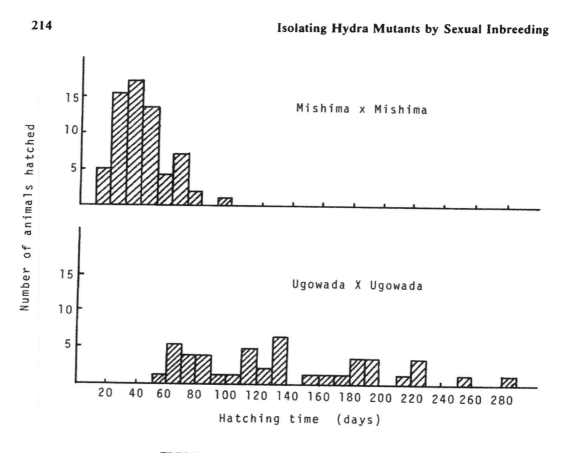

FIGURE 1. Hatching times of hydra eggs.

TYPES OF MUTANTS

Examine the progeny derived from each hatched embryo for their developmental and morphological characteristics as soon as they start to multiply. No rapid screening techniques have been developed. Therefore, examine individual specimens of each strain under a dissecting or a light microscope. Listed below are some examples of the types of mutants isolated.

Mini and Maxi Strains. The mini strain is smaller (about one-fifth in cell numbers), while the maxi is larger (about three to four times), than their wild-type parents (Fig. 2). Mini hydra grow vigorously by budding, whereas maxi hydra produce buds much more slowly.

Twisted Column Strain. This strain is temperature sensitive. Although its morphology is normal at 18° (Fig. 3a), the lower half of its body column

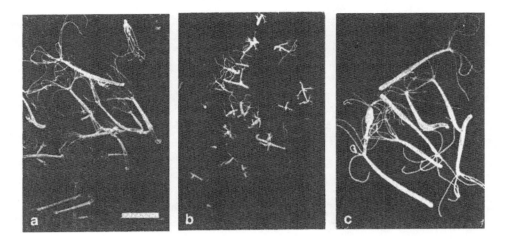

FIGURE 2. Photographs of (a) wild-type (strain 105), (b) mini-4, and (c) maxi-1 animals.

is grossly deformed at 23°C (Fig. 3b). This strain was originally found by Dr. K. Noda among a culture of wild-type animals.

Multiheaded Strains. One of the multiheaded strains is shown in Fig. 3c. With these strains, the new buds produced by parents frequently remain attached to (instead of detaching from) the parental polyps, thereby producing multiheaded animals.

Nematocyst-Deficient Strains. Many nematocyst-deficient strains of *H. magnipapillata* are found, such as nem-4, which lacks stenoteles (Fig. 4b); nem-3, which lacks holotrichous isorhizas (Fig. 4c); and nem-1, which contains deformed holotrichous isorhizas in their tentacles (Fig. 4d).

Regeneration-Deficient Strains. Hydra's capacity to regenerate is greatly reduced or altered in some mutants. For example, reg-19 regenerates its foot normally but frequently fails to regenerate its head after the head and foot are amputated (middle-row photographs in Fig. 5). Strain nem-10 frequently regenerates double-headed animals after the same treatment (bottom-row photographs in Fig. 5).

Strains with Altered Proportions of Cell Types. The normal proportion of cell types (Bode *et al.*, 1973) is greatly altered in some mutants (Table I). An extreme case is nf-1, which completely lacks the interstitial

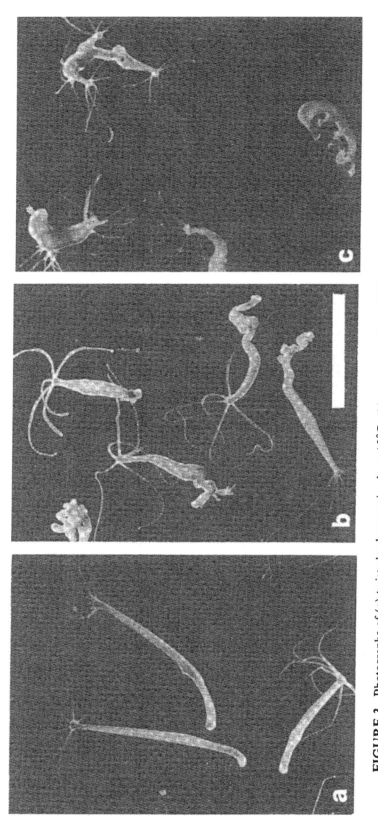
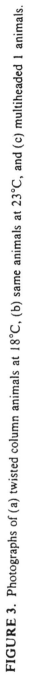

FIGURE 3. Photographs of (a) twisted column animals at 18°C, (b) same animals at 23°C, and (c) multiheaded 1 animals.

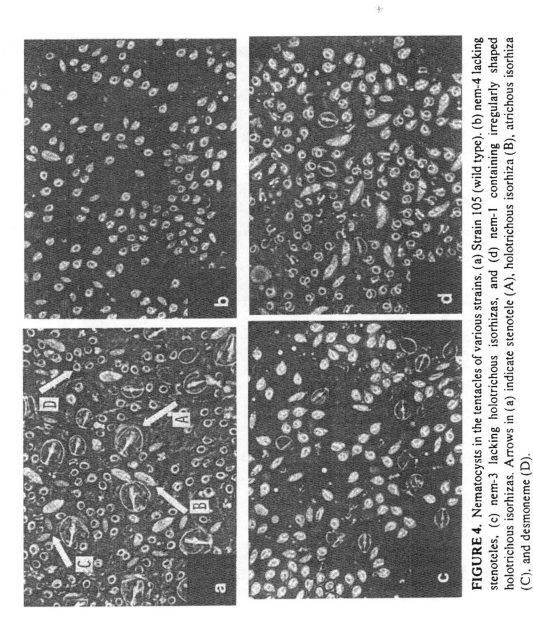

FIGURE 4. Nematocysts in the tentacles of various strains. (a) Strain 105 (wild type). (b) nem-4 lacking stenoteles, (c) nem-3 lacking holotrichous isorhizas, and (d) nem-1 containing irregularly shaped holotrichous isorhizas. Arrows in (a) indicate stenotele (A), holotrichous isorhiza (B), atrichous isorhiza (C), and desmoneme (D).

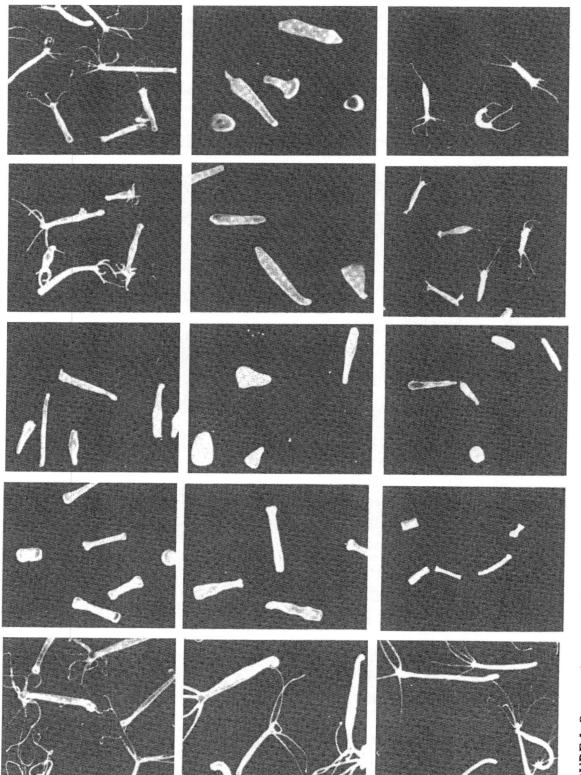

FIGURE 5. Regeneration process after head and foot amputation of strain 105 (wild type) (top row), reg-19 (middle row), and nem-10 (bottom row). Regeneration sequences are shown from left to right in the order of original animals, same animals immediately after amputation, 2 days later, 4 days later, and 6 days later.

TABLE I. Proportions of the Various types of Cells in Some Mutant Strains (%)

Strain	Epitheliomuscular	Digestive	Interstitial	Nematocyte and nematoblast	Nerve	Gland and mucous
105 (wild type)[a]	16.4	16.7	29.5	28.8	2.5	6.1
nem-3	29.6	29.5	13.9	16.0	3.2	7.8
nf-1	49.8	48.9	0	0	0	1.2
nf-11	16.4	16.8	42.0	23.4	0.4	1.0

[a] The cellular composition of four other wild-type strains tested was very similar to that of this strain.

cells and its derivative cell types (nematocytes and nerves). This strain, which requires forced feeding because it cannot feed by itself, is similar to the "nerve-free" hydra produced by means of colchicine treatment of wild-type hydra by Campbell (1976) (Chapter 36). Nem-3 has a low interstitial cell content, whereas nf-11 has a low nerve cell content.

Male Sterile Strains. These strains develop testes of normal appearance by the standard sex induction procedure, but the sperms contained in them cannot fertilize eggs. When examined under a microscope, these sperms show greatly reduced motility compared to the wild-type sperms, which exhibit a variety of highly active movements.

COMMENTS

The characteristics of the mutants described above are all stable, and are transmitted as such by asexual budding to the progeny. The screening program, however, often picks up many strains with unstable characters that gradually or suddenly disappear during the continued maintenance of the clones. If you encounter such strains, discard them.

The transmissal of mutant genotype through sexual reproduction is a requisite of Mendelian genetics. Such sexual transfer, however, is often difficult to observe with hydra for a variety of reasons. Some mutants such as nem-4 cannot be induced to form gonads; thus sexual progenies cannot be obtained. In the case of the mini strain, its phenotype is unexpressed in the F_1, but expressed in the F_2, generation, indicating that the gene(s) responsible for the mini trait is recessive.

In the case of the twisted column strain, its character is transmitted only to the asexual progenies but not to any of the sexual progenies examined (F_1, F_2, and F_1 back-cross). This strain therefore may be considered as an "epigenetic" mutant.

The mutant strains described above are all started from single polyps and propagated by asexual reproduction in the laboratory. These strains, therefore, can be considered as clonal lines. However, they should not be confused with genetically "pure" lines, which can be produced only through repeated inbreeding. Thus, no "congenic" lines are available to be used as controls; therefore, parental or sibling lines must be used as substitutes.

REFERENCES

Bode, H., Berking, S., David, C. N., Gierer, A., Schaller, H., and Trenkner, E. 1973. Quantitative analysis of cell types during growth and morphogenesis in hydra. *Wilhelm Roux Arch. Entwichlungsmech. Org.* 171:259–285.

Campbell, R. D. 1976. Elimination of *Hydra* interstitial and nerve cells by means of colchicine. *J Cell Sci.* **21**:1–13.

Fujisawa, T., and Sugiyama, T. 1978. Genetic analysis of developmental mechanisms in *Hydra*. IV. Characterization of a nematocyst-deficient strain. *J. Cell Sci.* **30**:175–185.

Lenhoff, H. M. 1965. Cellular segregation and heterocytic dominance in hydra. *Science* **148**:1105–1107.

Loomis, W. F., and Lenhoff, H. M. 1956. Growth and sexual differentiation of hydra in mass culture. *J. Exp. Zool.* **132**:555–574.

Moore, L. B., and Campbell, R. D. 1973. Non-budding strains of hydra: Isolation from sexual crosses and developmental regulation of form. *J. Exp. Zool.* **185**:73–82.

Sugiyama, T., and Fujisawa, T. 1977a. Genetic analysis of developmental mechanisms in *Hydra*. I. Sexual reproduction of *Hydra magnipapillata* and isolation of mutants. *Growth Dev. Differ.* **19**:187–200.

Sugiyama, T., and Fujisawa, T. 1977b. Genetic analysis of developmental mechanisms in *Hydra*. III. Characterization of a regeneration deficient strain. *J. Embryol. Exp. Morphol.* **42**:65–77.

Sugiyama, T., and Fujisawa, T. 1978a. Genetic analysis of developmental mechanisms in *Hydra*. II. Isolation and characterization of an interstitial cell deficient strain. *J. Cell Sci.* **29**:35–52.

Sugiyama, T., and Fujisawa, T. 1978b. Genetic analysis of developmental mechanisms in *Hydra*. V. Cell lineage and development of chimeric *Hydra*. *J. Cell Sci.* **32**:215–232.

Part VII

Manipulating Tissue Organization

Chapter 30

Grafting: A Rapid Method for Transplanting Tissue

Harry K. MacWilliams

PURPOSE

I present a fast and flexible method for transplantating tissue with which a single worker can routinely perform 80 transplantations in a day. It is thus practical to accumulate sample sizes large enough for quantitative studies of the hydra transplantation phenomena.

MATERIALS

Grafting Dishes

Draw out fine glass tubing (0.5–1.0 mm outer diameter) in the pilot flame of a Bunsen burner or in the flame of a burner made with a large-bore hypodermic needle. Hold the tubing in the flame until it sags, withdraw it, and, at that instant, pull; do not pull while the tubing is still in the flame or the tubing will melt through. The objective is to produce needles fine enough at one end to penetrate the gastrovascular cavity of hydra, and wide enough at the other end to act as a thicker shank; the shank allows easy manipulation.

Treat the finished needles with Siliclad or an equivalent hypodermic agent. The treated needles adhere to wax (see below) even when they are wet; untreated needles will not stick to wax in the presence of water.

Harry K. MacWilliams • Department of Anatomy, University of Massachusetts Medical Center, Worcester, Massachusetts.

Form Tackiwax (Central Scientific Co.) into the shape of a worm 3 mm in diameter and bend this back on itself to make a ring about 1 cm across. Flatten the ring onto the bottom of a 100-mm Petri dish (plastic or siliconized glass); use a hot metal needle to carve the inner edge into a smooth, craterlike profile. Do not allow overhanging edges to form as they may obstruct hydra from view.

Cut grooves across the ring and insert the shanks of one long and two shorter glass needles (Fig. 1A). Allow the long needle to project about two-thirds of the way across the dish; its end should project above the dish a distance equal to half the diameter of a hydra body column. Pass one of the short needles under and at right angles to the long one; have it *contact* the long one approximately at its midpoint. Check the positions of these two needles and seal both shanks in place with hot wax. Place the second short needle parallel to the first short one, but crossing *over* the long needle *without touching it*, and about 2 mm further toward the long needle's tip. The second short needle is to be movable; use a steel dissecting probe to fluff the wax ring to receive its shank.

Knives

Knives made from razor blade fragments give a clean cut that heals easily. Attach fragments to a serviceable handle. I recommend you use a Koh-i-noor Technigraph® drafting lead holder (Fig. 2A), which you can buy at an art supply store; this instrument can be used comfortably for hours.

The drafting lead holder requires blade fragments of a particular shape. Break razor blades into 2 × 5-mm parallelograms using electronic pliers that have smooth interior jaws (Fig. 2B). You can remove burrs from the jaws of a new pair of pliers by repeatedly gripping fine emery paper and pulling it from the jaws. To break the razor blade, twist the plier jaws about its long axis; motion about any other axis causes the blade to crumble.

If your blades bend but do not break, they have probably been heat treated ("coated") by the company so that the metal is too ductile to break cleanly. I use "uncoated" blades that I get directly from the metallurgy department of a major safety razor company.

Glass Probes

To produce fine probes for manipulating hydra fragments in the grafting dishes, draw out the tips of Pasteur pipets in the fine flame used to make glass needles.

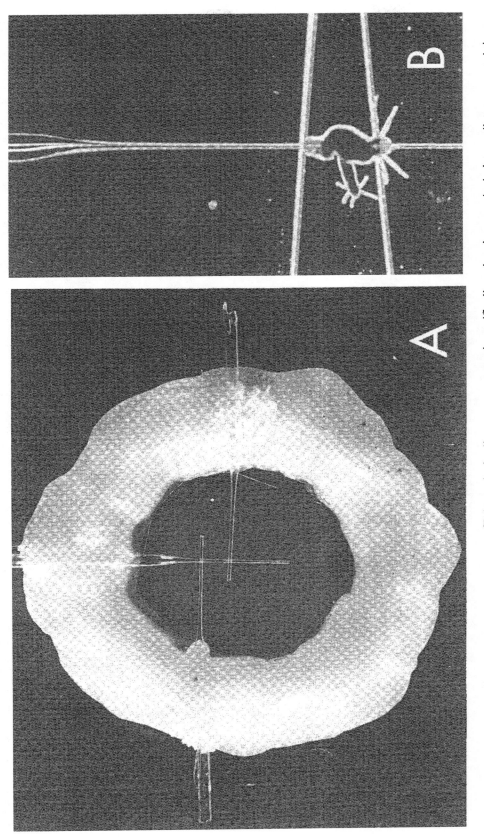

FIGURE 1. (A) A glass-needle jig for grafting hydra. This particular jig was constructed specifically to be photographed: the needles are several times thicker than those normally used. (B) Glass-needle jig in use in an axial transplantation. Closeup of center part of (A) showing hydra in place.

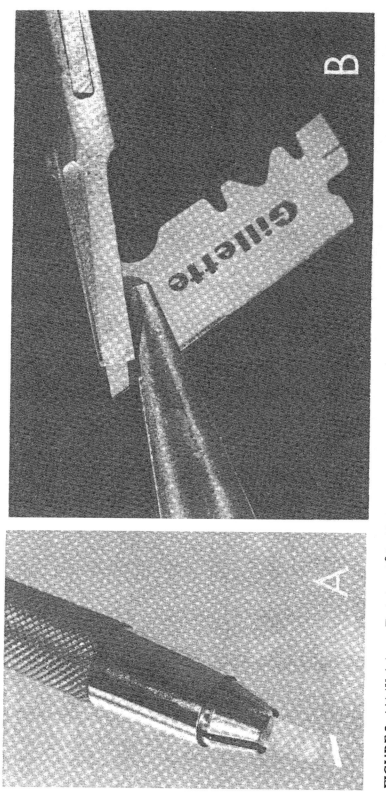

FIGURE 2. (A) (Koh-i-noor Technigraph® lead holder holding a razor blade fragment for cutting hydra. Note that the fragment is positioned between two opposed jaws. Since this positioning is impossible with three-jaw lead holders, only four-jaw holders are satisfactory. (B) Razor blade in position for breaking with pliers.

The Workplace

Cut, assemble, and examine hydra under a dissecting microscope (12–25×). For comfort and speed, use a microscope on a swinging arm stand and operate on the flat surface of the lab table. If you must operate on a microscope stage, use blocks or ramps to support your forearms; extreme dorsiflexion of the wrist to gain the height of a microscope is incompatible with a precision grip.

To obtain excellent lighting, fasten a fragment of mirror on the table surface under the microscope. Cover half of the mirror with black tape and position the microscope over the edge of the tape. Direct a focusable lamp down onto the microscope field from the side opposite the tape. Place the animals over the tape near its edge. Some of the rays of the lamp will illuminate the animals' upper surfaces directly; others, reflected by the mirror, will produce a dark-field effect rendering the epidermis bright and clearly visible.

PROCEDURES

Gathering Animals

Gather hydra from the mass cultures using a Pasteur pipet. Gently scrape the basal disk free from the culture disk before sucking an animal into the pipet; this procedure is faster than attempting to gather animals by suction alone. It also reduces tearing the hydra's basal disk; animals with torn disks remain contracted and cannot be cut accurately.

If you find manipulating the pipet bulb tiresome, replace it with a 30-cm length of rubber tubing fitted with a pinch clamp. Draw animals into the pipet by mouth suction combined with gentle pressure on the clamp. When you release the clamp (e.g., while searching for further animals), the tubing will be closed off and it will not be necessary to maintain mouth suction.

Cutting Technique

Cut hydra while they are in small (35 or 60 mm diameter) disposable plastic Petri dishes filled with culture medium. It is important to hold the knife (see Materials) with the edge parallel to the bottom of the dish and cut through the hydra and into the plastic slightly. If the knife edge is not parallel with the dish bottom, you will have cut deeply into the plastic, thereby dulling the blade and robbing the cutting blade of essential speed. Some workers cover the bottom of the cutting dish with rubber or block wax.

Hydra contract in response to almost any stimulus; contracted animals cannot be cut accurately. Therefore, put twice as many animals in the cutting dish as you will actually use, and cut the ones that are most extended. To get a higher percentage of extended hydra, some workers use relaxants (2% urethane, 10% ethanol) or viscous media [2.5% tylose MH 4000 (Hoechst)]. I find that using extra animals is just as convenient and does not raise unnecessary questions about extraneous factors affecting the animals.

Injured hydra tend to remain contracted, and may remain contracted in the vicinity of the injury even if the rest of the animal extends. If you are making more than one cut in an animal, make the one that requires the most accuracy first.

Lateral Transplantation

A lateral transplantation, that is, transplanting a small fragment into the side of an intact host, is the most common grafting procedure used. Minor adaptations are necessary for an axial transplantion. Isolate the transplant from the donor hydra with two parallel transverse cuts, producing an annulus of tissue with a central hole (the gastrovascular cavity). Prepare the host by making a transverse cut halfway across the body column at the desired transplantation site. Fill a grafting dish with culture medium and transfer host and transplant to the dish with a Pasteur pipet.

Using a glass probe, thread the transplant onto the projecting long needle so that the needle passes through the central hole. This process is rapid and effortless as long as the height of the needle's free end is correct. Push the host onto the same needle so that the needle passes into the transverse wound and out the mouth. Push host and transplant up the long needle until they are stopped by the fixed short needle. Lower the shank of the movable short needle making it contact the long needle so that it presses host and transplant together (Fig. 1B). Tease the apposing cut edges of host and transplant as necessary to assure that the cut gastrodermal edges are in contact.

Put the dish aside for 30 min; healing occurs in about 95% of cases in this period. Release the completed graft combination from the needles and transfer it to a separate dish for observation. The grafting dish may now be reused.

With practice the operations of cutting, assembly, and release of a single transplant should require less than 3 min. If one starts a new transplantation every 3 min and uses a 30-min healing period, 10 grafting dishes plus a few spares are required. With practice 80 transplantations require only half the working day with the rest of the day available to maintain cultures, repair grafting dishes, and record results.

RESULTS

Scoring Head and Foot Formation

Transplants may form heads (hypostome and tentacles) or feet (basal disks). Both types of structures appear within 48 hr in *Hydra littoralis* if the temperature is 18°C or higher; longer periods may be required at lower temperatures or in other species.

Heads are usually easy to recognize. Ambiguous "reduced" forms consisting of a single tentacle occur occasionally. In extreme cases the single tentacle is quite short but can be identified by an accumulation of battery cells in the ectoderm. The formation of single tentacles, commonest in experiments in which the overall frequency of head formation is low, is consistent with the idea that they are in fact "reduced heads."

Feet generally attach to the culture dish bottom, to the air–water interface, or to an air bubble. Transplants forming "reduced" feet may not stick to such surfaces, but their ectoderm should show a characteristic opalescence.

It is sometimes hard to decide whether a given transplant should be considered as a reduced form or scored as undifferentiated. In such cases, there is a danger that the experimenter's bias will determine how the result is recorded. If marginal cases occur with appreciable frequency, score the experiment blind or enlist the aid of a naive observer.

Influence of the Experimental Design

There are two basic types of transplantation in hydra.

1. In *lateral transplantation*, a small fragment of tissue is grafted into a wound made in a larger piece, often a whole animal. The small piece is the transplant and the larger piece the host.

2. In *axial transplantation*, two or more pieces, sometimes both large, are grafted together end to end. No consistent distinction of transplant and host is possible.

In analyzing lateral transplantation experiments, attention is usually focused on the differentiation of the transplant itself. It may form a head, form a foot, or remain undifferentiated. Formation of both heads and feet is rare.

In axial transplantation experiments, both head and foot formation may occur, sometimes within a single graft combination. This phenomenon is especially common when the combined graft tissues are substantially larger than a full-grown hydra. Thus, the results of axial transplantations are more complicated and may be harder to interpret.

A Special Precaution for Quantitative Work

Head- and foot-formation frequencies are not perfectly constant: a frequency for one kind of graft combination measured one day may differ significantly from the frequency determined for a comparable experiment measured a week earlier or later. These variations occur despite the best of efforts to maintain cultures in a constant state. As a consequence, two or more transplantation experiments performed on different days cannot be safely compared.

An effective way around this problem is to carry out experiments to be compared in an "interweaved" fashion; i.e., plan the entire series of experiments in advance, and perform each complete series of transplantations on each day of experimentation. Randomize, if possible, the order in which transplantations are performed.

Interleaving increases the amount of labor involved in a transplantation project, since an entire series of experiments must be repeated to add a single new data point. Nonetheless, spurious differences, usually misleading ones, almost always appear if this procedure is neglected. Furthermore, since all statistical tests necessarily presume the absence of systematic errors, failure to interleave renders all statistical tests performed on transplantation results meaningless. See Chapter 31 for procedures for interpreting results of transplantation experiments.

Quantitative Interpretation of Transplantation Phenomena

Harry K. MacWilliams

INTRODUCTION

What is the shape of the head activation gradient in hydra? With what kinetics does the hydra head inhibition change with time after the head is removed? These questions seem to be simple ones, but they require that transplantation phenomena be interpreted quantitatively. In this chapter I discuss some problems that arise when one attempts such interpretations and present what appear to me to be the best methods of dealing with them.

CONCEPTUAL BACKGROUND: ACTIVATING AND INHIBITORY PROPERTIES IN TRANSPLANTATION EXPERIMENTS

A small fragment of hydra tissue transplanted to an intact or near-intact host may do one of three things: it may form a head (hypostome and tentacles), form a foot (basal disk), or remain undifferentiated. The developmental behavior of transplants may be determined by the balance of intrinsic and long-range factors. For example, if tissue fragments from two different sources form heads with different frequencies when transplanted to a standard host, the fragments are concluded to differ intrinsically. On the

Harry K. MacWilliams ● Department of Anatomy, University of Massachusetts Medical Center, Worcester, Massachusetts.

233

other hand, if a standard transplant shows different head formation frequencies in two different kinds of hosts, the difference in transplant behavior can be considered due to a property of the host communicated over a long-range. It is well established that lateral transplants near a host's head do not develop into a head and that a transplant near the host's foot does not develop into a foot. These effects are clearly long-range ones. I refer to long-range effects in general as inhibitory. There is some justification for assuming that all long-range effects share a common mechanism (Cohen and MacWilliams, 1975; MacWilliams, 1983a).

The intrinsic property of transplants, which one can consider to oppose the long-range effect, may be considered to be "activating." One can distinguish between head and foot activating as well as head and foot inhibitory effects, although it is possible that the mechanisms responsible for the head and foot properties are not entirely distinct (Berking, 1979).

Hydra's body displays "morphogenetic gradients," i.e., gradations in the head and foot activating and inhibitory properties. The activating and inhibitory properties also change during head or foot regeneration. In the following pages I discuss quantitative methods for studying such gradients or developmental changes.

STATEMENT OF THE CENTRAL PROBLEM

Any study of the shapes of a gradient or the kinetics of developmental changes must begin with the results of transplantation experiments. A significant problem is that the quantities one can measure in transplantation experiments, namely, head- or foot-formation frequencies, are at best indirectly related to the values of the "fundamental parameters," which one presumes are actually responsible for activation and inhibition. These parameters might be interpreted to be concentrations of morphogenetic substances, electric field strengths, biochemical wave frequencies, etc. To appreciate the indirectness of the relationship, consider the following:

1. The head- or foot-formation frequencies are defined at the level of a population of experimental animals. Fundamental parameter values (e.g., morphogen concentrations) are defined within individuals.

2. Head- or foot-formation frequencies are restricted to values between 0 and 1; fundamental parameter values have no such artificial restrictions. Consider the following example which draws on this fact and strongly suggests that frequency and morphogen concentration cannot be linearly related. Imagine that a particular experiment gives a head-formation frequency of 50%. Increasing the concentration of an activating substance by a certain amount might raise the frequency to 80%. A second, equivalent

increase in activator concentration cannot cause a second, equivalent increase in the head-formation frequency, for such an increase would require a head-formation frequency greater than 1.

Experiments suggest that the relation between head-formation frequency and fundamental parameter values is not only indirect but inconsistent. Fig. 1A gives a rather mild example of this phenomenon: measurements of the head inhibition gradient in *Hydra attenuata* made with two different transplants give qualitatively different curves, one convex and one concave. Simple models (see below), in fact, lead one to expect this kind of inconsistency in raw data on head- or foot-formation frequency.

It thus seems likely that head- or foot-formation frequencies, although clearly determined by the values of the fundamental activating and inhibitory parameters, contain quantitative distortions which can give a misleading

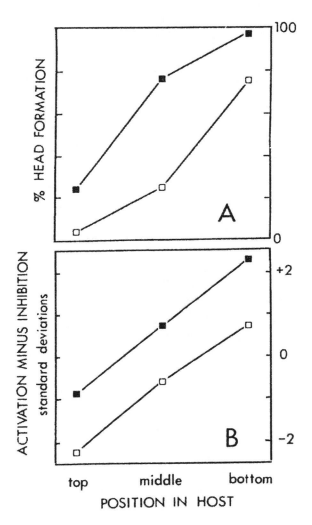

FIGURE 1. The head inhibition gradient in *Hydra attenuata* seen in two ways. (A) "Raw data" showing head formation frequencies obtained in tissue fragments transplanted to three positions. Transplants consisted of first (top curve) or second (bottom curve) eighths of the donor's body column, numbered starting at the apical end. Note that the two curves differ in shape. (B) Relative inhibition values calculated from the data of (A). In this form, the gradients appear roughly linear in both cases.

picture of the way the fundamental parameters change in space and time. It is necessary to correct these distortions if one wishes to look at the fundamental parameters themselves. Since the head- or foot-formation frequencies are the only available experimental data, schemes for correcting them can only be based on logic and inference; they cannot be proven valid. A reasonable approach is to contruct a model of the way the fundamental parameters might determine head- and foot-formation frequencies, and to apply this model in reverse to derive numbers from the transplantation data which could be directly and simply related to the fundamental parameter values. It turns out that when one follows this approach using what appears to be the simplest possible model, one gets numbers from frequency data which are consistent with one another and appear to make sense.

In the following pages I will describe this approach in enough detail to orient readers having only a general mathematical background. I will:

1. Describe a model of the determination of head or foot formation frequency in a transplantation experiment, thereby introducing a concept of activation and inhibition levels. These are abstract quantities that may be directly related to fundamental parameter values.
2. Discuss the effects of statistical error on activation and inhibition levels calculated from transplantation data.
3. Discuss the problem posed by head- or foot-formation frequencies near zero or one, thereby introducing a concept of the limited measuring range of a single transplant or host.
4. Discuss a mathematical optimization procedure which allows one to measure gradients or time courses whose range exceeds the measuring range of a single transplant or host.
5. Present a method for statistical evaluation of such optimization-derived "measurements" of gradients or developmental kinetics.

The experiments I discuss are all lateral transplantation experiments (see Chapter 30) in which there is a clear distinction between host and transplant. My methods can be applied to other sorts of data using the general concepts of "actor" and "setting" (see Cohen and MacWilliams, 1975). The models were originally designed to account for foot formation, but can be applied equally well to head formation.

THE ACTIVATION–INHIBITION MODEL

In a model proposed by MacWilliams *et al.* (1970), foot formation in individual transplantation experiments is controlled by two abstract parameters called activation and inhibition; these parameters describe the strengths of activating and inhibitory effects within individual hydra. The model posits that a given transplant forms a foot if and only if its foot activation is greater than the foot inhibition it experiences. The model posits that the activation level varies somewhat even in a group of supposedly identical transplants. Thus when an experiment is repeated, the relative magnitudes of activation and inhibition may change and the outcome may be different (one could just as well assume that the variability is in the inhibition level, or in both activation and inhibition levels). In experiments in which the mean activation level in the population of transplants equals the inhibition level that the transplants experience in the hosts, activation is expected to exceed inhibition in 50% of cases, giving a foot-formation frequency of 0.5. When the mean levels of activation and inhibition differ, the expected foot-formation frequency is determined by the difference in average levels and by the variability of this difference. The determination of a head-formation frequency by an identical mechanism is illustrated in Fig. 2.

SETS OF RELATIVE ACTIVATION OR INHIBITION LEVELS

The model of Fig. 2 can be used in reverse to derive the difference between mean activation and inhibition levels corresponding to any given head- or foot-formation frequency. One procedure for deriving this difference is to find, in a table of normal curve areas, the standard deviation value V such that the integral of the normal curve from minus infinity to V equals the observed frequency. The difference so determined is expressed in units equal to one standard deviation of the activation variability.

If this procedure is applied to the results of a set of experiments in which several different sorts of transplants were placed in a standard host, the calculated differences between activation and inhibition levels can be interpreted as "relative activation levels." Thus, if four transplants to a single host form feet with frequencies of 0.16, 0.50, 0.84, and 0.98, the corresponding differences between activation and inhibition levels are -1, 0, $+1$, and $+2$ standard deviations, respectively, and the transplants have relative activation levels of -1, 0, 1, and 2.

A similar provedure can be used to determine "relative inhibition levels" from the results of an experiment in which a standard transplant was placed into several different hosts.

Gradients and developmental time courses can in principle be mapped by calculating relative activation and inhibition levels. When interpreting sets of relative activation or inhibition levels, however, two important limitations must be kept in mind: (1) The absolute levels of activation and inhibition remain unknown. Thus, the activation levels in the example above could just

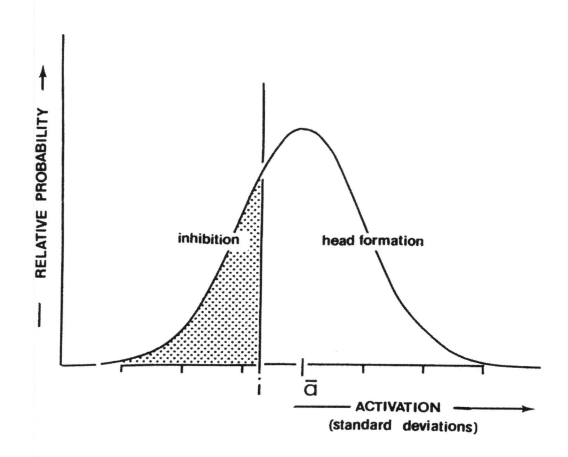

FIGURE 2. Determination of a head-formation frequency according to the activation–inhibition model. The model assumes that the activation level in a group of "identical" transplants is normally distributed (bell-shaped curve) with mean value $\bar{a}$. A head is formed if and only if the activation exceeds the inhibition level i. The head-formation frequency is given by the ratio of the area under the curve to the right of i (unshaded) to the total area under the cur e. Note that the head-formation frequency would not be affected by changing a and i by the same amount, but would be affected by a change in the difference between $\bar{a}$ and i or by a change in the standard deviation of the normal curve.

as well be quoted as 1, 2, 3, 4. This variability is troubling in some cases. For instance, one might want to know how close the foot inhibition level comes to zero after foot removal. The activation–inhibition model gives no direct way of answering this kind of question. (2) The relative activation levels of a set of transplants can only be compared with one another if one can assume that the variability of the activation level is the same in all transplants. Similarly, a set of relative inhibition levels is only valid if the inhibition variability in all transplants is the same. The assumption of constant variability is difficult to verify directly; it was found adequate in a large study of foot formation (Cohen and MacWilliams, 1975; see below), but questioned in more recent work on head formation (MacWilliams, 1983*b*).

Despite these problems, it remains possible that relative activation and/or inhibition levels are simply and directly related to the values of fundamental parameters, which control head and foot formation; raw frequencies of foot- or head-formation cannot be so related. The value of calculating activation and inhibition levels is illustrated in Fig. 1b, which shows relative inhibition gradients calculated from the two head-formation frequency gradients illustrated in Fig. 1a. The calculated curves agree quite closely in shape, although the raw curves are markedly different. Moreover, both of the calculated curves are close to linear, while neither of the experimental curves have so simple a shape. The ability of the activation–inhibition model to extract a simple and internally consistent interpretation from complex-appearing data has been confirmed several times (see Cohen and MacWilliams, 1975).

STATISTICAL UNCERTAINTY OF ACTIVATION AND INHIBITION VALUES

Experimentally observed head- or foot-formation frequencies can always be expected to differ from the "true" head- or foot-formation probabilities because of sampling errors. These errors cause uncertainties in calculated activation and inhibition values. To make the activation–inhibition model easier to use, I have prepared plots which allow one to estimate activation or inhibition levels and their associated uncertainties directly from head- or foot-formation frequencies (Fig. 3). Uncertainties are given in these plots as confidence intervals (Clopper and Pearson, 1934). These are ranges of values for the difference between activation and inhibition levels. The confidence intervals contain all values that are statistically compatible with the given head- or foot-formation frequency and sample size.

For example, given a head-formation frequency of 0.8 and a sample size of 100, the 95% confidence interval can be read from Fig. 3d as running from

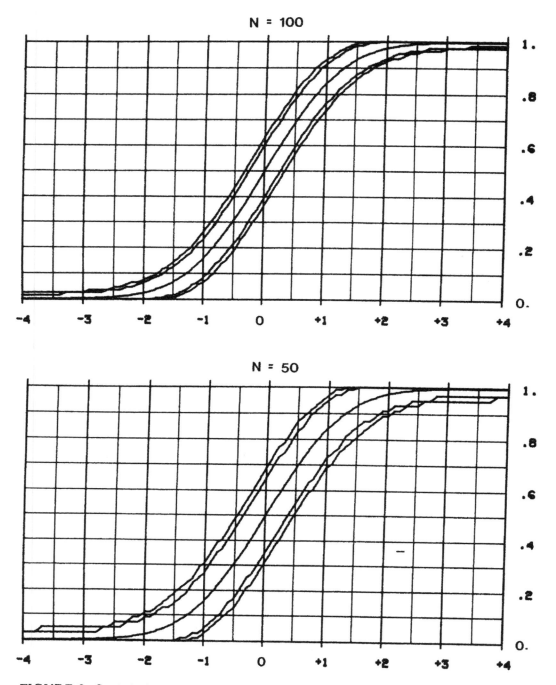

FIGURE 3. Statistical uncertainties for the difference between activation and inhibition for different head- or foot-formation frequencies and sample sizes. In each plot the smooth sigmoid curve gives the most likely value for the difference. The inner pair of rougher curves defines the 95% confidence interval, while the outer pair defines the 99% confidence interval for the difference between activation and inhibition. All values are given in standard deviations of the difference between mean activation and mean inhibition levels. To find a confidence interval for

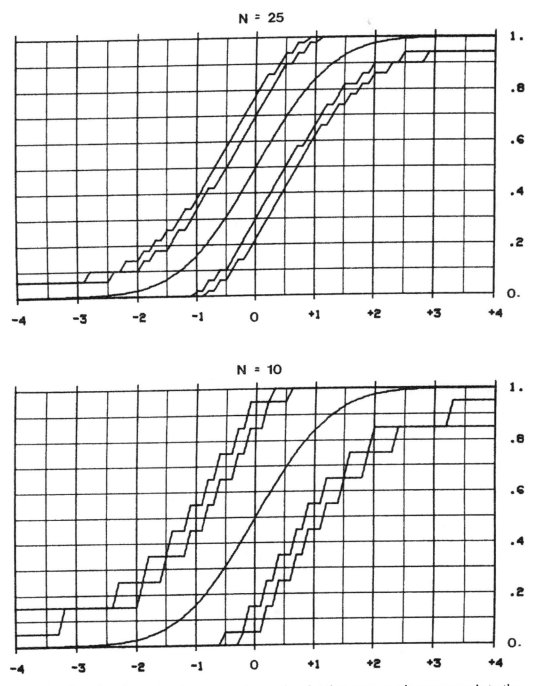

a given head- or foot-formation frequency, choose the plot that most nearly corresponds to the sample size. Locate the frequency on the right hand side of the plot and draw a horizontal line through it. Read down from the intersections with the confidence interval boundaries to determine the confidence limits. All curves were calculated directly from the binomial distribution.

0.5 to 1.1 standard deviations. The most likely value of the difference between activation and inhibition is 0.8, in the center of this range. If the difference is 0.5, the head-formation frequency will generally be less than 0.8, but a frequency of 0.8 or less will be observed 5% of the time. Differences between activation and inhibition outside the range of 0.5 to 1.1 are incompatible (at the 5% level) with a head-formation frequency of 0.8.

Limited Measuring Range of a Single Transplant or Host

Notice that the confidence intervals shown in Fig. 3 become larger for head- or foot-formation frequencies near zero or one, and that the confidence intervals at these frequencies have only one boundary. This pattern reflects that 100% head or foot formation in consistent with any large excess of activation over inhibition, while 0% head or foot formation may be observed in any case in which inhibition is substantially in excess. Thus, there are two consequences: (1) If two experiments both give 0% or 100% head or foot formation, one cannot conclude that the difference between activation and inhibition is the same in the two cases. A substantial difference may become apparent under slightly modified experimental conditions. (2) More generally, any given transplant or host has a limited useful "measuring range"— the range of activation or inhibition values over which it gives head- or foot-formation frequencies between about 5% and 95%. Experiments which give frequencies outside this range do not permit accurate estimates of the difference between activation and inhibition.

ESTIMATING RELATIVE ACTIVATION AND INHIBITION LEVELS BY OPTIMIZATION

The limited useful measuring range of any single transplant or host may make it necessary to use several transplants or several hosts to measure the entire course of a gradient or developmental change in a transplantation property of hydra. For example, the results of using a number of different transplants to measure the foot inhibition gradient in *Hydra viridis* (Fig. 4) indicate that no single one of the transplants can usefully measure the inhibition level over more than one-half of the animal's length. In order to obtain a profile of the gradient as a whole, one must combine the results obtained from several different transplants.

One way of combining results obtained with several different transplants would be to calibrate the transplants with respect to one another. Thus, the relative activation levels of transplants 1 and 2 could be determined from their foot-formation frequencies when transplanted to position 3; 3 could be

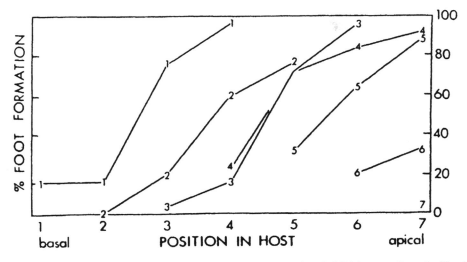

FIGURE 4. Partial results of an experiment to explore the foot inhibition gradient in *H. viridis* (MacWilliams, 1972; Cohen and MacWilliams, 1975). Seven different sorts of transplants, consisting of the first (1) to seventh (7) from basal body column eighth of donor animals, were transplanted to wounds made at equally spaced sites along the body column of hosts. Any given transplant demonstrates a gradient over at most a portion of the host's body column.

calibrated with respect to 2 at position 4; and 5 could be calibrated with respect to 3 at position 5. The calibrated set of transplants would then allow measurements of the inhibition level over the entire length of the animal. This procedure would work well in the absence of experimental error, but it handles uncertainties in the foot-formation frequencies in an awkward fashion: (1) The use of just one experimental result to calibrate a pair of transplants with respect to one another, although several results are available, makes calibration somewhat arbitrary and calibration errors larger than necessary. (2) Calibration errors accumulate by calibrating from end to end, so that uncertainties in the final inhibition levels are much greater in some positions than others.

An alternative method for finding activation and inhibition levels in experiments involving several different transplants and hosts involves mathematical optimization techniques. This method, which takes advantage of all available data and is statistically elegant, gives the best possible activation and inhibition values in a statistically meaningful sense. In addition to the activation and inhibition values, the method yields a measure of the statistical acceptability of the activation–inhibition model (applied to the given data set) as a whole. Specific hypotheses about the shapes of gradients or the kinetics of developmental changes can be tested directly against the data by constructing modified versions of the activation–inhibition model and testing these models by another round of mathematical optimization.

I present here the essence of the mathematical optimization method, applying it, as an example, to the experiment illustrated in Fig. 4.

Principle of Optimization

This method is simple in principle: seek the set of activation levels (for each kind of transplant in an experimental series) and inhibition levels (for each kind of host) that give the best possible prediction of the experimental data. By assuming any set of values at all for the activation and inhibition levels, you can calculate an expected head- or foot-formation frequency for any possible combination of transplant and host and thus can calculate a set of predicted results for an experimental series as a whole. For some sets of assumed activation and inhibition values the predicted results will correspond more closely to the real data than for others. The degree of difference between the predicted and actual results can be regarded as a mathematical function of the assumed activation and inhibition levels. Mathematical procedures can be applied to this function to find activation and inhibition values for which it assumes the smallest possible size. These are the "best" activation and inhibition values, and the degree of difference corresponding to these values can be interpreted statistically as a measure of the acceptability of the activation–inhibition model.

Uncertainty-Weighted Sum of Squared Deviations as a Difference Measure

A deviation is the difference between a predicted frequency and the corresponding experimental value. A simple measure of the difference between predicted and actual data sets is the sum of all deviations. When this sum is large, the predictions are poor; a small sum indicates a good "fit" between predictions and data.

A degree-of-difference measure, which is more commonly used in statistical procedures, is the sum of squared deviations. Squaring each deviation before summing puts proportionally more weight on the large deviations in accordance with the statistical principle that large deviations are much less likely to occur by chance than small ones. A further refinement, the uncertainty-weighted sum of squared deviations, can be calculated by dividing each deviation by the uncertainty of the corresponding experimental value before squaring and summing. You can estimate the uncertainties of head- or foot-formation frequencies by taking one-fourth of the corresponding 95% confidence intervals (Clopper and Pearson, 1934). The binomial uncertainty $(p - p^2)^{1/2}$, which appears tempting to use, gives misleading zero uncertainties for $p = 0$ and $p = 1$. When uncertainty weighting is employed, each data point contributes to the final result according to its certainty. Furthermore, the uncertainty-weighted sum of squared deviations is expected to have a chi-squared distribution. After the "best" activation and inhibition values have been found, one can thus determine how well the activation-inhibition model, or variants of it, account for the data simply by comparing the minimized value of the uncertainty-weighted sum of squared deviations with the appropriate entry of a chi-squared table.

Redundant Variables

The activation–inhibition model, applied to a typical series of experiments, contains more variables than are actually necessary to predict results for all of the experiments in the series. If the extra "redundant variables" are not tracked down and eliminated, optimization will be inefficient and statistical tests inaccurate.

One source of redundancy variables comes from the absolute levels of activation and inhibition having no effect on the predicted head- or foot-formation frequencies; only the relative levels matter. Thus an arbitrary constant can be added to all activation and inhibition values without changing the predictions of the model. This redundancy can be eliminated by holding one activation or inhibition level at a fixed value. The relative activation and inhibition levels are not constrained by this procedure, but the apparent number of variables in the model is decreased by one. It makes no difference which activation or inhibition value is fixed. In analyzing the data of Fig. 4, I set one value to zero; all other activation and inhibition levels were then expressed relative to this fixed one.

Redundancy can also arise when the predictions of the model do not change because all activation and inhibition values and the standard deviation (see Fig. 2) are multiplied by a single constant. In analyzing the data of Fig. 4, I eliminated this source of redundancy by fixing the value of the standard deviation at 1. All activation and inhibition values were then automatically expressed in units equal to one standard deviation of the variability of the difference between activation and inhibition.

Minimizing the Uncertainty-Weighted Sum of Squared Deviations

The best activation and inhibition values are those that give the smallest possible difference between the model's predictions and the actual experimental data. Accordingly, seek activation and inhibition values which minimize the uncertainty-weighted sum of standard deviations between predictions and data. There is unfortunately no direct formula for finding these values; it is possible, however, to search for them in an efficient manner using a computer. The search procedure is analogous to climbing a hill in the dark without being able to see: one makes local explorations (small changes in the values of the variables) to determine which direction is up (which "direction" in variable space decreases the weighted sum); one then heads in this direction, readjusting the course until one can go no higher. A number of "hill climbing" computer algorithms are available. I have used Rosenbrock's (1960) algorithm, which is probably outdated. Consult an applied mathematician about more recent developments in this field.

As might be expected from the analogy to climbing a physical hill, there is an important limitation to computerized hill climbing as a method for finding the minimum value of a function: the procedure is only guaranteed to work if the hill in question has but a single summit. If the hill is irregularly shaped and has subsidiary peaks, it is possible that the climber will end up on a subsidiary peak and think, since he cannot see, that he has found the true summit. Thus, it is only possible to guarantee that a hill-climbing routine has located the true minimum if the function in question has no other local minima. I have not been able to show formally that the weighted sum of squared deviations, expressed as a function of the parameters of the activation–inhibition model, has only a single minimum. I have, however, conducted computer experiments in which optimization was started from a number of different "positions" — different sets of values for the activation and inhibition levels. The minimum found by the hill-climbing routine was always the same.

Activation–inhibition models can be very closely approximated by models of quite different mathematical form, so-called log-linear models (Cohen and MacWilliams, 1975). Optimum values for the variables in log-linear models can be determined directly and are therefore not subject to uncertainties about multiple minima. Cohen and MacWilliams applied the log-linear approximation in a number of cases previously studied by hill climbing, and confirmed the hill-climbing result in every case.

Statistical Tests of Activation–Inhibition Models

A particular model is acceptable statistically if the differences between its predictions and the actual experimental data are small enough to be attributed to chance. To perform statistical tests one must therefore understand how large a difference is to be expected by chance. This test is fairly straightforward in the case of the activation–inhibition model if the model has been fitted by minimizing the uncertainty-weighted sum of squared deviations. Assuming that the activation–inhibition model is correct, and that the optimizing routine has located the correct activation and inhibition levels, the deviations between predictions and data are random variables with mean values of zero and standard deviations equal to the uncertainties of the experimental measurements. Dividing each deviation by the corresponding uncertainty gives a set of random variables with means of zero and standard deviations of 1. The sum of the squares of n such variables has a chi-squared distribution with n degrees of freedom. In principle one can determine the acceptability of an activation–inhibition model by comparing the weighted sum of squared deviations after optimization (henceforth the "residual weighted sum") with the appropriate line in a chi-square table.

In general the appropriate chi-square distribution will not have n degrees of freedom, but fewer because optimizing routines tend to find activation and inhibition levels that fit the experimental data even better than the correct activation and inhibition values would. The routines fit those aspects of the experimental data which are due to sampling error as well as those aspects which are "real." The residual weighted sum will therefore on the average be smaller that that chi-squared with n degrees of freedom. To compensate, one subtracts degrees of freedom: one for each (nonredundant) variable for which an optimum value was found. In the case of the data of Fig. 4, for example, there were 22 measured foot-formation frequencies and thus 22 terms in the sum of squared deviations. Values were found for seven activation and seven inhibition levels, but one of these was redundant; there were thus 13 optimized variables. The residual weighted sum would thus be compared to a chi-squared distribution with 22–13 or 9 degrees of freedom.

My actual analysis of the data of Fig. 4 (MacWilliams, 1972) included 18 additional foot-formation frequencies measured in hosts from which the feet had been removed; these are not shown in Fig. 4. There were thus 40 terms in the sum of squared deviations and 20 optimized variables (seven activation levels, seven inhibition levels in intact hosts, and seven inhibition levels in footless hosts, minus one redundant variable). The residual value of the weighted sum was 15.0, which is an acceptable value of chi-squared with 20 degrees of freedom ($p > .70$). The activation–inhibition model is thus satisfactory for these data.

Testing Hypotheses about the Shapes of Activation and Inhibition Profiles

The activation and inhibition levels obtained by optimization can be plotted against position or time to obtain pictures of gradients or developmental time courses. Figure 5, for example, shows the foot-activation gradient in *Hydra viridis*, derived as above, as well as two foot-inhibition gradients, one for intact and one for footless animals, which were determined in the same analysis. Examination of these gradients suggests that (1) both

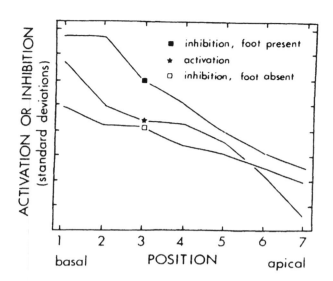

FIGURE 5. Relative activation and inhibition levels determined using the mathematical optimization from the data of Fig. 4 (and other data not shown) and plotted against position in the donor or host. Hypotheses about these gradients (for instance, that they are linear) can be tested by another round of optimization (see text).

inhibition gradients are roughly linear, (2) the inhibition gradient is steeper in intact than in footless hosts, and (3) the activation gradient is systematically nonlinear.

One can normally make a rough-and-ready test of such hypotheses by examining the error bars associated with the individual data points. Unfortunately, activation and inhibition levels determined by optimization cannot be given conventional error bars. It is possible, however, to use the optimization method to test a hypothesis directly against the original experimental values: construct an activation–inhibition model incorporating the relationship to be tested, find optimum values for its variables, and judge the residual weighted sum of squared deviations as above. MacWilliams (1972) and Cohen and MacWilliams (1975) tested the hypotheses suggested above in this manner. A thumbnail review of their findings illustrates the power of this technique.

1. The hypothesis that the two inhibition gradients are linear was tested by fitting a model in which the 14 inhibition levels were constrained to lie on two straight lines, one for intact and one for footless hosts. The 14 inhibition variables were thus represented in the optimization by 4 variables giving a slope and an intercept for each line. There were 11 optimized variables, one of which was redundant; the residual weighted sum was 27.9, which is an acceptable value of chi-squared with 30 degrees of freedom ($p > .50$).

2. The hypothesis that the inhibition gradients have different slopes was tested by fitting a model similar to (1) in which the two slopes were constrained to be the same. The hypothesis was rejected (residual weighted sum = 68.8; this sum is not an acceptable value of chi-squared with 31 degrees of freedom with $p < .001$).

3. The hypothesis that the activation gradient is nonlinear was tested by

fitting a model which assumed linearity; the seven activation values were thus replaced with two which gave a slope and an intercept. The model was rejected; the residual weighted sum was 41.8, which is not an acceptable value for chi-squared with 25 degrees of freedom ($p < .02$). This analysis suggests that the observed shape of the gradient—steeper at both ends than at the middle—is real, which is consistent with the idea that both head and foot influence the activation level.

These examples deal exclusively with the issue of gradient shape, but the same methods can be applied to the analysis of developmental changes of transplantation properties in hydra (see MacWilliams *et al.*, 1970).

REFERENCES

Berking, S. 1979. Analysis of head and foot formation in *Hydra* by means of an endogenous inhibitor. *Wilhelm Roux Arch. Entwichlungsmech. Org.* **186**: 189–210.

Clopper, C. J., and Pearson, E. S. 1934. The use of confidence or fiducial limits illustrated in the case of the binomial. *Biometrika* **26**:404–413.

Cohen, J. H., and MacWilliams, H. K. 1975. The control of foot formation in *Hydra viridis*. *J. Theor. Biol.* **50**:87–105.

MacWilliams, H. K. 1972. The control of foot formation in *Hydra viridis*. Doctoral dissertation, Harvard University.

MacWilliams, H. K. 1983a. Hydra transplantation phenomena and the mechanism of hydra head regeneration. I. Properties of the head inhibition. *Dev. Biol.* (in press).

MacWilliams, H. K. 1983b. Hydra transplantation phenomena and the mechanism of hydra head regeneration. II. Properties of the head activation. *Dev. Biol.* (in press).

MacWilliams, H. K., Kafatos, F. C., and Bossert, W. H. 1970. The feedback inhibition of basal disk regeneration in *Hydra* has a continuously variable intensity. *Dev. Biol.* **23**:380–398.

Rosenbrock, H. H. 1960. An automatic method for finding the greatest or least value of a function. *Comput. J.* **3**:175–184.

Chapter 32

Dissociating Tissues into Cells and the Development of Hydra from Aggregated Cells

Kristine M. Flick and Hans R. Bode

PURPOSE

To dissociate hydra tissue into a suspension of viable cells, and to form from those cells aggregates of tissue that will develop into viable whole hydra.

INTRODUCTION

This simple, rapid, and highly reproducible procedure was originally described by Gierer *et al.* (1972). It consists of soaking hydra tissue in a simple salt solution, mechanically dissociating the loosened tissue into a suspension of cells with a pipet, and centrifuging the cell suspension into clumps or aggregates of cells.

MATERIALS

Neubauer cell-counting chamber with 0.1 mm depth for phase microscope; phase microscope with 25× and 40× objectives; incubator set at

Kristine M. Flick and Hans R. Bode ● Developmental Biology Center and Department of Developmental and Cell Biology, University of California, Irvine, California.

TABLE I. Dissociation Medium

Stock solution	Component	Stock solution concentration (g/100 ml)	Final concentration in medium (mM)
1	$CaCl_2 \cdot 2H_2O$	1.47	5
	$MgSO_4 \cdot 7H_2O$	0.49	1
	KCL	4.18	2.8
	TES[a]	4.95	11
2	Na_2HPO_4	0.19	0.67
	KH_2PO_4	0.12	0.44
3	Na Pyruvate	1.10	5
	Na_3 Citrate $\cdot 2H_2O$	2.94	5

[a] TES = N–tris (hydroxymethyl) methyl-2-aminomethansulfonic acid (Sigma). HEPES can be substituted for TES. Make up stock solutions (which are 20X concentrated in distilled water), filter sterilize (0.22 μ or 0.45 μ Millipore; sterilization by autoclaving causes precipitation), and store frozen. In making up stock solution 1 it is important that the ingredients be added and dissolved one at a time to prevent precipitation. To make the dissociation medium, add 5 ml of each stock solution to 85 ml distilled water, and then adjust the pH to 6.9–7.0 with 2 N NaOH (usually 0.1 ml). Filter sterilized, the medium can be stored at 4°C.

20 ± 1°C; nylon cloth (Nitex, 53-μm mesh, Tobler, Ernst & Traber); clinical centrifuge with a swinging bucket rotor which will hold 15- or 40-ml centrifuge tubes and adapters for 0.5-ml microfuge tubes; plastic 0.5-ml microfuge tubes (Beckman) and 35- and 60-mm-diameter Petri dishes; glass 15- and 40-ml centrifuge tubes; 5- and 9-in. Pasteur pipets with rubber bulbs; Rifampicin and Gentamycin (Sigma Chemical Co.); flasks for stock solutions.

Do not wash the glassware with soap. Instead, simply rinse them with distilled water. Keep this glassware separate from all other laboratory glassware.

Make up stock solutions (which are 20X concentrated in distilled water) and sterilize them by filtering through 0.22 or 0.45 Millipore disks (sterilization by autoclaving causes precipitation). Store the solutions at $-18°$ C or below. In making up stock solution 1, add and dissolve the ingredients one at a time to prevent precipitation. To make the dissociation medium, add 5 ml of each stock solution to 85 ml distilled water, and then adjust the pH to 6.9–7.0 with 2 N NaOH (usually 0.1 ml). Sterilize the medium by filtering and store at 4°C.

PROCEDURES

Dissociating Hydra Tissue into a Cell Suspension

Collect 300–500 1-day-starved animals from a stock culture. Wash them twice in 500 ml hydra culture solution (e.g., M) by swirling, allow them to settle, pour off the medium, and repeat the washing process once more. To dislodge debris and exudate that may be attached to the hydra, stir them with a magnetic stirrer for 15–30 min in clean culture solution.

The following procedures are designed for using 300–500 hydra. When using 100 hydra or less, reduce the volume of the solution accordingly. Otherwise the dissociation process is harder to control, the cell yield is considerably lower, and the amount of cell debris is higher.

Transfer the clean animals to a 15-ml conical centrifuge tube and withdraw as much of the culture solution as possible with a narrow-bore 5-in. Pasteur pipet. Use a pipet whose orifice has been previously reduced one-third to one-half with a small flame. Add 5 ml cold (4°C) dissociation medium and thoroughly mix by pipeting the hydra up and down with a 5-in. Pasteur pipet. Allow the animals to settle, remove as much of the solution as possible, and add 5 ml fresh cold dissociation medium.

Place the tube containing the animals suspended in the medium in ice or in a refrigerator for 20–30 min. Soaking animals for less than 15 min results in incomplete dissociation, yielding large clumps of tissue and low yields of single cells. Extending this period to 60–120 min increases the fraction of single cells. If you want high yields of single cells, mince the animals with clean razor blades or scalpels before placing them in the dissociation medium. To mince them efficiently, place the animals on a piece of Teflon, plastic, or rubber and remove as much of the surrounding liquid as possible before cutting.

As a final cleaning step to remove nonhydra material that may have come loose during the soaking, do the following: Using a 5-in. Pasteur pipet, gently pipet the animals (whole or minced) up and down until the solution is just slightly turbid. Allow the animals to settle and remove as much of the turbid solution as possible.

To the clean animals, add 5 ml cold dissociation solution and begin to dissociate the tissue. Using a 5-in. Pasteur pipet with a normal or slightly narrowed bore, pipet the hydra up and down with a fair amount of velocity to promote turbulence, but not to the extent of blowing air bubbles through the solution. Pipet the suspension in this manner until it is turbid due to the cells being released from the tissue. Place the tube in ice for 2–4 min and let the large pieces settle out. Remove the turbid solution with a clean pipet and place it in a 40-ml conical centrifuge tube that is standing in ice and contains 5 ml of cold dissociation medium. Keep these diluted cells in the 40-ml tube at 4°C throughout the process; otherwise, much reaggregation will occur.

To any large pieces of tissue that settle out during the process, add 3–5 ml dissociation medium and carry out the dissociation procedure just described. Repeat this procedure four to six times to be certain that you obtain all the single cells available from your preparation. For the latter repetitions of these steps, use 2–3 ml of the dissociation medium and a 5-in. Pasteur pipet with a narrow bore. Add each portion of newly acquired cells to the 40-ml conical tube, and either swirl or gently bubble air (with a Pasteur pipet) through the suspension to keep the cells from settling out. This gentle mixing also reduces the reaggregation that occurs among cells settling to the bottom.

Collect all of the cell suspensions in the 40-ml conical tube and remove large clump of cells of one of two methods: Either let the cell suspension stand 5 min or filter it through a nylon cloth of ~50-μm mesh. If you use the first method, do not let the suspension stand much more than for 5 min; if it stands longer than 10 min, single cells are lost in large numbers. The resulting cell suspension should consist primarily of single cells of all types except for the epithelial cells. About 40–50% of these occur as single cells; another 40–50% occur in clumps of two to five cells, and the remainder in larger clumps.

Formation of Aggregates

Use only suspended cells. If you prepared your suspension by the "standing" procedure, use only the cell suspension above the conical part of the tube and transfer it to a second tube. If you obtain the cell suspension by filtering it through a nylon mesh, use the entire cell suspension. If the cell suspension contains a great deal of cellular debris (i.e., if the debris and cells occur in roughly equal amounts), centrifuge the suspension in a clinical centrifuge at 1000–1200 rpm (170–200g) for 2–3 min and resuspend the collected cells in the same or a smaller volume of dissociation medium. Note that the cell suspensions always will form reaggregates. Therefore, gently disburse such pellets into single cells. Be careful not to centrifuge and resuspend the cells more than twice; otherwise the cells will lose their capacity to aggregate.

To control the size of the aggregates when using 0.5-ml microfuge tubes, use cell suspensions containing about 300,000 cells/ml. Too few cells form a layer instead of a pellet and cannot be recovered as a coherent clump of cells. An excess of cells, on the other hand, results in a large pellet which breaks up into several smaller, yet perfectly usable clumps. Determine the concentration of cells in suspension with a Neubauer cell-counting chamber or simply centrifuge several concentrations of the cell suspension in 0.5-ml microfuge tubes and examine the size of the pellet. With a little practice you will be able to recognize the pellet size(s) which forms a single aggregate capable of development. Then adjust the concentration of the cell suspension appropriately either by diluting it or by centrifuging it and resuspending the pellet cells in a smaller volume.

To form an aggregate, place 0.5 ml of the cell suspension into a 0.5-ml microfuge tube using a 9-in. Pasteur pipet. The 9-in. Pasteur pipet has a smaller orifice diameter than a 5-in. one and will reach to the bottom of the microfuge tube. Fill the tubes with cell suspension medium from bottom to top to prevent an air bubble from existing at the bottom of the tube, as the bubble sometimes prevents proper pellet formation.

To centrifuge the cells, place a number of such microfuge tubes containing cells in a test tube, but beforehand fill each test tube with sand or paper up to a distance from the top equal to the length of the microfuge tube. Put as many microfuge tubes in the test tube as required to hold all of them firmly in place. Put in each centrifuge bucket and centrifuge at 1000–1200 rpm (170–200g) for 3–5 min.

To dislodge the pellet of the cells from the microfuge tubes, try one of two methods. In the first, simply stand the microfuge tubes upside down. The pellet usually dislodges from the conical part of the tube and falls to the meniscus of the solution within 10–20 min. Then simply remove it with a Pasteur pipet and transfer it (see below) to a 35-mm Petri dish containing 1–2 ml of dissociation medium. Alternatively, lower a 9-in. Pasteur pipet into the microfuge tube to a spot just above the pellet. Expel a small amount of solution sharply at the pellet. Remove the loose pellet with the pipet and transfer it to a Petri dish. If pellets tend to fall apart with this latter method, either let the pellets stand in the microfuge tube for 15–30 min before attempting to remove them or use the first method.

Regardless of the method used to dislodge the pellet of cells, now called "aggregates," transfer them gently as they are quite fragile at this stage. After all the aggregates have been collected in one or more dishes, incubate them at 20°C. If you desire small aggregates, cut a large one into smaller pieces with a scalpel.

Development of Aggregates into Hydra

Once the aggregates are in the dish they will proceed to develop through the stages shown in Fig. 1. All that need be done is to change the medium by one of two ways: the "single change" method or the "dilution" one. The single-change method is simple and works when the animals and aggregates appear to be in the best of condition. By this method, simply place the

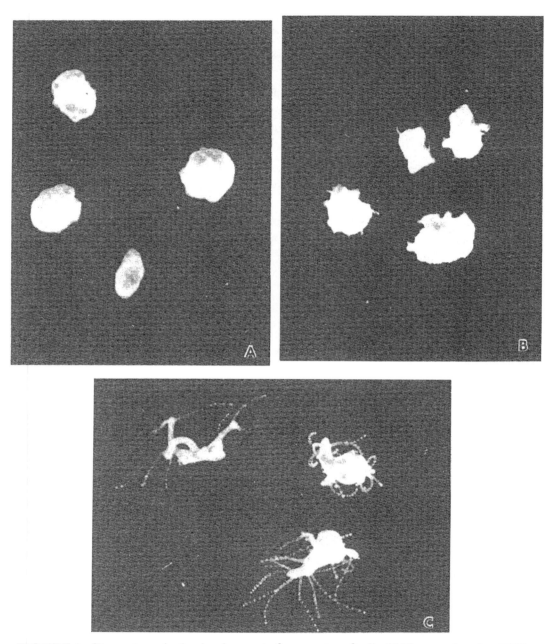

FIGURE 1. Three stages in the development of aggregates of cells (×15, reproduced at 85%). (A) 1-day: Smooth, hollow spheres. (B) 3-day: Hollow spheres with single tentacles as well as hypostomes with tentacle bumps. (C) 6-day: Several axes with developed hypostomes, tentacles, and body columns.

aggregates after 6–8 hr (step 1) directly into culture solution (e.g., M) and allow them to develop. We find that aggregates from healthy hydra develop rapidly by this procedure.

By the dilution method, change the medium around the aggregates in accord with particular stages of development as follows.

1. At 6–8 hr after the aggregates are first transferred, examine them using a dissecting microscope. By this time the cells on the ragged surgace of the pellet should have coalesced into a smooth continuous sheet. At this point, place the aggregates in clean Petri dishes containing dissociation medium diluted 1:1 with hydra culture solution (e.g., M).

2. By 18–23 hr the aggregates should begin to hollow out; that is, a fluid-filled space should become visible in the aggregates (Fig. 1a). Once they are visible, place the aggregates in fresh dissociation medium diluted 1:3 with culture solution.

3. By 28–32 hr the aggregates should be considerably more hollow. The first tentacle bumps may appear. Debris, extruded from the interior of the aggregate, may be observed alongside the aggregate. Place these aggregates, especially when they show tentacle bumps, directly in culture solution. If the aggregates are developing more slowly, adjust the dilution schedule accordingly.

4. Following stage 3, replace the culture solution daily or every 2–3 days. During the next week or so, the aggregates should develop as follows: By 40–60 hr tentacles should appear (Fig. 1b), while the hypostomes with surrounding tentacles should be seen by 3–4 days. By 7–10 days each aggregate should develop several hydranths (Fig. 1c), which eventually should separate from one another to form complete hydra. The number of hydranths formed in an aggregate should be proportional to its initial size. Aggregates can be fed by the 4th or 5th day of their development when the hydranths are sufficiently formed.

COMMENTS

Bacterial Infection

Often, successful development of aggregates does not occur if either the hydra or the resultant aggregates are heavily contaminated with bacteria. Aggregates made from cells of infected hydra develop slowly, if at all. Such aggregates form a smooth outer layer but may never hollow out and eventually disintegrate. If the aggregates become infected, they usually develop to the hollow sphere stage, rarely further, and then disintegrate. The incidence of disintegration in aggregates is greatly lowered by adding the antibiotic Rifampicin and/or Gentamycin to a final concentration of 50 μg/ml to the solution in which the aggregates develop. These antibiotics have no observable effects on the development of aggregates or of intact animals. Treatment of infected hydra with the antibiotics does not always prevent disintegration of the resultant aggregates.

C. D. David (Chapter 33) has used a clever alternative method to combat the bacteria infesting aggregates. He employs the commensal protozoa which are present in moderate numbers around hydra to feed on the bacteria in solution. By his method, 6–10 hydra are placed in 5–10 ml hydra medium in a 60-mm Petri dish at the start of an aggregation experiment. At the time when the aggregates are to be placed in hydra culture solution, David would add them to the dish containing the hydra. He found that those dishes having many ciliates and flagellates moving around on the bottom of the dish, as seen with a dissecting microscope, gave aggregates that developed normally. This method is not foolproof either.

Substitute Dissociation Medium

If aggregate development does not appear quite normal or is a little slow, try substituting the original complex dissociation medium (Gierer *et al.*, 1972; Trenkner *et al.*, 1973) for the simple one given in Table I.

Viability of Cells in Suspension

A constraint on the method is the period of time the cells can be maintained as a suspension and subsequently still form aggregates which will develop normally. The length of that time has not been examined extensively, but cells can remain as cell suspensions for up to 4 hr at room temperature without loss of their ability to aggregate. Cell suspensions maintained at 4°C retain for at least 8 hr the capacity to form aggregates that develop normally; on the other hand, they lose their ability to form clones in the aggregates if previously they have been in suspension for over an hour.

Species of Hydra and Chemical Treatment of the Animals

This method was developed using *Hydra attenuata*, but has also been successful with *Hydra viridis* (P. Bode, personal communication). Aggregates made from cells of animals subjected to treatments with chemicals which drastically alter the cell composition, such as colchicine (Campbell, 1976) or nitrogen mustard (Diehl and Burnett, 1964; David and Murphy, 1977), will also develop at the normal rate. In the former case the animals forming from the aggregates have the altered morphology typical of colchicine-treated hydra (P. Vincent and H. Bode, unpublished results).

REFERENCES

Campbell, R. D. 1976. Elimination of *Hydra* interstitial and nerve cells by means of colchicine. *J. Cell Sci.* **21**:1–13.

David, C. D., and Murphy, S. 1977. Characterization of interstitial stem cells in *Hydra* by cloning. *Dev. Biol.* **58**:372–383.

Diehl, F. A., and Burnett, A. L. 1964. The role of interstitial cells in the maintenance of *Hydra*. I. Specific destruction of interstitial cells to normal, asexual, and non-budding animals. *J. Exp. Zool.* **155**:253–259.

Gierer, A., Berking, S., Bode, H., David, C. N., Flick, K., Hansmann, G., Schaller, H., and Trenkner, E. 1972. Regeneration of *Hydra* from reaggregated cells. *Nature (London) New Biol.* **239**:98–101.

Trenkner, E., Flick, K., Hansmann, G., Bode, P., and Bode, H. 1973. Studies on *Hydra* cells *in vitro*. *J. Exp. Zool.* **185**:317–326.

Chapter 33

Culturing Interstitial Stem Cells in Hydra Aggregates

Charles N. David

PURPOSE

To investigate the growth and differentiation of interstitial stem cells of hydra, we have developed a method for culturing those cells within aggregates of cells taken from hydra previously treated with nitrogen mustard (NM) (David and Murphy, 1977; Sproull and David, 1979).

INTRODUCTION

When small numbers of cells are seeded in such NM aggregates, which serve as "feeder layers," individual stem cell clones can be identified and counted. In addition, the feeder layer technique is suitable for following the differentiation of interstitial cells committed to become nerve cells or nematocytes (Gierer *et al.*, 1972; Venugopal and David, 1981; Fujisawa and David, 1981; Yaross *et al.*, 1982).

GENERAL COMMENTS

The procedure for culturing stem cells in NM aggregates is outlined schematically in Fig. 1. Treat hydra with NM to destroy endogenous

Charles N. David ● Department of Molecular Biology. Albert Einstein College of Medicine, Bronx, New York.

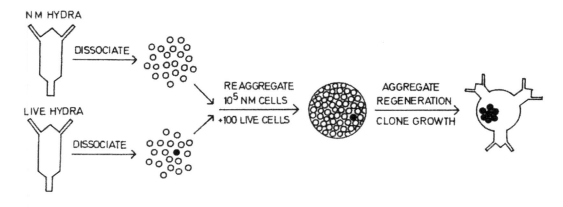

FIGURE I. Schematic representation of method for cloning interstitial stem cells in aggregates of NM-treated cells. (●) Stem cell.

interstitial cells (see Chapter 40). Dissociate the treated hydra to yield a cell suspension (see Chapter 32). Likewise, dissociate sample of untreated hydra tissue. Mix an aliquot of the untreated cell suspension containing an appropriate number of stem cells with ~200,000 NM-treated cells and centrifuge the mixture to form a cell aggregate. During incubation of the aggregate over the next few days (see Chapter 32), stem cells from the untreated sample will proliferate to form interstitial cell clones. To visualize such clones, stain the aggregates with Toluidine Blue. Interstitial cells and differentiating nematoblasts in clones stain darkly and can be easily identified against the lightly stained epithelial cells of the host tissue.

About 0.6% of total hydra cells give rise to interstitial cell clones in NM aggregates (David and Murphy, 1977). Since about 50% of the cells used to form the aggregates are sloughed during the cloning procedure, about 2 times 0.6% or 1.2% of hydra cells are estimated to be stem cells by the cloning assay. Since the fraction of stem cells in intact hydra estimated from cell flow analysis is 4% (David and Gierer, 1974), the apparent cloning efficiency of stem cells in NM feeder layers is about 25%. This estimate is a minimum one since some stem cells differentiate in NM aggregates instead of forming clones.

MATERIALS

Polyethylene centrifuge tubes (0.4 ml) with smooth, conical bottoms and 100-ml pear-shaped centrifuge bottles with graduated tips.

Prepare cell culture medium (Chapter 4) in large batches and store it frozen. Do not sterilize the medium since the tissue used in experiments is not sterile.

"Ecology" dishes are Petri dishes in which hydra have been cultured for 2–3 days. In addition to hydra, they contain amoebae, flagellates, and other protozoa which normally coexist with hydra in our cultures. They are the best "antibiotic" available for developing aggregates.

PROCEDURES

Preparing NM-Treated Host Tissue

Treat about 2000 hydra with 0.01% NM for 10 min. Feed and wash the hydra 1 day after NM treatment and use them for cloning experiments 5–6 days later. By this time the tissue is essentially free of endogenous interstitial cells. Note that the NM treatment must be done very carefully because only one live untreated hydra, which contains 1000 stem cells, among 1000 NM-treated hydra, can contribute a significant background of stem cell clones to the NM host tissue.

Dissociating Cells

Dissociate NM-treated hydra in cell culture medium and collect the cells by centrifuging (200g; 6 min) them in 100-ml pear-shaped centrifuge bottles. Discard the supernatant and resuspend the cell pellet in 30 ml fresh medium per 0.2 ml cell pellet. This suspension corresponds to a cell concentration of about 5×10^5/ml; 0.4-ml aliquots, on centrifugation, yield aggregates containing 200,000 cells.

To dissociate the small amounts of tissue (5–10 hydra) required for cloning experiments, add 100–200 NM-treated hydra as carrier to the live tissue and dissociate the mixture. Typically such suspensions contain 200–500 clone-forming cells (CFU) per milliliter, so that about 2 μl of the suspension per aggregate is sufficient to yield an average of one clone per aggregate.

Preparing Aggregates

To prepare aggregates, mix an aliquot of NM host suspension with a sample of the live cell suspension such that the mixture contains ~2.5 CFUs/ml. Distribute the mixture to 0.4-ml polyethylene centrifuge tubes with a Pasteur pipet. The suspension is held in the tubes by capillarity so the tubes can be put on their side and otherwise handled rather roughly. Place 15–20 such tubes into large 50-ml tubes and centrifuge them at 100g for 6 min to pellet the cells.

After centrifugation, remove the small tubes from the centrifuge and stand them upside down in a 100-ml beaker. The cell pellets come off the bottom of the tubes after 5–15 min and fall to the meniscus from which they can easily be dropped into a Petri dish with fresh medium. Allowing the pellets to come off the bottom in this matter minimizes cell loss due to handling.

Dilute the cell culture medium in twofold steps over the next 18 hr (see Chapter 32) and then transfer aggregates to "ecology" dishes for further incubation. Two to three hundred aggregates can be conveniently processed in an experiment using the procedure outlined above.

After 5–6 days of clone growth, fix aggregates with ethanol, stain with 0.1% of Toluidine Blue and prepare whole mounts (Diehl and Burnett, 1964). Clones are easily identified as groups of darkly staining interstitial cells and differentiating nematoblasts. By focusing up and down through an aggregate, it is possible to identify clones throughout an aggregate.

Quantitatively Estimating Clone-Forming Cells

Before using the NM feeder layer technique to assay CFUs, it is useful to estimate the number of CFUs in the sample to be assayed. To do this, determine the total cell number in a parallel sample of tissue using maceration (Chapter 20) and multiply this number by 0.006 to obtain an estimate of the number of CFUs in the sample. Then prepare several sets of 30 NM aggregates with dilutions of the live cell suspension estimated to yield 0.5–2.0 CFUs/aggregate. Score the total number of clones in each set after 5–6 days of clone growth.

To determine the actual number of CFUs present in the sample, (1) count the total number of clones in a set of 30 aggregates. This value equals the number of CFUs in the sample used to prepare the aggregates. (2) Calculate the fraction of the aggregates which contain clones and use the Poisson distribution to estimate the average CFUs/aggregate (n): (aggregates with clones)/(total aggregates) $= 1 - e^{-n}$.

Both methods should yield comparable results. The variability between replicate assays done on the same day and equivalent assays performed on different days is ±30%.

Rapid CFU Assay

To improve on the speed and accuracy of the cloning assay, we have developed an alternative procedure in which large numbers of CFUs are seeded in NM aggregates and the total size of the interstitial cell population is determined by maceration after 4 days of clone growth (David and Plotnick, 1980). Since the growth rate of stem cell clones is independent of clone density up to 100 clones per aggregate (Sproull and David, 1979), the number of interstitial cells (1s+2s) on day 4 is linearly proportional to the number of CFU seeded in the aggregates on day 0. The proportionality constant is 19 $(1s+2s)_{day\ 4}/CFU_{day\ 0}$.

To use this procedure inoculate NM aggregates with 5–50 CFUs each. After 4 days of clone growth (the clones are confluent and individual clones cannot be distinguished), macerate five aggregates (Chapter 20) and count the total number of interstitial cells (1s+2s) per aggregate. Divide this number of 19 to determine the number of CFUs in the inoculum.

PRECAUTIONS

Because bacterial contamination can overtake and destroy aggregates, add streptomycin (50 μg/ml) to the medium with each daily medium change. In addition, maintain aggregates in "ecology" dishes so that the protozoa present will consume much of the contaminating bacteria.

To achieve good cloning, complete an experiment rapidly. Stem cells are not viable in culture medium for more than a few hours, and the ability of host tissue to form good aggregates also decays with time. It is best to complete an experiment from the start of dissociation to centrifugation of aggregates in less than 1 hour. For this reason the procedure as outlined above contains no cell-counting steps or other delays.

Carry out the entire procedure at 20°C. At higher temperatures cell losses are greater and aggregates survive poorly.

REFERENCES

David, C. N., and Murphy, S. 1977. Characterization of interstitial stem cells in hydra by cloning. *Dev. Biol.* 58:372–383.

David, C. N., and Plotnick, I. 1980. Distribution of interstitial stem cells in *Hydra. Dev. Biol.* 76:175–184.

Diehl, F., and Burnett, A. L. 1964. The role of interstitial cells in the maintenance of hydra. I. Specific destruction of interstititial cells in normal, sexual and non-budding animals. *J. Exp. Zool.*155:253–259.

Fujisawa, T., and David, C. N. 1981. Commitment during nematocyte differentiation in hydra. *J. Cell Sci.* 48:207–222.

Gierer, A., Berking, S., Bode, H., David, C. N., Flick, K., Hansmann, G., Schaller, C., and Trenker, E. 1972. Regeneration of hydra from reaggregated cells. *Nature (London) New Biol.* 239:98–101.

Sproull, F., and David, C. N. 1979. Stem cell growth and differentiation in *Hydra attenuata*. I. Regulation of self-renewal probability in multi-clone aggregates. *J. Cell Sci.* **38**:155–169.

Venugopal, G., and David, C. N. 1981. Nerve commitment in hydra. I. Role of morphogenetic signals. *Dev. Biol.* **83**:353–360.

Yaross, M., Baca, B., and Bode, H. 1982. Commitment of hydra interstitial cells to nerve cell differentiation must be initiated during S-phase. *Dev. Biol.* (in press).

Chapter 34

Separating Viable Tissue Layers

Georgia E. Lesh-Laurie

PURPOSE

Each of the two tissue layers of hydra possesses a unique and characteristic cellular composition. Therefore, viable separate layers can be used in a variety of physiological and developmental studies. I describe here three commonly used methods for isolating viable hydra endoderm and ectoderm.

INTRODUCTION

Isolated tissue layers must be free from contaminating cells of the other tissue layer. An extensive series of histological and ultrastructural investigations (Haynes and Burnett, 1963; Burnett *et al.*, 1966; Davis *et al.*, 1966; Davis 1970*a*,*b*) documents the purity of hydra endoderm isolated by the procedure described below. Isolated ectoderm, on the other hand, has not been scrutinized with transmission electron microscopy. Neither has isolated tissue layer been examined, to date, with scanning electron microscopy.

The definitive work on the isolation of the endoderm has been performed on *Hydra viridis* (Haynes and Burnett, 1963; Davis *et al.*, 1966), whereas the isolation of ectoderm has been most successful using *Hydra oligactis* or *Hydra pseudoligactis* (Lowell and Burnett, 1969).

Georgia E. Lesh-Laurie ● Department of Biology, Cleveland State University, Cleveland, Ohio.

MATERIALS

Haynes solution (Davis *et al.*, 1966): 0.1% NaCl, 0.2% $CaCl_2 \cdot 2H_2O$, 0.01% $KHCO_3$, and 0.03% $MgSO_4 \cdot 7H_2O$. M solution (Muscatine, 1961; Chapter 4); reduce pH of final solution to 2.5 with HCl.

The supply items necessary for tissue layer separation include routinely available glassware plus watchmaker's #5 forceps. In addition, if the perfusion method for separating ectoderm is selected, modify #33 hypodermic needles for the perfusion process as follows: Using a fine grinding wheel, make a hole in the side of the needle $\sim 1/3$ in. from the tip and seal the tip with an epoxy adhesive.

PROCEDURES

Isolation of Endoderm and Formation of New Ectoderm

Allow the hydra to relax approximately 1 min in M solution of pH 2.5 (Muscatine and Lenhoff, 1963). Excise the hypostome (with tentacles) and peduncle (with basal disk) and transfer the remaining cylinder of tissue to Haynes solution. Shortly after being placed in Haynes solution the ectoderm should contract until it forms a small ring surrounding a column of extended endodermal tissue. Remove the ectodermal annulus with watchmaker's forceps and place the isolated endodermal fragments into small quantities (~ 1.5–2 ml per fragment) of fresh Haynes solution (Haynes and Burnett, 1963; Burnett *et al.*, 1966; Davis *et al.*, 1966).

To observe the formation of a new ectoderm, transfer the regenerating fragments to fresh Haynes solution daily. Depending upon the temperature at which the fragments are kept, new ectoderm should form in 2–8 days (Davis *et al.*, 1966). The greatest survival of isolated endodermal fragments should occur at 8–10°C, with new ectoderm forming in 7–8 days; at room temperature the ectoderm should elaborate in 2–4 days.

Once ectoderm is evident, place the fragments in a mixture of three parts Haynes solution to one part normal hydra culture water (e.g.,see Chapter 4). On day 2, transfer the reconstitute to a solution with a ratio of Haynes to hydra culture water of 1:1; on day 3 to a 1:3 mixture; and on day 4 to hydra culture water only. Allow the fragments to continue regenerating ectoderm at room temperature. As soon as tentacles appear, start feeding the regenerates.

Because fragment sizes may vary at all steps during the isolation and reconstitution process, it is difficult to prescribe the exact amount of Haynes solution into which the fragment should be placed. We find it convenient to maintain individual fragments in spot plates with depressions holding 1.5–2 ml, until tentacles appear.

Isolation of Ectoderm: Perfusion Method
(Lowell and Burnett, 1969, 1973)

Thread a hydra onto a modified #33 hypodermic needle. The sealed tip should enter the basal disk of the animal and emerge through its mouth with the hole on the side of the needle positioned in the animal's gastrovascular cavity. To maintain the animal in this position, force a small piece of parafilm over the needle tip.

Perfuse the impaled hydra with Haynes solution at 10–15°C by attaching any convenient reservoir to the hypodermic needle. No specific rate of flow needs to be maintained; it is necessary only to keep the perfusate flowing until separation is apparent. Between 30 min and 2 hr after beginning perfusion the tissue layers should begin to separate at some point between the tentacle ring and the basal disk. The separation should proceed as a wave in all directions to give a fluid-filled space between the two layers. Normally the layers do not separate in the hypostome and tentacles, basal disk, or developing buds, and do so only partially in the peduncle. Observe the process through a dissecting microscope. If the hydra's mouth closes during perfusion, the animal may swell considerably; once the mouth opens, however, the pressure is apparently equalized and no adverse effect is noted.

Remove the separated ectoderm with watchmaker's forceps. Once manipulated the ectoderm tends to collapse, but with practice you should easily peel it away from the underlying endoderm. Some curling of the isolated ectodermal fragments may occur, presumably the result of epitheliomuscular fibers contracting. Place the isolated fragments in 3–5% Haynes solution diluted with hydra culture water (i.e., 3–5 ml Haynes solution, 95–97 ml hydra culture water).

Observe the formation of a new endoderm while maintaining the ectodermal fragments at room temperature and changing the culture medium daily. After the second day omit Haynes solution from the medium and allow the fragments to develop in hydra culture water. The temporal sequence of regeneration depends somewhat upon the region of the animal from which the ectoderm is isolated. In general, regeneration will be completed within 1 week.

Isolation of Ectoderm: Mechanical Method (Burnett *et al.*, 1973)

Place a hydra into culture water containing $10^{-5} M$ reduced glutathione to induce mouth opening. Insert a watchmaker's forceps into the mouth and through the gastrovascular cavity; then grasp the basal disk. Pull the grasped basal disk up through the mouth, everting the animal, and place it in a solution of 2% urethane (ethyl carbamate) made up in culture water. Amputate the hypostome (including tentacles) and basal disk, leaving a cylinder of everted hydra. Put one or more such everted cylinders in a vial and shake by hand; the endoderm should peel off in approximately 30 sec. Quickly place the contents of the vial in culture water, retrieve the ectodermal fragments, and with watchmaker's forceps turn them back to their original orientation, i.e., outside out.

COMMENTS AND PRECAUTIONS

The mechanical procedure is simpler and reportedly gives larger pieces of separated ectoderm than the perfusion method. It was originally performed using nitrogen-mustard-treated *H. pseudoligactis*; no confirmation of its accuracy and/or effectiveness has been published by other workers using untreated animals. The preliminary histological data presented, however, support the authors' contention that the epidermal pieces are free of gastrodermis (Burnett *et al.*, 1973).

The published methods presented for isolating ectoderm have not been as rigorously tested as have those for isolating endoderm. Take care to establish that isolated ectoderm is totally free of endodermal cells.

REFERENCES

Burnett, A. L., Davis, L. E., and Ruffing, F. E. 1966. A histological and ultrastructural study of germinal differentiation of interstitial cells arising from gland cells in *Hydra viridis*. *J. Morphol.* 120:1-8.

Burnett, A. L., Lowell, R. D., and Cyrlin, M. 1973. Regeneration of a complete *Hydra* from a single, differentiated somatic cell type, In: *Biology of Hydra* (A. L. Burnett, ed.) Academic Press, New York, pp. 255-267.

Davis, L. E. 1970a. Cell division during dedifferentiation and redifferentiation in the regenerating isolated gastrodermis of *Hydra*. *Exp. Cell Res.* 60:217-132.

Davis, L. E. 1970b. Further observations on dividing and nondividing cnidoblasts in the regenerating isolated gastrodermis of *Hydra*. *Z. Zellforsch.* 105:526-537.

Davis, L. E., Burnett, A. L., Haynes, J. F., and Mumaw, V. R. 1966. A histological and ultrastructural study of dedifferentiation and redifferentiation of digestive and gland cells in *Hydra viridis*. *Dev. Biol.* 14: 307-329.

Haynes, J. F., and Burnett, A. L. 1963. Dedifferentiation and redifferentiation of cells in *Hydra viridis*. *Science* 142:1481-1483.

Lowell, R. D., and Burnett, A. L. 1969. Regeneration of complete hydra from isolated epidermal fragments. *Biol. Bull.* 137:312-320.

Lowell, R. D., and Burnett, A. L. 1973. Regeneration from isolated epidermal explants, In: *Biology of Hydra* (A. L. Burnett, ed.) Academic Press, New York, pp. 223-232.

Muscatine, L. 1961. Symbiosis in marine and fresh water coelenterates, In: *The Biology of Hydra* (H. M. Lenhoff and W. F. Loomis, eds.), University of Miami Press, Coral Gables, Fla., pp. 255–268.

Muscatine, L., and Lenhoff, H. M. 1963. Symbiosis: On the role of algae symbiotic with hydra. *Science* **142**:956–958.

Chapter 35

Preparing Ectoderm/Endoderm Chimeras

Nancy Wanek

PURPOSE

To produce chimeric hydra consisting of ectoderm from one strain and endoderm from a different strain. The procedure involves vital staining, grafting, and microsurgery. Nitrogen mustard-treated host animals are used to support the growth of small chimeras.

INTRODUCTION

This method makes use of normal epithelial tissue movements in hydra. In grafts between two different strains, such movements produce small chimeric regions near the graft junction. The chimeric region is visible when a polyp with vitally stained ectoderm and endoderm is grafted to an unmarked polyp. Tissue recruitment into regions of morphogenetic activity (e.g., tentacle bases, budding region) sometimes results in a displacement of the tissue layers relative to one another (Campbell, 1974). When this displacement occurs in the grafted specimens, the stained ectoderm of one polyp can be seen overlying the unmarked endoderm of the other polyp (see Fig. 1). In this procedure, the chimeric region is excised and allowed to regenerate and form a whole chimeric animal.

Nancy Wanek ● Developmental Biology Center and Department of Developmental and Cell Biology, University of California, Irvine, California. Current Address: Department of Biology, and Health Science, Chapman College, Orange, California.

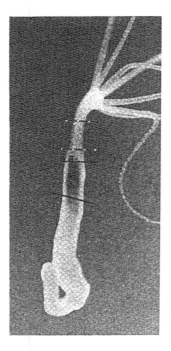

FIGURE 1. Tissue displacement in grafted vitally stained animals to form chimeric region. This photograph was taken 10 days after a vitally stained ring of normal *H. attentuata* was grafted into an unmarked *twisted column* polyp (Chapter 29). The ectoderm (speckled black marks) has moved distally relative to the endoderm (diffuse gray marks). Lines indicate where cuts should be made to isolate chimeric regions. The tissue between the dotted lines consists of normal ectoderm/ twisted column endoderm. The tissue between the unbroken lines consists of twisted column ectoderm/normal endoderm.

When the chimeric region is very small, it is useful to graft it to a nitrogen mustard-treated (NM-treated) host animal. These hydra are able to feed and build up food reserves. In such host animals, the graft tissue proliferates while the NM-treated tissue does not. Eventually, the graft tissue overgrows the host tissue.

MATERIALS

India ink; glass micropipets; polyethylene tubing; microscalpels; watch-maker's forceps; fish line, 12 lb; polyethylene tubing, P.E. 20; sticky wax; 2% urethan in M solution.

For vital staining with India ink, see Chapter 24; for grafting, see Chapter 30.

PROCEDURES

Grafting

These procedures routinely yield a workable percentage of chimeric regions. The most optimal location for the graft junction, however, varies with different strains of hydra. Thus, for a particular combination of strains make the grafts at different levels on the body column to determine the best location.

Example: Chimera of Strain A Ectoderm/Strain B Endoderm. Mark with India ink (Chapter 24) the ectoderm of the upper one-fourth to one-half of the gastric region of 20 polyps of strain A 1 day prior to grafting. It is important to mark the ectoderm in a complete ring around the body. Now mark the endoderm by injecting India ink into the gastric cavity shortly after the animal has ingested food. Allow ink to remain in the gastric region for 1 hr; then flush both food and ink from the cavity. This procedure gives a lightly marked endoderm. Using microscalpels, make two cuts within the marked region on a polyp of strain A. Be sure that the ectoderm of the ring of tissue is entirely marked. Make a single cut in the "neck" or subhypostomal region of a strain B polyp. String the strain B head, strain A ring, and strain B body onto the fish line. Push all the pieces together using a polyethylene sleeve at each end. Keep the pieces on the fish line for 1 hr, or until the graft junctions have healed. Examine them daily for chimeric regions. The rate of formation of chimeric regions varies. Chimeric regions which are 0.5 mm or longer are suitable for isolation.

Isolating Chimeric Region

Relax the hydra by placing it in a small, low dish, such as a cover of a 35 × 10-mm Petri dish, filled with 2% urethan (Macklin, 1976) in M solution. After about 1 min, carefully check the location of ink marks all around the body column. The chimeric regions will probably be uneven. Using a microscapel, isolate a small ring by making two cuts within the chimeric region. As soon as the cuts have been made, transfer the isolate to M solution.

Regeneration of Chimeric Region

Isolates which are 0.5 mm or longer will regenerate tentacle bumps within about 4 days after isolation. Feed these regenerates fragments of *Artemia* nauplii using glass micropipet.

Use of NM-Treated Hosts

If an isolate is smaller then 0.5 mm, the regenerate will be so tiny that it will be almost impossible to feed. Thus, implant such small isolates onto NM-treated host animals almost immediately after isolating the chimeric region.

Place a small piece of sticky wax on the bottom of a Petri dish. Fill the dish with M solution. Make a groove about the width of a hydra in the wax with a forceps. Transfer the isolated chimeric region into the dish. Select a host animal (Chapter 40 and below) and cut a slit in the gastric region. Be sure the slit is about the same size as the piece to be implanted. Place the host animal in the groove. Carefully position the implant into the slit. With the forceps, pinch a flap of wax from one side of the groove and bend it to cover over the host and implant, as with a blanket, to hold the implant in place while the tissue heals. Remove host and implant from the wax groove within about a half-hour.

The implant does not have to be reisolated. The NM blocks any further cell divisions in the host hydra. The implant cells will continue to divide and grow. Eventually the NM-treated tissue will be sloughed off of the hydra and the polyp will consist entirely of the chimeric tissue (Wanek and Campbell, 1982).

Nitrogen Mustard Treatment

The maximum concentration of NM that the hydra will survive varies among different strains of hydra. Select a range of concentrations and treat different groups of animals. The directions given are for *Hydra attenuata* fasted 24 hr before treatment. For details of the method, reagents, and supplies, see Chapter 40.

Place 10 ml M solution into a 50-ml beaker. Add 30 μl 10% NM solution. Check the pH with litmus paper. Use 0.1 N NaOH to adjust to pH 7.0. Add hydra to the beaker and treat them for 10 min. Transfer the hydra to a 50-ml beaker filled with M solution, swirl them, and transfer them to the next beaker. Wash the animals with three fresh changes of M solution. One hour later, repeat the washing procedure three times.

Use treated animals as hosts for implants at any time after treatment. Set aside control animals from each treatment and care for them as you do for host animals.

One week after the treatment, macerate (see Chapter 20) several control animals to examine for interstitial cells. The absence of interstitial cells indicates that the treatment was sufficient to block further cell divisions in the epithelial cells (R. Campbell, personal communication).

A more rigorous evaluation of the effectiveness of the NM treatment can be done 2 weeks after the treatment. Inject several control animals with a single pulse of 50 μCi/ml [^{3}H]thymidine. Macerate the tissue and prepare the cells for autoradiography (see Chapter 21). The epithelial cells of the NM-treated animals should not incorporate any [^{3}H]thymidine.

PRECAUTIONS

When using NM, wear plastic gloves and use the hood. Place everything that touches nitrogen mustard into a wash beaker of 2% $Na_2S_2O_3$ for 24 hr. Such items can then be discarded or washed with water.

REFERENCES

Campbell, R. D. 1974. Cell movements in *Hydra. Am. Zool.* **14**:523–535.

Macklin, M. 1976. The effect of urethan on hydra. *Biol. Bull.* **150**:442–452.

Wanek, N. and Campbell, R. D. 1982. Roles of ectodermal and endodermal epithelial cells in hydra morphogenesis: construction of chimeric strains. *J. Exp. Zool.* **221**:37–47.

Part VIII

Manipulating Cellular Composition
in Vivo

Eliminating All Nonepithelial Cells Using Colchicine

Beverly A. Marcum and Richard D. Campbell

PURPOSE

To eliminate the interstitial cell population of hydra using colchicine treatments (Campbell, 1976; Marcum and Campbell, 1978). The resulting viable animals consist only of two layers of epithelial cells plus the noncellular mesoglea. These animals are termed epithelial hydra.

INTRODUCTION

Species of hydra respond differently to extended exposures to colchicine with regard to losing their interstitial and nerve cells. The animals most amenable to this colchicine treatment belong to the group that includes *Hydra attenuata* and *Hydra magnipapillata* (Chapter 3). It is possible to reduce the number of interstitial cells in *Hydra viridis* using alternate treatments with colchicine and hydroxyurea (Chapter 39), but epithelial hydra have not yet been produced in any of these other groups of hydra using colchicine. Our method, thus far, applies to *Hydra attenuata*. Perhaps other species will respond to modifications in colchicine concentration, treatment time and spacing, or culture medium. Colcemid, an analog of colchicine, can also be used to eliminate cell types from *H. attenuata*.

Beverly A. Marcum ● Department of Biological Sciences, California State University, Chico, California . Richard D. Campbell ● Department of Developmental and Cell Biology, University of California, Irvine, California.

MATERIALS

Colchicine (Sigma Chemical Co.), stored as powder in the dark until ready for use [culture medium, M solution (Chapter 4)], containing 50 μg/ml Rifampicin antibiotic (Sigma). A stock solution of 500 μg/ml Rifampicin in M solution may be stored several weeks at 4°C and diluted daily for use. Maceration fluid and supplies (Chapter 20).

PROCEDURES

Single Colchicine Treatment

Prepare a fresh 0.4% solution of colchicine in culture medium (a 0.04% solution of colcemid is effective). Place hydra in the colchicine solution in a Petri dish at a density of 5 hydra per milliliter or less. As many as 500 hydra in one vessel have been successfully treated in our laboratory. After 8 hr,

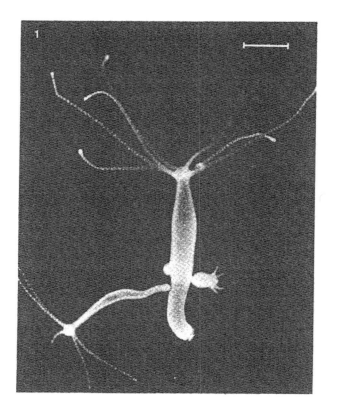

FIGURE 1. Control *H. attenuata*. Bodies are elongated with prominent hypostomes. Tentacles are long and contain batteries of nematocytes. Scale bar: 1 mm.

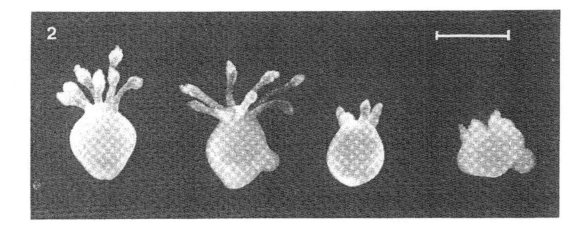

FIGURE 2. *H. attenuata* after 8 hr of colchicine treatment. Bodies are contracted and beginning to swell. Notice cellular debris at the hypostome (far right) from cell sloughing within the gastric cavity. Scale bar: 1 mm.

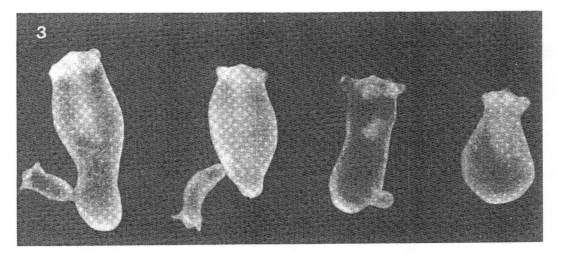

FIGURE 3. *H. attenuata* 1 day following colchicine treatment. Bodies are swollen, and cellular debris accumulates in the gastric cavity. Tentacles are short knobs. Scale bar: 1mm.

wash hydra by serial transfer five times with fresh medium. Finally transfer to culture medium containing Rifampicin and wash the animals twice a day for 5 days. Without Rifampicin the hydra become infected with bacteria and die.

Observations

Treatment with colchicine causes the hydra's tentacles to shorten, bodies to round up, and cells to slough off as shown in Figs 1–3. Some cellular debris will accumulate in the gastric cavity and will be periodically expelled into the surrounding medium. After approximately 1 week the hydra will begin to regenerate tentacles and the body column will elongate somewhat. The tissue will appear transparent and the animals will become slightly swollen. The tentacles will appear thin and will lack nematocytes.

Double Treatment with Colchicine

The first treatment eliminates 95–99% of all nonepithelial cells. The remaining ones may be eliminated by treating the same hydra with colchicine a second time 10–15 days later. The time of the second treatment may vary according to the state of recovery of the animals from the first treatment.

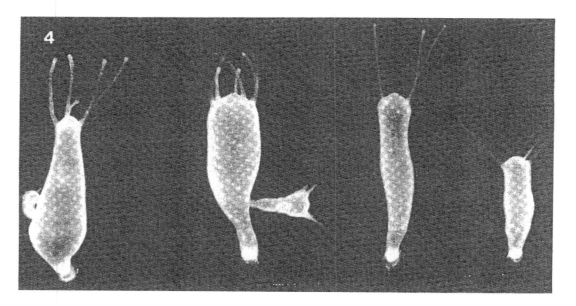

FIGURE 4. Epithelial *H. attenuata* 1.5 weeks after 2nd colchicine treatment. Tentacles have regenerated but are thin and devoid of nematocytes. These animals have been fed daily since the 5th day after the 1st colchicine treatment. Scale bar: 1mm.

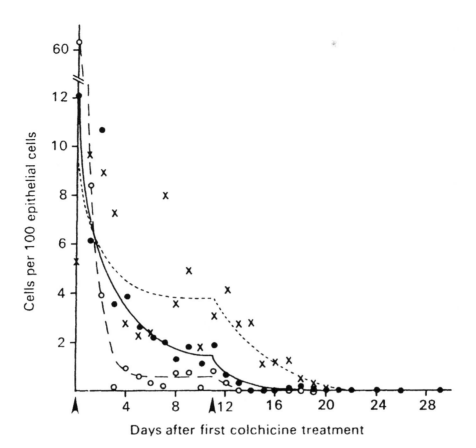

FIGURE 5. Time course of cell disappearance following colchicine treatment. The population levels of nerve cells (●, solid line), interstitial cells (○, broken line), and endodermal gland cells (X, dotted line) are expressed relative to epithelial cell number. Colchicine treatments (0.4%, 8 hr) were given on days 0 and 11 (arrows). From Marcum and Campbell, 1978.

Apply the second treatment after the hydra have regenerated tentacles and have ceased sloughing cells. Their response to the second tretment and their patterns of recovery should be similar to those of the first. Treated animals may be fed during the period of time between treatments if large budding animals are desired (Chapter 37). However, feeding is not necessary to obtain healthy epithelial animals. Unfed hydra 1.5 weeks after a double colchicine treatment are shown in Fig. 4.

Monitoring Cell Loss

Monitor cell elimination by periodically (e.g., daily) macerating several polyps (Chapter 20) and counting the number of cells present. Figure 5 illustrates typical changes in cell abundance in *H. attenuata* of interstitial cells, nerve cells, and endodermal gland cells relative to the epithelial cell number.

Establishing Clones of Epithelial Hydra

Force feed (Chapter 37) daily a few treated hydra beginning on day 5 after the first colchicine treatment. Discontinue feeding for the first 3 days immediately following the second colchicine treatment. Within 1–2 weeks the animals should begin to bud. Feed new buds as soon as they develop a mouth, and continue until each parent has produced two to three buds. Keep each clone in a separate dish. Macerate individual buds of each clone on separate microscope slides (Chapter 20). Examine at least 2000 cells of each bud; continue culturing and sampling only those clones having buds showing no interstitial cells upon maceration. If three successive buds in a clone are found to be free of all nonepithelial cells, then that clone can be considered as an epithelial one. Sample a bud from each clone for nonepithelial cells once monthly thereafter. The double colchicine treatment should completely eliminate the interstitial cells in at least 50% of the *H. attenuata* treated.

REFERENCES

Campbell, R. D. 1976. Elimination of *Hydra* interstitial and nerve cells by means of colchicine. *J. Cell Sci.* **21**:1–13.

David, C. N. 1973. A quantitative method for maceration of hydra tissue. *Wilhelm Roux Arch. Entwicklungsmech. Org.* **171**:159–268.

Marcum, B. A., and Campbell, R. D. 1978. Development of hydra lacking nerve and interstitial cells. *J. Cell Sci.* **29**:17–33.

Chapter 37

Culturing Epithelial Hydra

Beverly A. Marcum

PURPOSE

To culture and care for epithelial hydra, i.e., animals that cannot capture or ingest prey independently and cannot digest or eliminate particulate waste normally.

INTRODUCTION

Epithelial hydra can be produced by a variety of methods, including colchicine treatment and gamma irradiation (Campbell, 1976, Fradkin *et al.*, 1978; Chapters 36, 38–41) and inbreeding (Sugiyama and Fujisawa, 1978). These hydra consist of ectodermal and endodermal epithelial cells separated by the acellular mesoglea. They completely lack nerve cells, nematocytes, interstitial cells, gland and mucous cells, and gametes (Wanek, *et al.*, 1980). Without nematocytes and nerve cells, epithelial hydra cannot capture prey or coordinate feeding behavior, and without gland cells digestion is reduced. It is possible, however, to rear these animals by force-feeding them with brine shrimp nauplii. Also, because they cannot contract, they cannot force out any undigested material from their gastric cavities. The accumulated wastes lead to excessive bacterial growth, and if not flushed out, these hydra die. Both the force-feeding and the flushing procedure can be accomplished utilizing a simply constructed mouth pipet with a polyethylene tip.

Beverly A. Marcum ● Department of Biological Sciences, California State University, Chico, California.

MATERIALS

Brine shrimp nauplii–use animals less than 1 day old because they have more yolk granules (Chapter 6); polyethylene tubine (Clay Adams, Inc. Intramedic) (inner diameter 0.047 in., outer diameter 0.067 in.; mouth pipet–15 in. of Tygon tubing (inner diameter 1/16 in.) slipped over a polished Pasteur pipet; M solution (Chapter 4) containing $50\mu g/ml$ rifampicin antibiotic (Sigma Chemical Co.).

PROCEDURES

Preparing the Feeding Pipet

Cut a short length (2–3 in.) of polyethylene tubing. Hold it briefly over a very small flame. Draw the tubing into a fine strand by gently pulling on the two ends. Cut the strand where it has the proper diameter to accommodate the tail end of a brine shrimp nauplius, but where it is not wide enough to allow the head to pass. Connect the feeding tip to a mouthpiece, such as a Pasteur pipet, using about 12–14 in. of Tygon tubing.

Force-Feeding Epithelial Hydra

Opening the Mouth. Place hydra in a Petri dish and observe it using a dissecting microscope. Gently grasp the base of the hydra with fine jeweler's forceps (#5 point) in one hand. This process usually causes the animal to contract and open its mouth. If the mouth does not open at first, apply a little more pressure or poke the hydra. If the mouth still does not open, place the tip of the feeding pipet on the hypostome, apply gentle suction, and pull on the hypostome. As soon as the mouth opens, blow a gentle stream of culture solution into the gastric cavity. This stream cleans the gastric cavity, causes the hydra to swell, and opens its mouth wider.

Inserting the Shrimp (Fig. 1). When the hydra is in the proper position (contracted and mouth open) quickly pick up a shrimp nauplius, break the exoskeleton, and open the yolk sac by slightly crushing the shrimp against the forceps with which you are still holding the hydra. Insert the shrimp into the gastric cavity and release it from the feeding tip by gently blowing into the mouth pipet. The yolk sac must be broken to release yolk particles into the gastric cavity; otherwise none of the material will be digested. Also, the

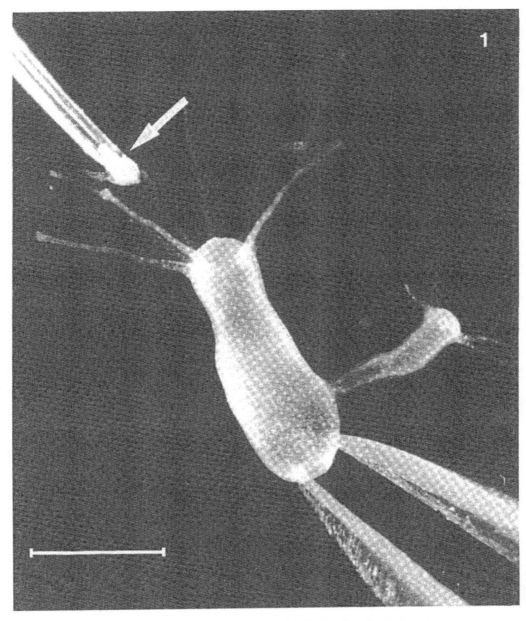

FIGURE 1. Feeding technique for epithelial hydra. Scale bar: 1 mm.

shrimp must be deposited entirely inside the hydra or it will slip back out through the mouth.

Quantity of Food. Feed adult hydra as many shrimp (5–15) as will fit inside a gastric cavity. Feed new buds as soon as possible after they have developed a mouth. Usually, one well-crushed shrimp suffices for a single feeding of new buds. When feeding many shrimp to one hydra, insert the shrimp into the gastric cavity rapidly while the hydra is contracted. Once the animal begins to elongate, it is more difficult to push the shrimp through the mouth.

Removing Undigested Food. Use a mouth pipet apparatus and a polyethylene tip with a slightly larger bore than that used for feeding. Insert the pipet tip into the hydra's mouth and blow a gentle stream of culture medium into the gastric cavity until all food debris has been expelled.

Maintaining a Health Epithelial Hydra. Health epithelial hydra have long tentacles and a translucent body column. Whenever the tentacles become short or opacity develops in the body, postpone feeding and continue to flush the hydra daily with culture solution containing Rifampicin. Continue this treatment until the animals recover. If animals are to be maintained without feeding, the gastric cavity should still be flushed daily to remove accumulated cell debris, relieve osmotic pressure, and prevent bacterial infection. Maintain the cultures at 18°C; at this temperature animals, if flushed daily, survive without food for up to 3 weeks.

REFERENCES

Campbell, R. D. 1976. Elimination of *Hydra* interstitial and nerve cells by means of colchicine. *J. Cell Sci.* 21:1–13.

Fradkin, M., Kakis, H., and Campbell, R. D. 1978. Effect of irradiation of hydra: Elimination of interstitial cells from viable hydra. *Radiat. Res.* 76:187–797.

Sugiyama, T., and Fujisawa, T. 1978. Genetic analysis of developmental mechanisms in hydra. II. Isolation and characterization of an interstitial cell-deficient strain. *J. Cell Sci.* 29:35–52.

Wanek, N., Marcum, B. A., and Campbell, R. D. 1980. Histological structure of epithelial hydra and evidence for the complete absence of interstitial and nerve cells. *J. Exp. Zool.* 212:1–11.

Chapter 38

Reducing Populations of Interstitial Cells and Nematoblasts with Hydroxyurea

Hans R. Bode

PURPOSE

To lower selectively and reversibly the number of interstitial cells and nematoblasts in live hydra.

INTRODUCTION

Hydroxyurea (HU) kills cells in the S phase of the cell cycle and blocks the transition of cells from G_1 to S in many different cell types (Sinclair, 1965). Since 50% of the interstitial cell cycle is S phase (Campbell and David, 1974) compared to 20% of the epithelial cell cycle (David and Campbell, 1972) in hydra, HU can be used to reduce the interstitial cell population selectively. In theory, by treating the hydra with a regime in which they are exposed to three 24-hr cycles of HU followed by 12 hr in culture solution, all of the interstitial cells and 70% of the epithelial cells should be killed. In fact, this regime reduces the interstitial cell population to 1–5% of normal and leave the number of epithelial cells practically unaffected (Bode *et al.*, 1976).

Hans R. Bode ● Developmental Biology Center and Department of Developmental and Cell Biology, University of California, Irvine, California.

MATERIALS

HU made to 0.1 M in culture solution; this stock solution can be stored indefinitely at 4°C.

PROCEDURES

Prepare culture solution containing 0.01 M HU. Place specimens of *Hydra attenuata* in the HU-culture solution and feed and wash the animals for the duration of the treatment. After the animals are washed with fresh culture solution, add sufficient stock HU to bring its concentration back to 0.01 M. Animals can be exposed to HU for 1–3 days or by using an alternating regime in which the animals are exposed to HU for 24 hr followed by 12 hr in culture solution. 2–3 cycles are normal. These hydra should remain healthy and continue to feed and bud normally.

Results of a typical experiment (Fig. 1) show that the populations of all cell types, except the epithelial ones, decreased to some extent and later recovered. The interstitial cell population was reduced to 1–5% of normal between 6 and 8 days of treatment; after this time it eventually returned to normal. Dividing nematoblasts, which are more sensitive to HU, were reduced to zero within 3 days of treatment. The nematoblast population dropped almost as fast. Subsequently, nematocytes dropped in number, which is to be expected as they are derived from nematoblasts. Recovery of all three populations followed that of the interstitial cell population. The nerve cell population was less affected since nerves turn over relatively slowly.

COMMENTS

The cellular effects of treating *Hydra attenuata* with HU have been examined extensively by Bode *et al.* (1976). It greatly reduces DNA synthesis. On removal of HU, DNA synthesis resumes. Similarly, mitotic activity ceases by the 2nd day after the hydra are exposed to HU, and resumes on removal of the drug. Dividing nematoblasts are more sensitive to lower concentrations of HU than dividing epithelial or interstitial cells.

Hydra exposed to a long nonalternating treatment of HU, say, for 4 days, are affected irreversibly. These animals cease to feed and bud within a few days after the end of the treatment. They acquire the bloated appearance typical of animals free of both interstitial cells and nerve cells as obtained with colchicine treatment (Chapter 20). A 5-day HU treatment produces hydra having no interstitial cells.

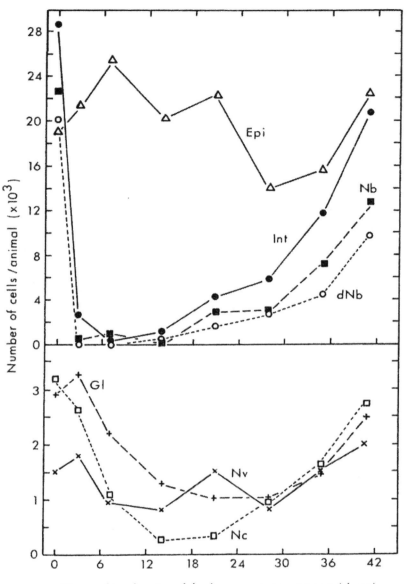

FIGURE 1. Change in cell populations size of seven cell types with time after a 2-day alternating regime of hydroxyurea treatment. Epithelial cells (△. solid line); interstitial cells (●, solid line); dividing nematoblasts (○. dotted line); nematoblasts (■, broken line); nematocytes (□, dotted line); nerve cells (×, solid line); gland cells (+, broken line). Numbers are for whole animal minus the head and buds which were removed. Reprinted from Bode *et al.* (1976) with permission.

The effects of a given treatment occasionally vary and probably depend on the health of the animals. Less healthy animals are more severely affected in terms of decrease and/or loss of the interstitial cell population than are healthy animals. Animals devoid of interstitial cells have been obtained with the alternating HU regime (Sacks and Davis, 1979). In our hands this treatment occasionally resulted in no, or a very slow, recovery of the interstitial cell population in all the treated animals.

REFERENCES

Bode, H. R., Flick, K. M., and Smith, G. S. 1976. Regulation of interstitial cell differentiation in *Hydra attenuata*. I. Homeostatic control of interstitial cell population size. *J. Cell Sci.* 20:29–46.

Campbell, R. D., and David, C. N. 1974. Cell cycle kinetics and development of *Hydra attenuata*. II. Interstitial cells. *J. Cell Sci.* 16:349–358.

David, C. N., and Campbell, R. D. 1972. Cell cycle kinetics and development of *Hydra attenuata*. I. Epithelial cells. *J. Cell Sci.* 11:557–568.

Sacks, P. G., and Davis, L. E. 1979. Production of nerveless *Hydra attentuata* by hydroxurea treatments. *J. Cell Sci.* 37:189–203.

Sinclair, W. I. 1965. Hydroxyurea: Differential lethal effects on cultured mammalian cells during the cell cycle. *Science* 150:1729–1731.

Chapter 39

Preparing *Hydra viridis* with Nerve Cells and No Interstitial Cells, or with Neither of These Cell Types

Patricia Novak

PURPOSE

To prepare specimens of *Hydra viridis* that either contain the normal number of nerve cells and no interstitial cells, or lack nerve cells as well as i cells and their derivative cells.

INTRODUCTION

Hydra viridis does not respond to colchicine to give epithelial animals as does *Hydra attenuata* (Chapter 36). By using a modification of the hydroxyurea (HU) method of Bode (Chapter 38) in combination with the colchicine method of Marcum and Campbell (Chapter 36), it is possible to produce either of the types of hydra described above.

MATERIALS

Standard laboratory glassware, microscopes, 0.1 M HU made up in M solution, and 0.5 M colchicine made up in M solution.

Patricia Novak ● Department of Developmental and Cell Biology, University of California, Irvine, California.

PROCEDURE

Grow the hydra at 10°C for at least 4 weeks so that they will increase in size (Hecker and Slobodkin, 1976). Place these hydra in a Petri dish, draw off all the M solution with a pipet, add 0.1 M HU made in M solution so that the density is 5–10 hydra/ml solution, and let the hydra remain in that solution for 6 hr.

Wash the animals in several rinses of M solution and place them for an additional 6 hr in the Petri dish now containing M solution. Repeat this alternating regime of 6 hr in HU and 6 hr in M solution for 6–7 days.

At the end of this period, the animals should have retained all of their nerve cells, whereas their interstitial cells should have dropped from 35% to 0.2% of the total cell population with a small percentage of nematocytes still remaining.

To also eliminate the nerve cells, on day 7 or 8, treat these animals for 8 hr with 0.5% colchicine made in M solution (Chapter 4).

COMMENTS

Hydra viridis are normally about one-fourth the size of the average brown hydra. Usually after hydra have been treated to remove their i cells and/or nerve cells, the animals become extremely small and are difficult to maintain. Thus, that is why we grow the green hydra at cold temperatures to increase their size before treating them with HU or colchicine.

To test the effectiveness of your procedures, remove sample animals at various times during treatment and determine the number of each cell type present using the maceration technique (Chapter 20).

These animals appear to repopulate themselves with i cells when they are force-fed (Chapter 37) within 4 weeks; therefore, it is advisable to use them for experiments as soon as they look healthy enough to manipulate following the treatment with colchicine.

REFERENCES

Bode, H. R., Flick, K. M., and Smith, G. S. 1976. Regulation of interstitial cell differentiation in *Hydra attenuata*. I. Homeostatic control of interstitial cell population size. *J. Cell Sci.* 20:29–46.

Campbell, R. D. 1976. Elimination of *Hydra* interstitial and nerve cells by means of colchicine. *J. Cell Sci.* 21:1–13.

David, C. N. 1973. A quantitative method for maceration of hydra tissue. *Wilhelm Roux Arch. Entwicklungsmech. Org.* 171:257–268.

Hecker, B., and Slobodkin, L. B. 1976. Responses of *Hydra oligactis* to temperature and feeding rate. In: *Coelenterate Ecology and Behavior* (G. O. Mackie, ed.), Plenum Press, New York, pp. 175–183.

Marcum, B. A., and Campbell, R. D. 1978. Development of hydra lacking nerve and interstitial cells. *J. Cell Sci.* **29**:17–33.

Chapter 40

Eliminating Interstitial Cells with Nitrogen Mustard

Charles N. David

PURPOSE

To remove interstitial cells and differentiating nematoblasts from hydra leaving a shell of epithelial and gland cells.

INTRODUCTION

Treatment of hydra with nitrogen mustard (NM) causes the rapid elimination of interstitial cells and differentiating nemotoblasts from the tissue (Diehl and Burnett, 1964). Such hydra have been used to investigate the role of interstitial cells in budding and regeneration (Diehl and Burnett, 1965a,b). In addition, NM-treated hydra have been used as feeder layers for the culture of interstitial cells added to them by grafting (Diehl and Burnett, 1966) or reaggregation techniques (David and Murphy, 1977). The method, described here for *Hydra attenuata*, is essentially that of Diehl and Burnett (1964), who used *Hydra pseudoligactis* and *Hydra pirardi*.

Charles N. David ● Department of Molecular Biology, Albert Einstein College of Medicine. Bronx, New York.

COMMENTS

NM is a potent alkylating agent capable of adding ethyl residues to nucleic acids including DNA (see Goodman and Gilman, 1974, for review). It is strongly cytotoxic to proliferating cells; nonproliferating or slowly proliferating cells appear to be less affected.

NM acts on cells at any stage of the cell cycle. Progression through the cycle, however, is usually blocked in the G_2 (premitotic) phase. Cells blocked in G_2 continue synthesizing RNA and protein and often become enlarged due to unbalanced growth.

Treatment of hydra with 0.01% NM for 10 min leads to the disappearance from hydra tissue of interstitial cells and differentiating nematoblasts over the next 4–8 days. This process can be easily monitored by observing interstitial cells in whole mounts of hydra stained with Toluidine Blue (Diehl and Burnett, 1964) or by counting interstitial cells in macerations of treated animals (David, 1973). Subsequently the number of differentiated nerves and nematocytes also declines. By comparison, the epithelial and gland cell populations appear to be less affected. Five days after NM treatment, hydra consist of a shell of epithelial and gland cells, and in this condition they survive for 4 weeks or longer.

The effects of NM on hydra cells are best explained with reference to the proliferation kinetics of hydra cell types. Interstitial cells are rapidly proliferating cells with generation times of 18–27 hr (Campbell and David, 1974). They are rapidly killed by NM and eliminated from hydra tissue, probably by phagocytosis by epithelial cells. Epithelial cells have cell generation times of 3 days in well-fed hydra and more than 6 days in starving hydra (David and Campbell, 1972). They are also killed by NM, but because of their longer cell cycle they survive longer than interstitial cells and thus give rise to animals consisting only of epithelial cells. Gland cells have a similar cell cycle to that of epithelial cells and also survive for long periods in NM-treated hydra.

MATERIALS

Two percent (w/v) sodium thiosulfate and 0.01% NM (Sigma Chemical Co.,). *Special precaution*: NM is toxic and should be handled with care. Carry out as much of the procedure as possible in a fume hood. In addition, have 1–2 liters of 2% sodium thiosulfate solution available to detoxify any spilled NM solution as well as any unused reagent.

PROCEDURES

Because NM is unstable in water, prepare the reagent from the dry powder immediately before use. Add NM to hydra at a final concentration of 0.01%. Mix the solution thoroughly by stirring with a pipet, taking care that all hydra are in suspension and not stuck to the sides of the dish. After 10 min allow the hydra to settle, decant the solution and fill the dish with fresh medium. Repeat the washing procedure four times to stop the action of NM on the hydra. Thereafter wash the hydra at least once each day in order to remove dead hydra and debris from the dish.

After NM treatment hydra can be fed for about a week until their nematocytes are depleted (Diehl and Burnett, 1964). However, feeding stimulates cell cycling and accelerates the death of treated animals. If the purpose of NM treatment is to prepare hydra free of interstitial cells, then one feeding after NM treatment appears to optimally stimulate the disappearance of interstitial cells without adversely affecting the survival of the host animal.

A final concentration of 0.01% NM is usually effective in completely eliminating interstitial cells from tissue without immediately destroying the animals. However, the precise concentration of NM required to eliminate interstitial cells varies slightly between batches of NM. Thus, it is useful to test several concentrations when using a freshly opened bottle of NM. If, after prolonged use, the NM in a bottle loses some of its potency, increase the concentration of NM used in experiments. However, do not use more NM than necessary because it does destroy epithelial cells and thus may noticeably shorten the survival of treated animals.

SPECIAL APPLICATIONS

NM-treated hydra free of interstitial cells are useful hosts in which to study the fate of interstitial cells added to them by grafting or reaggregation techniques. When normal hydra tissue is grafted into NM-treated tissue, interstitial cells migrate from the normal tissue into the NM tissue, where they proliferate and differentiate normally (Diehl and Burnett, 1966). Interstitial cells can also be introduced into NM tissue by preparing aggregates from dissociated NM-treated hydra (David and Murphy, 1977). Such aggregates regenerate normal hydra structures. When small amounts of normal tissue are dissociated and added to such NM aggregates, the added interstitial cells proliferate and differentiate normally. The number of cells seeded in such aggregates can be easily controlled, and the aggregates function effectively as tiny tissue culture dishes (see Chapter 33).

REFERENCES

Campbell, R. D., and David, C. N. 1974. Cell cycle kinetics and development of *Hydra attenuata*. II. Interstitial cells. *J. Cell Sci.* **16**:349–358.

David, C. N. 1973. A quantitative method for maceration of hydra tissue. *Wilhelm Roux Arch. Entwicklungsmech. Org.* **171**:259–268.

David, C. N., and Campbell, R. D. 1972. Cell cycle kinetics and development of *Hydra attenuata*. I Epithelial cells. *J. Cell Sci.* **11**:577–568.

David, C. N., and Murphy, S. 1977. Characterization of interstitial stem cells in hydra by cloning. *Dev. Biol.* **58**:372–383.

Diehl, F., and Burnett, A. L. 1964. The role of interstitial cells in the maintenance of hydra. I. Specific destruction of interstitial cells in normal, sexual and non-budding animals. *J. Exp. Zool.* **155**:253–259.

Diehl, F., and Burnett, A. L. 1965*a*. The role of interstitial cells in the maintenance of hydra. II. Budding. *J. Exp. Zool.* **158**:283–298.

Diehl, F., and Burnett, A. L. 1965*b*. The role of interstitial cells in the maintenance of hydra. III. Regeneration of hypostome and tentacles. *J. Exp. Zool.* **158**:299–318.

Diehl, F., and Burnett, A. L. 1966. The role of interstitial cells in the maintenance of hydra. IV. Migration of interstitial cells in homografts and heterografts. *J. Exp. Zool.* **163**:125–140.

Goodman, L. S., and Gilman, A. 1974. *The Pharmacological Basis of Therapeutics.* Macmillan, New York.

Chapter 41

Altering Cell Population Levels by Gamma Irradiation

Cheng-Mei Fradkin

PURPOSE

To produce viable hydra with few or no interstitial cells and interstitial cell derivatives (Fradkin *et al.*, 1977).

INTRODUCTION

Advantages of gamma irradiation over chemical treatments for the removal of interstitial cells are: (1) The treatment itself is simple. (2) There are few harmful side effects on the animals. In comparison, colchicine treatment (Chapter 36) leaves the hydra in a depressed state for several days, whereas gamma irradiation has no apparent immediate effects on the hydra's physiological state. No discernible long-lasting effects on the epithelial cells are detected. (3) It is a simple procedure to produce many animals free of interstitial cells, and it can also be used to produce hydra containing nerve cells but no interstitial cells.

Cheng-Mei Fradkin ● Department of Developmental and Cell Biology, University of California, Irvine, California.

303

MATERIALS

The source of gamma rays should deliver 3–8 krad. We use Model M38-2 gammator (Isomedix Inc., Parsippany, NJ 07059). The irradiation source in this model is ^{137}Cs. *Hydra attenuata* or related species can be used.

PROCEDURES

Place hydra in groups of 10 animals in 35-mm plastic Petri dishes containing 5 ml of culture fluid. Irradiate with doses in the range of 3.5–5.5 krad at a rate of 1 krad/min. After irradiating the hydra, place them in larger dishes and culture them normally.

After 2 weeks examine the cultures for three classes of animals: (1) Hydra with a normal appearance, including normal coloration and long, mobile tentacles with nematocysts. These hydra will recover. (2) Hydra permanently contracted, richly colored, with short, stubby, nematocyst-laden tentacles. These hydra will die. (3) Hydra which are thin, swollen, and nearly transparent, with slender tentacles lacking nematocysts (see Fig. 4 of Chapter 36). These are viable hydra with few or no interstitial cells. Culture them in separate dishes using the method of force feeding (Chapter 37). As each polyp gives rise to a clone by budding, macerate a few individuals (Chapter 20) to determine whether the clones are free of interstitial cells.

When trying this method on a species other than *H. attenuata*, find the highest dose of irradiation that will produce several of these i-cell-free hydra and at the same time will not destroy most of the animals.

PRECAUTIONS

Because different species and strains do not respond to gamma irradiation in the same way, try a range of doses. Two successive treatments (of 2-week intervals) may be more effective than a single treatment. The dosage is affected by the age of the gamma source and the distance of the source to the animal. The effectiveness of irradiation is also affected by the rate of irradiation.

REFERENCES

Fradkin, M., Kakis, H., and Campbell, R. D. 1977. Effects of gamma-irradiation of *Hydra*: Elimination of interstitial cells from viable hydra. *Radiat. Res.* 76:187–197.

Chapter 42

Reducing Number of Nematocytes
in the Tentacles

G. Scott Smith and Hans R. Bode

PURPOSE

To reduce the number of all types of nematocytes in the tentacles of many hydra or, using a few hydra, the number of those nematocytes housing only stenotele nematocysts.

INTRODUCTION

Since more than 95% of all nematocytes are mounted in the tentacles (Bode and Flick, 1976), the methods for reducing their numbers focus on their removal from the tentacles. The methods are based on means that induce the discharge of the nematocysts and the subsequent sloughing of the spent nematocytes. There is an extensive literature on agents that will cause nematocyst discharge (see Pantin, 1942; Picken and Skaer, 1966; Mariscal, 1974). Our two methods take advantage of a finding by Lentz and Barnett (1962), who showed that fructose-1,6-diphosphate specifically enhanced the discharge of stenoteles. One is highly specific for stenotele discharge, but is slow because it requires treatment of individual animals. The other is rapid and easily applied to a large number of animals, but is less specific in the number and type of nematocysts discharged.

G. Scott Smith and Hans R. Bode Developmental Biology Center and Department of Developmental and Cell Biology, University of California, Irvine, California.

MATERIALS

M solution; Hydra medium consisting of 1×10^{-3} M $CaCl_2$, 1.25×10^{-5} M Na_2 EDTA, and 1×10^{-3} M $NaHCO_3$, pH 7.5-8.0; 2.4×10^{-2} M fructose-1,6-diphosphate (Ba^+ salt, Nutritional Biochemicals; Lucite chamber for electric shock (Fig. 1); and square-wave stimulator (Grass, Model SD9, Grass Instruments).

Prepare shrimp extract as follows. Collect nauplii of the brine shrimp *Artemia salina* on filter paper by vacuum filtration with a Buchner funnel. Transfer 3 g wet weight of the larvae to a glass homogenizer, dilute them with an equal volume of distilled water, and homogenize the suspension. Centrifuge the extract at 2400 rpm ($410g$) in a clinical centrifuge for 2 min to remove large pieces. Remove the supernatant below the "lipid" pellicle and dilute it about fivefold. Add about 1 ml of the resultant shrimp extract to the culture medium in the chamber. Prepare this extract fresh each time before use.

PROCEDURES

Specific Reduction of Stenoteles

Place animals that have not been fed for 1 day in M solution containing 2×10^{-4} M fructose-1,6-diphosphate. Using a glass rod, stroke the tentacles of individual animals for about 8 min per tentacle. Repeat the process two more times during the same day. This method should reduce the stenotele population of the tentacles by 90% while the population of other nematocytes should remain unaffected (Zumstein and Tardent, 1971; Zumstein, 1973).

Reduction of Nematocyte Populations by Electric Shock

Place up to 100 hydra that have been without food for 1 day in M solution in the chamber shown in Fig. 1. When an additional component is added to the M solution, place the animals in the modified medium in the chamber 15 min before beginning of treatment. Have the chamber connected to the Grass square-wave stimulator. Deliver twin pulses of current (95 V, 5 mA, 13-msec duration per pulse, 9-msec delay between pulses) to the solution every 5 sec for a set period of time. Count the number of nematocytes in the tentacles before and after the treatment using the procedures described in Chapter 23, Method III. To eliminate 10–50% reduction of all nematocytes, shock the animals for 60 min. To reduce the stenotele population 70%, add fructose-1,6-diphosphate to M solution to

FIGURE 1. Chamber for electric shock treatment. Cut chamber into a Lucite block (11.5 × 5.5 × 2.5 cm). Cement silver wire electrodes (se) into holes drilled through the block into the ends of the chamber. Separate the electrodes, kept 10 cm apart, from the central chamber (8.0 × 4.0 × 2.0 cm) by sintered glass barriers (sg, 0.2 × 4.0 × 2.5 cm). The latter reduce or delay electrolysis products from entering the central chamber. To clean the electrodes after treating the hydra, rinse the chamber with 0.1 M HCl followed by distilled water.

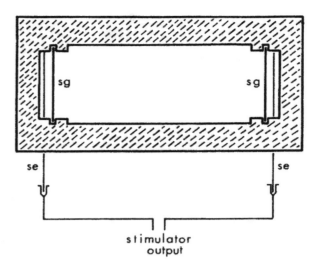

give a final concentration of 8.4×10^{-5} M, and shock the hydra for 30 min. To get a 90% reduction in stenoteles, and up to 50% reduction in the other types of nematocysts (desmonemes, atrichous, and holtrichous isorhizas) shock the animals for 2 hr in the fructose-1,6-diphosphate solution (Smith *et al.*, 1974). To reduce the number of all types of nematocytes in the tentacles, place the animals in culture medium containing 1 ml shrimp extract and shock them for 20–22 hr.

Hydra subjected to the shock treatment for up to several hours show no obvious damage and feed normally 1 hr after the end of the treatment. After treatments animals treated for 20–22 hr, will appear contracted, but should seem normal and feed within 12 hr after the end of the treatment.

REFERENCES

Bode, H. R., and Flick, K. M. 1976. Distribution and dynamics of nematocyte populations in *Hydra attenuata*. *J. Cell Sci.* **21**:15–34.

Lentz, T. L., and Barnett, R. J. 1962. The effect of enzyme substrates and pharmacological agents of nematocyst discharge. *J. Exp. Zool.* **149**:33–35.

Mariscal, R. N. 1974. Nematocysts. In: *Coelenterate Biology, Reviews and New Perspectives* (L. Muscatine and H. M. Lenhoff, eds.), Academic Press, New York, pp. 129–165.

Pantin, C. F. A. 1942. The excitation of nematocysts. *J. Exp. Biol.* **19**:249–310.

Picken, L. E. R., and Skaer, R. J. 1966. A review of researches on nematocysts. In: *The Cnidaria and Their Evolution* (W. J. Rees, ed.), Academic Press, New York, pp. 19–50.

Smith, S., Oshida, J., and Bode, H. 1974. Inhibition of nematocyst discharge in hydra fed to repletion. *Biol. Bull.* **147**:186–202.

Zumstein, A. 1973. Regulation der Nematocyten Produktion bei *Hydra attenuata*. Pall. *Wilhalm Roux Arch. Entwicklungsmech. Org.* **173**:295–318.

Zumstein, A., and Tardent, P. 1971. Beitrag zum Problem der Regulation der Nematocyten Produktion bei *Hydra attenuata* Pall. *Rev. Suisse Zool.* **78**:705–715.

Part IX

Assay and Isolation of Substances Controlling Morphogenesis in Hydra

Chapter 43

Assay and Isolation of Substances Controlling Morphogenesis in Hydra

H. Chica Schaller, Cornelis J. P. Grimmelikhuijzen, and
Tobias Schmidt

PURPOSE

To assay and isolate morphogens from hydra.

INTRODUCTION

Hydra has two centers of organization, head and foot; gradients of induction and inhibition extend from both toward the opposite ends (Webster, 1971; Shostak, 1974; MacWilliams *et al.*, 1970). These gradients in biological properties might be due to an unequal distribution along the body axis of the animal of substances that activate or inhibit head and foot formation. So far four such substances have been found: an activator and an inhibitor of head formation (Schaller, 1973; Berking, 1977; Schaller *et al.*, 1977), and an activator and an inhibitor of foot formation (Grimmelikhuijzen and Schaller, 1977; Schmidt and Schaller, 1976).

H. Chica Schaller, Cornelis J. P. Grimmelikhuijzen, and Tobias Schmidt • Max-Planck-Institut für medizinische Forschung, Abteilung Biophysik, Heidelberg, Federal Republic of Germany.

MATERIALS

Animals. Culture *Hydra attenuata* in mass in a medium derived from that of Lenhoff and Brown (1970) consisting of 1 mM $CaCl_2$, 0.1 mM KCl, 0.1 mM $MgCl_2$, and 1 mM NaH_2PO_4/Na_2HPO_4, pH 7.6. Keep the water temperature at $19\pm2°C$. Feed animals daily with nauplii of *Artemia salina* and wash them 6–8 hr later. Use only animals starved at least for 24 hr for all experiments.

Crude Extract. Sonicate hydra for 1–2 min in distilled water with a Branson B12 ultra sonicator. Use the absorption at 280 nm to estimate the concentration of the crude extract. The extract from one hydra without buds corresponds to an absorbance of approximately 0.15.

Statistical Analysis. The significance of activation or inhibition can be ascertained by means of the t-test or the χ^2 test.

PROCEDURES

Biological Assays for the Four Morphogens

The assays for the four substances are based on their morphogenetic properties: The head factors specifically influence head and not foot formation, and the foot factors influence foot and not head formation (Schaller *et al.*, 1979). In most of the assays, therefore, the stimulating or inhibiting effect of the four substances on head or foot regeneration is measured. Because the head factors influence bud induction and bud outgrowth (Schaller *et al.*, 1979), activation or inhibition of bud formation is also used in some assays.

Assay for Head Activator
Standard Assay. Select 24-hr starved hydra without buds from the mass culture. Cut off and discard the hypostome and tentacles at time 0. Incubate 25–30 of the remaining body columns for the first 6 hr after cutting, in a Petri dish (6-cm diameter) containing 10 ml of hydra medium or hydra medium to which the extract to be assayed is added. For each concentration, use three dishes. After 6 hr, exchange the medium with fresh hydra medium without extracts. At 48 hr after cutting determine the average number of

tentacles regenerated per head. Figure 1 shows the effect of an aqueous homogenate (crude extract) of hydra on the tentacle number. Activation (A, in %) is defined as

$$A = [(T - C)/C] \times 100$$

where C is the average number of tentacles in the control and T that in the treated sample. At the concentration of crude extract corresponding to half a homogenized hydra per milliliter (or 0.07 $O.D._{280}/ml$) we obtain a 6% activation. We define as one biological unit (BU) the amount of material necessary to obtain this effect in 10 ml of medium and under the described conditions.

Fast Assay. This assay can only be used with purified head activator, because the presence of head inhibitor interferes. Select large, well-fed animals without buds from the mass culture and incubate them with and without factor. Record the number of animals that develop a bud after 3 hr incubation (Fig. 2a). Activation (A, in %) (Fig. 2b) is defined as

$$A = [(T - C)/C] \times 100$$

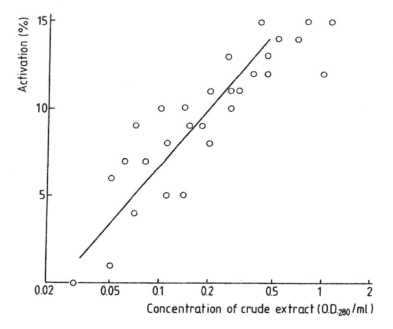

FIGURE 1. Standard head-activator assay. Dose–response curve of crude extracts of hydra on stimulating the tentacle number in animals regenerating a head.

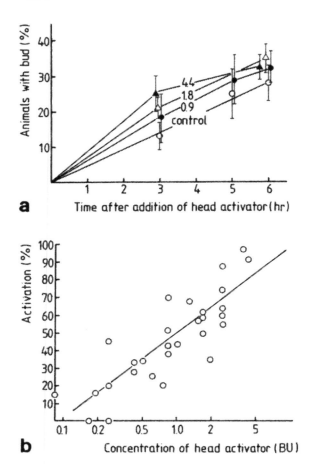

a Time after addition of head activator (hr)

b Concentration of head activator (BU)

FIGURE 2. Fast head-activator assay. (a) Activating effect of different concentrations of purified head activator on bud outgrowth. The concentrations are given in BU as determined in the standard assay. (b) Dose–response curve of purified head activator on bud outgrowth.

where C is the percentage of animals with buds in the control and T that in the treated sample at exactly 3 hr after the initiation of the experiment. We obtain an activation of 50% with a concentration corresponding to 1 BU of head activator as defined in the standard assay.

Assay for Head Inhibitor

Standard Assay. Select large, well-fed hydra from the mass culture. Cut off the hypostome and tentacles at time 0 to stimulate bud outgrowth. Transfer the remaining body columns immediately after cutting and incubate them with and without factor. Record the number of buds that develop (Fig. 3a). Bud inhibition (I, in %) is expressed as

$$I = [(C - T)/C] \times 100$$

where C is the percentage of animals with buds in the control and T that in the treated sample at exactly 8 hr after cutting (Fig. 3b). We obtain 50%

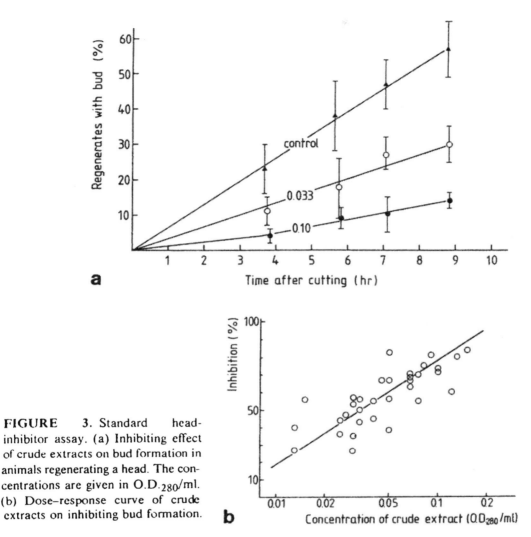

FIGURE 3. Standard head-inhibitor assay. (a) Inhibiting effect of crude extracts on bud formation in animals regenerating a head. The concentrations are given in O.D.$_{280}$/ml. (b) Dose–response curve of crude extracts on inhibiting bud formation.

inhibition with the extract of one-fifth of a hydra per milliliter (or 0.03 O.D.$_{280}$/ml) and define this activity as 1 BU.

Alternative Assay for Head Inhibitor

Select small animals without buds from the mass culture. Cut off the head at time 0 and incubate the remaining body columns with and without factor. Starting from 20 hr after cutting, note and record at roughly 2-hr intervals the number of regenerates with clearly visible outgrowth of at least two tentacles (Fig. 4a). When 75% of the control animals have tentacle bumps, we define inhibition (I, in %) as

$$I = (75 - T)/75$$

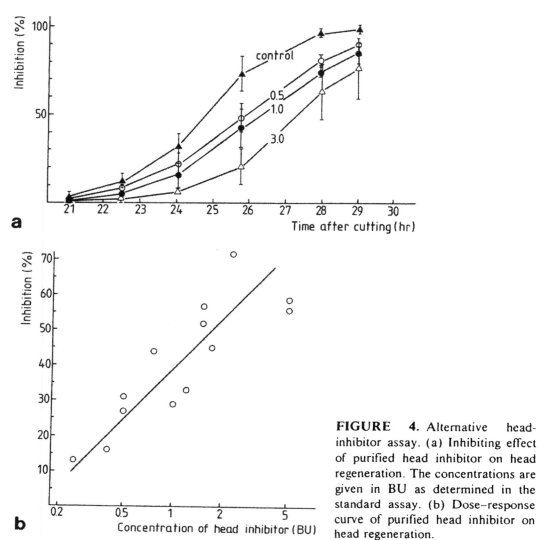

FIGURE 4. Alternative head-inhibitor assay. (a) Inhibiting effect of purified head inhibitor on head regeneration. The concentrations are given in BU as determined in the standard assay. (b) Dose–response curve of purified head inhibitor on head regeneration.

where T is the percentage of animals with tentacle bumps in the treated sample (Fig. 4b). We find that a significant inhibition of 25% can be obtained with 0.5 BU of the head inhibitor.

Assay for Foot Activator

Select hydra without buds and cut them transversely into two parts of equal length. Wash the upper halves and transfer them to Petri dishes containing medium with and without factor. After 3 hr of incubation wash the regenerates again and transfer them to new dishes containing fresh medium. Repeat this procedure again 19 hr after cutting. Starting at 20 hr after cutting, at roughly hourly intervals, count the number of animals that have regenerated a foot (Fig. 5a). We consider foot regeneration to be complete

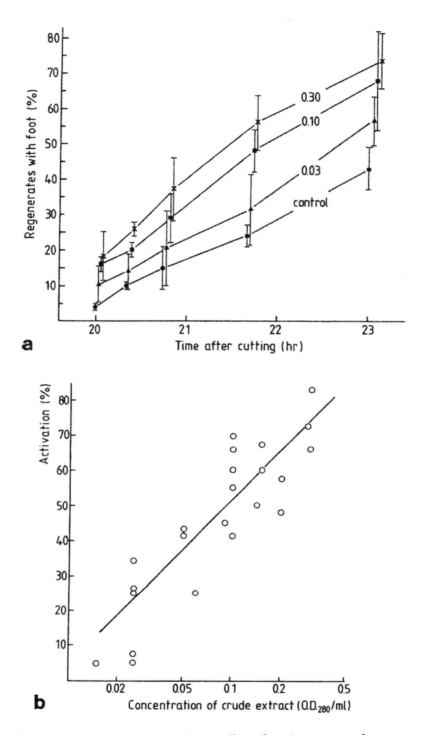

FIGURE 5. Foot-activator assay. (a) Stimulating effect of crude extract on foot regeneration. The concentration of crude extract is given as O.D.$_{280}$/ml.(b) Dose–response curve of crude extracts on stimulating foot formation.

when the animals are able to stick with their feet (basal disk) to the surface of either the dish or the water. We determine activation (A) percentage when 30% of the control animals have regenerated a foot. Thus, activation (A, in %) is defined as

$$[(T - 30/30] \times 100$$

where T is the percentage of animals that have regenerated a foot in the treated sample (Fig. 5b). We obtain a 50% activation using the extract from about half a hydra per ml (or 0.09 O.D.$_{280}$/ml). This effect is significant and is defined as 1 BU.

Assay for Foot Inhibitor

Select and cut hydra as described in the foot activator assay. After a 20 hr incubation period, wash the regenerates and transfer them to new dishes containing fresh medium. Measure foot formation at roughly hourly intervals (Fig 6a). We determine inhibition when 75% of the control animals have regenerated a foot. Thus, inhibition (I, in %) is defined as

$$[(75 - T)/75] \times 100$$

where T is the percentage of animals that have regenerated a foot in the treated sample (Fig. 6b). A 25% inhibition is significant. We achieve this effect with a crude extract of four-fifths of a hydra per milliliter (or with 0.12 O.D.$_{280}$/ml). We define the amount of extract necessary to achieve this effect as 1 BU.

Purification of the Four Morphogens

To obtain the four morphogenetic substances in a relatively pure state and free of contamination by each other, use the following isolation procedure:

1. Homogenize hydra in excess methanol, centrifuge the suspension at 3000g for 5 min, and reextract the pellet three times with methanol. Concentrate the pooled supernatants by rotary evaporation and extract this three times with petrol ether.

2. Concentrate by evaporation the methanol–water phase and apply it to a Sephadex G-10 column with distilled water as eluent. We find that the two inhibitors and the foot activator appear in the exclusion peak, and the head activator is retarded (Fig. 7a). Collect and concentrate the fractions containing the head activator and chromotograph them on Sephadex G-10 with 0.1 M NaCl and 0.01 M tris-HCl, pH 7.6, as eluent (Fig. 7b); on Biogel P-2

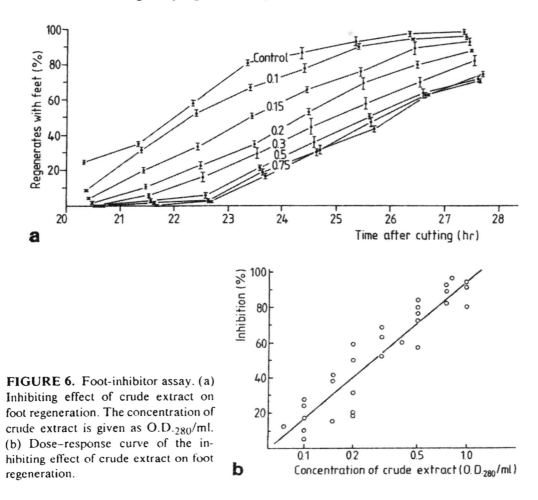

FIGURE 6. Foot-inhibitor assay. (a) Inhibiting effect of crude extract on foot regeneration. The concentration of crude extract is given as O.D.$_{280}$/ml. (b) Dose–response curve of the inhibiting effect of crude extract on foot regeneration.

with the same eluent (Fig. 7c); and on Sephadex G-10 with distilled water as eluent (Fig. 7d).

3. Pool the fractions containing the two inhibitors and the foot activator, concentrate them, bring them to pH 7.6 with NaOH, and apply this to a Sephadex DEAE A-25 column equilibrated with 35 mM tris-HCl, pH 7.6 (Fig. 8a). The two inhibitors do not bind and can be eluted with 35 mM tris-HCl, pH 7.6. The foot activator does bind and elutes between 0.28–0.45 M NaCl when a linear NaCl gradient is applied. The eluted fractions containing the foot activator can be desalted on a Sephadex G-10 column.

4. Lyophilize the pooled fractions containing the two inhibitors, dissolve them in methanol, and apply the solution to a Sephadex LH-20 column with methanol as eluent (Fig. 8b). The head inhibitor should elute before the foot inhibitor and can be further purified by chromatography on Biogel P-2 (Fig. 8c). Purification and yield of the four substances are summarized in Table I.

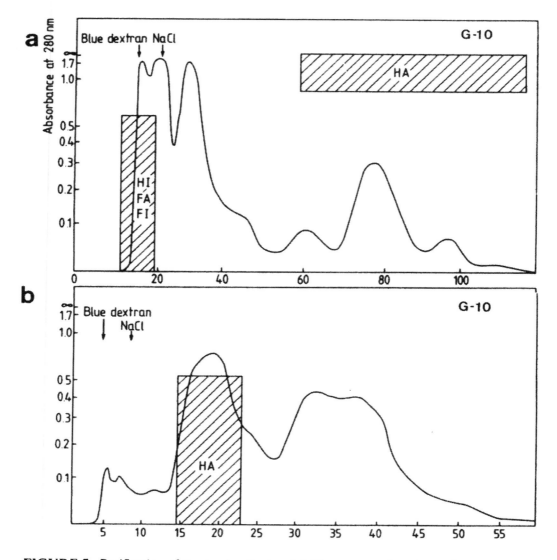

FIGURE 7. Purification of the head activator. (a) Chromatography of a methanol extract of hydra on Sephadex G-10 with distilled water as eluent (column size, 2.8 × 50 cm; volume, 340 ml; fraction size, 9 ml). The amount applied to the column corresponds to 100,000 hydra. Hatched areas indicate fractions in which the biological activity was found. HA stands for head activator, HI for head inhibitor, FA for foot activator, and FI for foot inhibitor. (b) Chromatography of fractions 60–120 of Fig. 7a on Sephadex G-10 with 0.1 M NaCl, 0.01 M Tris-HCl, pH 7.6, as eluent (column size 1.5 × 16 cm; volume, 25 ml; fraction size, 1.9 ml). The amount applied corresponds to 250,000 hydra. (c) Chromatography of fractions 15–23 of Fig. 7b on Biogel P-2 with 0.1 M NaCl, 0.01 M Tris-HCl, pH 7.6, as eluent (column size, 1.3 × 47 cm; volume 40 ml; fraction size, 1.9 ml). The amount applied corresponds to 250,000 hydra. (d) Chromatography of fractions 12–16 of Fig. 7c on Sephadex G-10 with distilled water as eluent (column size, 0.9 × 10 cm; volume, 5 ml; fraction size, 1.9 ml). The amount applied corresponds to 500,000 hydra.

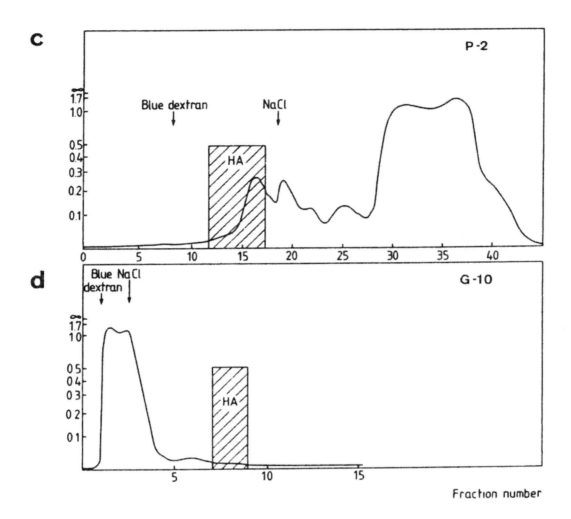

FIGURE 43 (*Continued*)

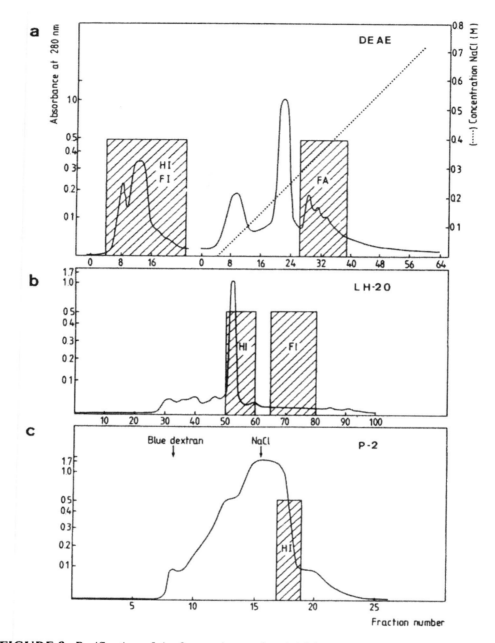

FIGURE 8. Purification of the foot activator, foot inhibitor, and head inhibitor. (a) Chromatography of fractions 11–12 of Fig. 7a on Sephadex DEAE A-25 with 35 m*M* tris-HCl, pH 7.6, as eluent (left panel) and with linear NaCl gradient (right panel); column size, 1.5 × 16 cm; volume, 28 ml; fraction size, 3.5 ml); The amount applied corresponds to 60,000 hydra. (b) Chromatography of fractions 4–25 (exclusion peak) of Fig. 8a on Sephadex LH-20 with methanol as eluent (column size, 1.2 × 150 cm; volume, 180 ml; fraction size, 2 ml). The amount applied corresponds to 50,000 hydra. (c) Chromatography of fractions 50–60 of Fig. 8b on Biogel P-2 with distilled water as eluent (colume size as described in Fig. 7c). The amount applied corresponds to 500,000 hydra.

TABLE I. Purification and Yield of the Four Morphogenetic Substances

Substance	Specific activity of crude extract (BU/mg protein)	Specific activity of purified factor (BU/mg protein)	Purification (X-fold)	Yield (%)
Head activator	4.2	$\gg$ 100,000	$\gg$ 25,000	75
Head inhibitor	9.6	$-^a$	$-^a$	70
Foot activator	3.9	13,000	3,300	80
Foot inhibitor	2.6	$-^a$	$-^a$	80

^{a} Since in contrast to the two activators (Schaller. 1973: Grimmelikhuijzen, 1979) the two inhibitors are neither proteins nor peptides (Berking, 1977: Schmidt and Schaller, 1980). it is unrealistic to express their specific activities as BU/mg protein. We believe that their degrees of purity are of the same order as, or better than, that of the foot activator.

SPECIAL PRECAUTIONS

The assays give reproducible results only if the animals are healthy and kept under strictly standardized conditions. Precise and fast cutting is also a necessary prerequisite, as is fast transfer immediately after cutting. Due to the biological variability of the test animals, the assays can be evaluated quantitatively only if enough points are collected to construct dose–response curves.

REFERENCES

Berking, S. 1977. Localization and purification of a substance which inhibits bud formation in hydra. *Wilhelm Roux Entwicklungsmech. Org. Arch.* **181**:215–225.

Grimmelikhuijzen, C. J. P. 1979. Properties of the foot activator from hydra. *Cell Differ.* **8**:267–273.

Grimmelikhuijzen, C. J. P., and Schaller, H. C. 1977. Isolation of a substance activating foot formation in hydra. *Cell Differ.* **6**:297–305.

Lenhoff, H. M., and Brown, R. D. 1970. Mass culture in hydra: An improved method and its application to other aquatic invertebrates, *Lab. Anim.* **4**:139–154.

MacWilliams, H. K., Kafatos, F. C., Bossert, W. H. 1970. The feedback inhibition of basal disc regeneration in hydra has a continuously variable intensity. *Dev. Biol.* **23**:380–398.

Schaller, H. C. 1973. Isolation and characterization of a low-molecular-weight substance activating head and bud formation in hydra. *J. Embryol. Exp. Morphol.* **29**:27–38.

Schaller, H. C., Schmidt, T., and Grimmelikhuijzen, C. J. P. 1977. Analysis of morphogenetic mutants from hydra: I. The aberrant. *Wilhelm Roux Entwicklungsmech. Org.* **183**:193–206.

Schaller, H.C., Schmidt, T., and Grimmelikhuijzen, C. J. P. 1979. Separation and specificity of action of four morphogens from hydra. *Wilhelm Roux Entwicklungsmech. Org.* **186**:134–149.

Schmidt, T., and Schaller, H. C. 1976. Evidence for a foot-inhibiting substance in hydra. *Cell Differ.* **5**:151–159.

Schmidt, T., and Schaller, H. C. 1980. Properties of the foot inhibitor from hydra. *Wilhelm Roux Arch. Entwicklungsmech. Org.* **188**:133–139.

Shostak, S. 1974. The complexity of hydra: Homeostasis, morphogenetic controls and integration. *Q. Rev. Biol.* **49**:287–310.

Webster, G. 1971. Morphogenesis and pattern formation in hydroids. *Biol. Rev.* **46**:1–46.

Part X

Isolation and/or Properties of Acellular Mesoglea and Nematocysts

Chapter 44

Isolating Mesolamellae

Robert M. Day and Howard M. Lenhoff

PURPOSE

To isolate intact the acellular material that separates the two epithelial cell layers. This material, called mesoglea in general and mesolamella in hydra, provides a useful substrate for the *in vitro* attachment of hydra cells (Day and Lenhoff, 1981).

INTRODUCTION

The acellular mesolamellae of hydra has been shown to have some of the chemical characteristics of mammalian basement membrane (Barzansky *et al.*, 1975; Barzansky and Lenhoff, 1974). The method we describe allows for the rapid and simple isolation of large numbers of mesolamellae, material that may prove useful for investigating the mechanisms and specificity of the interactions of epithelial cells in general with their basement membranes. It is already known, for example, that hydra epithelial cells readily attach and spread out on hydra mesolamella, whereas insect cells and those from normal and tumorous mammalian cells that have been tried do not (Day and Lenhoff, 1981).

Robert M. Day and Howard M. Lenhoff ● Department of Developmental and Cell Biology, University of California, Irvine, California.

MATERIALS

Detergents, such as 0.2% Sarkosyl NL-97 (CIBA-Geigy Co.), 0.1% Nonidet P-40 (Particle Data Labs., Inc.), or 0.5% N-lauroyl sarcosine (Sigma Chemical Co.); 6.5×10^{-3} M dithiothreitol, pH 8.7 (Sigma Chemical Co.); 35-mm-diameter plastic tissue culture dishes (Falcon Co.); acetone–dry-ice bath; Pasteur pipets.

PROCEDURES

Place 100–200 hydra in distilled water in a 3-ml conical centrifuge tube for 30 min. Drain off most of the water around the animals and replace it with detergent solution. Freeze the suspension rapidly in an acetone–dry-ice bath. Thaw the preparation and transfer the hydra into a Petri dish of distilled water using a Pasteur pipet with a fire-polished tip. To dislodge the adherent dead cells from the mesolamellae, gently draw the hydra back and forth through the pipet. During these dislodging steps, observe the suspension through a dissecting microscope. When the mesolamellae appear free of cells, transfer them to another Petri dish of distilled water, rinse them quickly, and transfer them to another Petri dish of distilled water, rinse them quickly, and transfer them for 5–15 min to test tubes containing 5 ml of 1 mg/ml dithiothreitol to dissolve any adhering nematocysts (Chapter 46). Rinse again in distilled water.

To prepare batches of mesolamellae for chemical extractions and analyses, centrifuge the tubes containing large numbers of mesolamellae for 20 min at about 3000g, pour off the supernatant, resuspend the pelleted mesolamellae in your experimental solution, centrifuge the mesolamellae again, and remove the pellet. You may use mesolamellae immediately or store them lyophilized or in fluid at −25°C or lower.

To prepare mesolamellae for studies of cell adhesion, omit the centrifuging step and instead transfer the mesolamellae individually in a pipet to the center of a tissue culture dish containing 0.5–1.0 ml distilled water. Carefully draw off the water so that the mesolamellae will settle onto the plastic. Air dry the preparation just until the mesolamellae adhere to the plastic and use immediately; excessive drying may lead to a decrease in cell attachment (Day and Lenhoff, 1981). To store the preparation, put a drop of distilled water on the attached mesolamellae and freeze them.

PRECAUTIONS

Isolated mesolamellae are sticky and will adhere to surfaces unless you keep them actively moving in suspension. If they stick to surfaces, try to dislodge them with forced streams of fluid from a pipet. Isolated mesolamellae appear to stick less if they remain in dilute detergent solutions. They stick less to polypropylene centrifuge tubes than to glass or polystyrene ones. Some species and strains of hydra yield more intact mesolamellae than others. Excellent results have been obtained with *Hydra pseudoligactis* and *Hydra attenuata*, whereas *Hydra viridis* usually yield fragmented mesolamellae by this method.

REFERENCES

Barzansky, B., and Lenhoff, H. M. 1974. On the chemical composition and developmental role of the mesoglea of hydra. *Am. Zool.* **14**:579–581.

Barzansky, B., Lenhoff, H. M., and Bode, H. 1975. Hydra mesoglea: Similarity of its amino acid and neutral sugar composition to that of vertebrate basal lamina. *Comp. Biochem. Physiol.* **50B**:419–424.

Day, R. M., and Lenhoff, H. M. 1981. Hydra mesoglea: A model for investigating epithelial cell-basement membrane interactions. *Science* **211**:291–294.

Chapter 45

Isolating Undischarged and Discharged Nematocysts from Acontiate Sea Anemones

Richard S. Blanquet

PURPOSE

The ability to obtain large quantities of isolated nematocysts provides material for the study of problems related to nematocyst discharge mechanisms and for the isolation and analysis of nematocyst toxins and capsule components (see Chapters 46, 47, and 48). To date, no satisfactory method has been developed for hydra. The procedure described is for isolating pure nematocyst suspensions from the acontia of some sea anemones.

INTRODUCTION

Isolated nematocysts can be easily obtained by placing acontia threads in various media which induce the active liberation of nematocysts from the epithelial cells, a process referred to as "extrusion" (Parker and Van Alstyne, 1932; Yanagita, 1959; Blanquet, 1968). Though these solutions are effective extrusion media for acontial nematocysts, they are usually ineffective for tentacle nematocysts even when the nematocysts are of the same type. The mechanism of extrusion and the reason for this difference is not known.

Richard S. Blanquet ● Department of Biology, Georgetown University, Washington, D.C.

MATERIALS

Sodium citrate, 1.0 M; clean, fine scissors; cheesecloth. The sea anemone *Aiptasia* can be grown in the laboratory according to methods described by D. A. Hessinger and J. A. Hessinger (1981).

PROCEDURES

Induce expanded anemones to contract by gently prodding them with the blunt end of a clean glass rod. This prodding usually results in the ejection of acontia threads from the mouth or cinclides (small openings in the body wall). Snip the threads from the anemones with a clean pair of fine scissors and transfer them to a solution of 1.0 M sodium citrate by means of a wide-mouthed pipet. Rough handling or exposure of the threads to the air will cause many nematocysts to discharge. Nematocyst extrusion is associated with a marked curling of the acontia and is normally complete within 15 sec after the acontia are placed into the citrate solution. Swirl the solution several times to liberate any nematocysts still adhering to the threads.

To remove the acontia, pour the suspension through several layers of cheesecloth and collect the filtrate containing the suspended nematocysts. Nematocysts can be collected by centrifuging at 1000g for 15 min. Suspend the resulting pellet in clean citrate solution and repeat several times. This procedure, for *Aiptasia*, should give large numbers of undischarged nematocysts almost entirely of a single type, the microbasic mastigophore (Fig. 1).

To discharge the nematocysts, add distilled water to the final pellet of washed nematocysts. Centrifuge at 1000g for 15 min to separate the discharged capsules from the supernatant, which can serve as a source of purified toxin (Blanquet, 1968). Resuspend the discharged nematocyst pellet and wash it several times in distilled water or other appropriate media to remove the sodium citrate. Discharged capsules can then be used for analyses of the capsule components (see Chapter 46).

COMMENTS

The procedure outlined here is that reported by Blanquet (1968) for the sea anemone *Aiptasia*. The procedure also works well for other acontiate species such as *Metridium* (Goodwin and Telford, 1971) and *Diadumene* (Yanagita, 1959). In the case of *Diadumene*, substitute glycerol for sodium citrate.

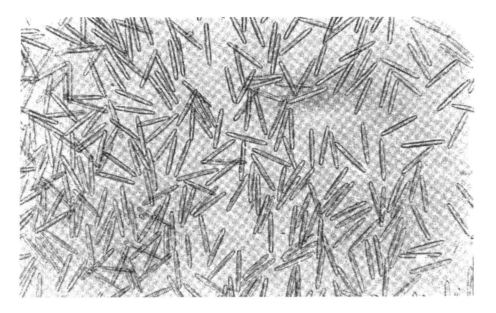

FIGURE 1. Purified suspension of undischarged microbasic mastigophore nematocysts from acontia of *Aiptasia pallida*. They are 80–86 μm long and about 10 μm at their widest point.

REFERENCES

Blanquet, R. 1968. Properties and composition of the nematocyst toxin of the sea anemone, *Aiptasia pallida*. *Comp. Biochem. Physiol.* **25**:893–902.

Goodwin, M. H., and Telford, M. 1971. Nematocyst toxin of *Metridium*. *Biol. Bull.* **140**:389–399.

Hessinger, D. A., and Hessinger, J. A., 1981. Method for rearing sea anemones in the laboratory. *In: Laboratory Animal Management: Marine Invertebrates* (Committee on Marine Invertebrates, *eds.*) National Resource Council, National Academic Press, Washington, D.C. pp. 153–179.

Parker, G. H., and Van Alstyne, M. A. 1932. The control and discharge of nematocysts, especially in *Metridium* and *Physalia. J. Exp. Zool.* **63**:329–344.

Yanagita, T. M. 1959. Physiological mechanism of nematocyst responses in sea anemone. VII. Extrusion of resting cnidae–Its nature and its possible bearing on the normal nettling response. *J. Exp. Biol.* **36**:478–494.

Chapter 46

Dissolving the Nematocyst Capsule Wall and Identifying its Protein Component(s)

Richard S. Blanquet

PURPOSE

Since the properties of the nematocyst capsule and thread undoubtedly play a significant role in the mechanism of nematocyst discharge, solubilization of these structures facilitates the chemical and physical analyses of some of their components. Analyses show that nematocysts contain a collagenlike protein (Lenhoff *et al.*, 1957) linked by disulfide bonds (Blanquet and Lenhoff, 1966).

INTRODUCTION

Solubilization of nematocyst capsule and thread proteins, through the reduction of disulfide cross-links, has been accomplished by the addition of various thiols such as thioglycolate, mercaptoethanol, dithiothreitol (DTT), and dithioerythritol (DTE) in an alkaline medium (Yanagita, 1959; Blanquet and Lenhoff, 1966; Mariscal, 1971). Due to their low oxidation–reduction potentials, high water solubility, and lack of a disagreeable odor, DTT or DTE (Cleland, 1964) is recommended for solubilizing nematocysts.

Richard S. Blanquet • Department of Biology, Georgetown University, Washington, D. C.

MATERIALS

Thiol Solution

DTT or DTE, 10^{-2} M (both from Sigma Chemical Co., St. Louis, MO 63178), buffered in 0.2 M carbonate–bicarbonate buffer, pH 10.5, should be freshly prepared before use.

Disk Electrophoresis Stock Solutions

1. Acrylamide, 14.0 g; bisacrylamide, 0.4 g, and distilled water to make 100 ml.

2. *N,N,N',N'*-Tetramethylethylenediamine (TEMED), 0.06 ml; tris base, 9.05 g; 1 *N* HCl, 12.0 ml, and distilled water to make 50 ml.

3. Ammonium persulfate, 0.14 g and distilled water to make 100 ml. Prepare fresh as needed.

4. TEMED, 0.23 ml; tris base, 3.0 g; 1 *N* HCl, 24.0 ml (to pH 6.7), and distilled water to make 50 ml.

5. Acrylamide, 10.0 g; bisacrylamide, 2.5 g, and distilled water to make 50 ml.

6. Riboflavin, 2.0 g, and distilled water to make 50 ml.

7. Coomassie Brilliant Blue, 0.5 g, and distilled water to make 50 ml.

8. Sucrose, 5.0 g, with distilled water to make 100 ml.

9. Trichloracetic acid (TCA), 12.5 g (12.5%) or 10.0 g (10%), with distilled water to make 100 ml.

10. Bromophenol Blue, 0.1 g, with distilled water to make 100 ml.

Other

Disk electrophoresis apparatus such as the Buchler Polyanalyst.

PROCEDURES

Qualitative Analysis of "Squash" Preparations (*Hydra littoralis*)

Place individual hydra on a microscope slide and remove excess water with a pipet. Add two drops of thiol solution, place a cover slip on top of the hydra, and apply pressure sufficient to disrupt the cells. Observe the liberated nematocysts for at least 30 min using bright field or phase contrast microscopy.

The first indication of nematocyst dissolution is a distinct wrinkling of the capsule followed by a rapid disappearance of both capsule and everted thread. Once initiated, dissolution of stenoteles is complete within 30 sec. A thin membrane delineating the original capsule wall should persist for several minutes before dissolving. The large stylets present on the stenotele butte do not dissolve. Undischarged nematocysts are more resistant to dissolution. Holotrichous and atrichous isorhizas, both discharged and undischarged, require 8–10 min to dissolve.

Dissolving Purified Discharged Nematocyst Capsules

Place isolated, discharged nematocysts (see Chapter 46) in at least 10 times their volume of thiol solution. Agitate the medium to keep the nematocysts in suspension. Remove small aliquots of the suspension immediately and then periodically to determine the degree of solubilization.

After solubilization is achieved, centrifuge the solution to remove any particulate material remaining. Dialyze the solution for at least 24 hr against an appropriate medium (the medium used will depend on the type of assay to be conducted) with three changes of the medium.

Test for Purity and Composition of Solubilized Components

The components of the solubilized nematocyst can be separated using standard acrylamide gel and disk electrophoretic techniques. Prepare the following two working solutions of acrylamide from stock solutions (see Materials) and bring to room temperature just before use:

1. *Separation gel.* Mix equal parts of stock solutions 1 and 2. The pH should be 8.9 ± 0.1. The resultant gel has a 7% cross-linking and allows resolution of proteins ranging from 10^3 to 10^5 molecular weight with maximum resolution between 3×10^3 and 3×10^4.

2. *Stacking gel.* Mix one part each of distilled water and stock solutions 1, 2, and 3. The pH should be 6.7 ± 0.1.

Mix equal parts of the separation gel working solution and stock solution 3. Within 5 min add about 2.0–2.5 ml of this solution to vertical glass electrophoresis tubes (5 mm ID × 12 cm) sealed at one end with Parafilm or a suitable plug. Carefully layer with a small amount of water and allow the gel to polymerize for 1 hr.

Remove the water layer with a syringe and add 0.15 ml of the stacking gel working solution over the polymerized separation gel. Again carefully layer some water on the stacking gel solution. Irradiate for 30 min with a fluorescent lamp placed close to the stacking gel solution to cause polymerization.

Place tubes containing the gels in the electrophoresis chamber and fill the upper and lower chambers with 0.4 M tris-glycine buffer, pH 9.3. Make sure no air bubbles are trapped in the electrophoresis tubes. Add approximately five drops of tracking dye (0.1% Bromophenol Blue) to the upper chamber.

Add about 100–200 μg of nematocyst protein in a 5% sucrose solution to each tube. Run the electrophoretic separation at a constant amperage of about 2–5 mA per tube. After completing electrophoresis, remove the gels from the tube and stain them for 1 hr in stock solution 7 diluted 1:20 with 12.5% TCA. Place the gels in a 10% TCA solution. Over a period of 24 hr the bands intensify and sharpen. Count and quantify the stained bands using standard techniques of densitometry or spectrophotometry. Maximum absorbance of the stain occurs at 750 nm. This procedure applied to the discharged mastigophores of the sea anemone *Aiptasia* gives a single protein band (Blanquet and Lenhoff, 1966).

Those unfamiliar with acrylamide electrophoretic techniques should consult the articles of Davis (1964) and Gordon (1972).

PRECAUTIONS

Reoxidation of the sulfhydryl groups of solubilized hydra nematocysts protein has not been studied. If subsequent analysis is delayed, it may be advisable to refrigerate the samples and keep them in the dark to prevent possible photo-oxidation.

When employing mercaptoethanol or thioglycollate as thiol-reducing agents for nematocyst solubilization, use a hood. When working with acrylamide, note the *warning label* printed on the bottle.

The concentration of reducing agent, pH, and time required for complete solubilization of the nematocysts varies with the species of cnidarian and nematocyst type tested (Blanquet and Lenhoff, 1966; Fishman and Levy, 1967; Mariscal, 1971). Proper conditions, in each case, may be determined quickly and fairly accurately through the use of squash preparations. The observed differences in solubilization times may, to some extent, be artifacts. For example, in squash preparations, mucus or other substances may affect the reducing agent directly or prevent the agent from reaching the nematocysts (Mariscal, 1971).

Studies designed to characterize the chemical and physical nature of the proteins which make up the nematocyst capsule and thread require pure suspensions of discharged nematocysts, preferably of a single type. Methods for obtaining such suspensions are yet to be developed for hydra.

REFERENCES

Blanquet, R., and Lenhoff, H. M. 1966. A disulfide-linked collagenous protein of nematocyst capsules. Science 154:152–153.

Cleland, W. W. 1964. Dithiothreitol, a new protective reagent for SH groups. *Biochemistry* 3(4):480–482.

Davis, B. J. 1964. Disc electrophoresis. II. Method and application to human serum proteins. *Ann. N.Y. Acad. Sci.* 121:404–427.

Fishman, L., and Levy, M. 1967. Studies on the nematocyst capsule protein from the sea anemone *Metridium marginatum*. *Biol. Bull. Woods Hole Mass.* 133:464–465.

Gordon, A. H. 1972. Electrophoresis of proteins in polyacrylamide and starch gels. In: *Laboratory Techniques in Biochemistry and Molecular Biology*, vol. 1, part 1 (T. S. Work and E. Work, eds.), North Holland, Amsterdam.

Lenhoff, H. M., Kline, E. S., and Hurley, R. 1957. A hydroxyproline-rich collagen-like protein of *Hydra* nematocysts. *Biochim. Biophys. Acta* 26:204–205.

Mariscal, R. N. 1971. Effect of a disulfide reducing agent on the nematocyst capsules from some Coelenterates, with an illustrated key to nematocyst classification. In: *Experimental Coelenterate Biology* (H. M. Lenhoff, L. Muscatine, and L. V. Davis, eds.), University of Hawaii Press, Honolulu, pp. 157–168.

Yanagita, T. M. 1959. Physiological mechanism of nematocyst responses in sea anemone. I. Effects of trypsin and thioglycolate upon isolated nematocysts. *Jpn. J. Zool.* 12:361–375.

Chapter 47

Purifying an Inhibitor of Succinoxidase Activity from *Hydra littoralis*

Edward S. Kline and Vaman S. Waravdekar

PURPOSE

To purify a potent inhibitor of succinoxidase activity from homogenates of *Hydra littoralis*. This inhibitor may represent one of the components of the nematocyst venom.

INTRODUCTION

The succinoxidase inhibitor, though purified from whole homogenates, may be one of the components of the venom present in the stenotele nematocysts. Evidence supporting this view was obtained when we showed inhibitor activity in the water surrounding hydra that had been stimulated electrically to discharge their nematocysts (Kline and Waravdekar, 1960; Glaser and Sparrow, 1909). Absolute proof, however, must await investigation of the internal components of purified, undischarged stenoteles. The succinoxidase inhibitor activity may represent a specific action of a more general property of the inhibitor. For example, the inhibitor may act

---

Edward S. Kline ● Department of Biochemistry, Medical College of Virginia, Virginia Commonwealth University, Richmond Virginia. Vaman S. Waravdekar   Microbiological Associates, Bethesda, Maryland.

generally to dissociate membrane components and thereby indirectly affect succinoxidase activity. (Other properties of components of nematocyst venom from the sea anemone *Aiptasia pallida* are given in Chapter 48.)

The initial extractions of the hydra homogenates with *n*-butyl alcohol were necessary to remove lipid components which appeared to either complex the inhibitor or render it inactive (Morton, 1955).

MATERIALS

Approximately 2.5 g of a lyophylized homogenate of *Hydra littoralis* are used for purification. Do not feed the animals for at least 1 day before the purification begins. Wash the hydra thoroughly by serial transfers through numerous changes of fresh culture solution just prior to the purification. For the enzymatic and toxicity experiments, we use the CAF_1 mouse strain, fed *ad libitum*. Fiddler crabs are also used for toxicity experiments.

Reagents for the purification include distilled *n*-butyl alcohol, dry acetone, diethyl ether, 0.02 *M* sodium phosphate buffer (pH 8.0), HCl, osmium tetroxide, and dialysis tubing.

Equipment for the purification includes Potter-Elvehjem all-glass or glass–Teflon homogenizers; a variable-speed stirring motor (for homogenizing); the Spinco Model L preparative ultracentrifuge; a freeze-dry apparatus; and a refrigerated centrifuge.

PROCEDURES

Measurement of Activity of Succinoxidase Inhibitor

One unit of activity is defined as the amount of succinoxidase inhibitor which produces 10% inhibition of succinoxidase activity in 5 mg of mouse liver homogenate. Specific activity is units/mg protein nitrogen. Use the succinoxidase assay of Schneider and Potter, with minor modifications (see Umbreit *et al.*, 1957), to determine this activity in mouse liver. Choose conditions for assaying the inhibitor so that the percentage inhibition of succinoxidase activity as a function of inhibitor concentration is linear to at least the 50% inhibitory level (Kline and Waravdekar, 1960; Kline, 1960).

Purification of the Enzyme Inhibitor (Table I)

Homogenize the hydra in cold distilled water and lyophilize the homogenate. Rehomogenize the dry material (2.5 g) in distilled, cold *n*-butyl

TABLE I. Fractional Separation of Succinoxidase Inhibitor from Hydra Lyophylized Homogenate

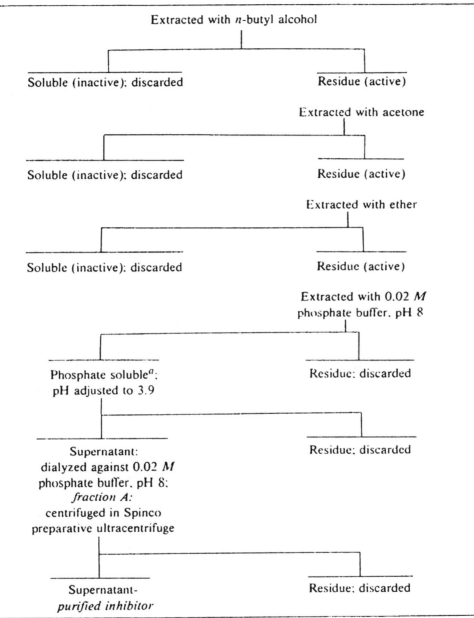

Extracted with *n*-butyl alcohol

Soluble (inactive): discarded   Residue (active)

Extracted with acetone

Soluble (inactive): discarded   Residue (active)

Extracted with ether

Soluble (inactive): discarded   Residue (active)

Extracted with 0.02 *M* phosphate buffer, pH 8

Phosphate soluble[a]: pH adjusted to 3.9   Residue: discarded

Supernatant: Residue: discarded
dialyzed against 0.02 *M* phosphate buffer, pH 8;
fraction A: centrifuged in Spinco preparative ultracentrifuge

Supernatant-   Residue: discarded
purified inhibitor

[a] Usually dialyzed for activity measurement, a procedure which may alter the observed activity.

alcohol. Store this mixture overnight in the cold to ensure thorough extraction of alcohol soluble matter. Centrifuge and discard the supernatant. Reextract the residue several times with cold *n*-butyl alcohol and discard each supernatant. Extract the residue several times with cold, dry acetone and, finally, with cold ether. Stop these extractions of lipids when the final ether extract produces less coloration than a 1:15,000 dilution of sesame oil, when tested with osmium tetroxide. Very little inhibitory activity should be lost in these steps.

Take up the remaining residue in cold 0.02 *M* phosphate buffer, pH 8.0. Most of the inhibitory activity should be solubilized by the phosphate, and the solution should be light brown. Repeat this extraction several times and discard the residues although they may contain some inhibitory activity. Add HCl to this phosphate-soluble preparation to give a pH of 3.9; a large amount of flocculation should result. Centrifuge and save only the clear supernatant containing most of the inhibitory activity. Dialyze the supernatant thoroughly in the cold against the pH 8 phosphate buffer. Discard the dialysate. Centrifuge the dialysand (*fraction A*) in the Spinco analytical ultracentrifuge at 35,000 rpm. You should obtain a single slow-moving peak if the fractionation proceeded well.

Fraction A may, in certain preparations, contain a second, fast-moving peak; the protein giving this latter peak may be removed by centrifuging the preparation in the Spinco preparative ultracentrifuge at a centrifugal force similar to that used in the analytical model, e.g., at 89,000*g*. The supernatant, following centrifugation in the preparative ultracentrifuge, should be the purified succinoxidase inhibitor (*purified inhibitor*). From the lyophylized homogenate the overall purification should be about 13-fold, with about 70% of the original inhibitory activity recovered.

Properties of the Purified Inhibitor

The *purified inhibitor* should show (1) a schlieren pattern with a single peak and a sedimentation constant of less than 2; (2) an ultraviolet absorption spectrum with a maximum absorbance at 280 nm with no absorbance in the visible range; (3) atypical qualitative test for carbohydrate and a negative test for DNA; (4) a positive test with protein reagents (Biuret and Folin–Ciocalteu); and (5) following acid hydrolysis, the appearance of ninhydrin-positive spots on paper chromatograms. Additionally, trypsin should destroy the succinoxidase inhibitory activity, even though the inhibitor may contain nonprotein moieties.

COMMENTS

Current information indicates that the inhibitor interrupts a step subsequent to the succinate dehydrogenase portion of succinoxidase and prior to the reoxidation of cytochrome C by the cytochrome C oxidase portion of succinoxidase (Kline, 1960; Kline, 1961; Slater, 1949; Umbreit *et al.*, 1957). The *purified inhibitor* is toxic to both mice and fiddler crabs, often killing these animals. In the fiddler crab, at a dose of 10 μg/g injected at the base of a walking leg, the inhibitor produces almost immediately signs of toxicity, including sluggishness and reduction or loss of righting ability, in a number of the animals. Eventually some die. In contrast, the same dose of boiled *purified inhibitor* produces no obvious effect.

PRECAUTIONS

The use of dry organic solvents and well-dried lyophylized homogenates of hydra should minimize denaturation of the succinoxidase inhibitor during the initial stages of the purification.

Osmium tetroxide and its vapors are dangerous. Safeguards are necessary when the container is opened and used. The use of less dangerous methods, such as iodine number, to test for lipid is recommended, particularly if safeguards can not be provided.

Although the discarded residue remaining after extraction with 0.02 M phosphate buffer, pH 8.0, has succinoxidase inhibitory activity, it is grossly contaminated with nematocysts, nematocyst capsules, and other cellular debris.

ACKNOWLEDGMENTS. This method was devised while the authors were in the Biochemistry Branch, Armed Forces Institute of Pathology, Washington, D.C.

REFERENCES

Glaser, O. C., and Sparrow, C. M. 1909. The physiology of nematocysts. *J. Exp. Zool.* 6:361–382.

Kline, E. S., and Waravdekar, V. S. 1960. Inhibitor of succinoxidase activity from *Hydra littoralis. J. Biol. Chem.* 235:1803–1808.

Kline, E. S. 1961. Chemistry of nematocyst capsule and toxin of *Hydra littoralis.* In: *The Biology of Hydra* (H. M. Lenhoff and W. F. Loomis, eds.), University of Miami Press, Coral Gables, Fla., pp. 153–168.

Kline, Edward S. 1960. Studies on a succinoxidase inhibitor from *Hydra*. Ph.D. thesis, George Washington University.

Morton, R. K. 1955. Methods of extraction of enzymes from animal tissues. In: *Methods in Enzymology*, vol. 1 (S. P. Colowick and N. O. Kaplan, eds.), Academic Press, New York, pp. 25–51.

Slater, E. C. 1949. A comparative study of the succinic dehydrogenase-cytochrome system in heart muscle and in kidney. *Biochem. J.* 45:1–8.

Umbreit, W. W., Burris, R. H. and Stauffer, J. F. 1957. In: *Manometric Techniques*, 3rd ed. (W. W. Umbreit, R. H. Burris, and J. F. Stauffer), Burgess, Minneapolis, Minn., pp. 173–176.

Chapter 48

Assays for Activities of Nematocyst Venoms and Their Components

David A. Hessinger

PURPOSE

A number of bioassays and biochemical tests for components of the nematocyst venom of the sea anemone *Aiptasia pallida* are described here in the anticipation that some or all may apply to components of the venom of the penetrant nematocysts (i.e., stenoteles) of hydra. They include assays for toxicity in representative vertebrates (mice) and crustaceans (fiddler crabs), hemolysis of red blood cells, phospholipase activity, and neurotoxicity on crayfish nerve.

INTRODUCTION

A proteinaceous material which inhibits succinoxidase activity has been purified from hydra (Chapter 47) and is presumed to be a component of the nematocyst venom. Absolute proof that the inhibitor is present in the nematocyst venom must await analysis of the venom isolated from pure, undischarged hydra stenoteles. Because the succinoxidase activity is associated with mitochondrial membranes, and because all of the known actions of the toxic components of the venom from sea anemone and Portuguese man-of-war (*Physalia* sp.) nematocysts act on membranes, the following assays may apply to the venom obtained from hydra stenoteles.

David A. Hessinger ● Department of Physiology and Pharmacology, School of Medicine, Loma Linda University, Loma Linda, California.

ASSAY FOR LETHALITY

COMMENTS

It appears that cnidarian venoms contain two types of toxins, one especially toxic to crustaceans and another more toxic to vertebrates. Standard bioassay procedures for both types of toxicities are described below.

MATERIALS

Crustaceans such as crayfish or crabs may be collected or purchased (Monterey Bay Hydroculture Farms, Santa Cruz, CA, and Pacific Bio-Marine Supply Co., Venice, CA 90291, respectively), whereas female Dublin white mice (25 $\pm$ 2 g) should be purchased (Flow Laboratories). Glass or disposable plastic 0.25-ml or 1-ml Tuberculin syringes (Tomac, American Hospital Supply) equipped with 27-gauge, 0.5-in. needles are used to inject the samples. A standard restraining device is needed to hold the mice during injections. Adequate cages supplied with water, chow, and litter are needed to maintain both kinds of animals under standardized conditions.

PROCEDURES

Crustacean Lethality Bioassay

Several different species of crabs can be used. Crabs seem to be especially sensitive to the protein neurotoxins which have been reported in several cnidarian species (Shapiro, 1968; Hessinger *et al.*, 1973; Rathmayer *et al.*, 1975). We use fiddler crabs, *Uca pugilator*, because of their availability. The minimum lethal dose ($LD_{100\%}$) is defined as the lowest amount of venom per gram of animal weight necessary to kill all animals tested within 30 min of injection. Use female crabs (2.0 0.2 $\pm$ g) because males possess one large claw whose variability in size significantly affects total body weight.

Immobilize the animals ventral side up by securing them with rubber bands to a wooden block while viewing under a dissecting microscope. Inject sample solutions into the body cavity through the membrane between the base of the left front walking leg and the thorax using strong 50-μl micropipets.

For the sea anemone venom the $LD_{100\%}$ is about 0.3 μg protein/g of crab. The legs of crabs injected with venom usually quiver immediately and gradually become rigid; the unrestrained crabs then assume an upright position. The legs eventually fall off (autotomy), and the animal shows progressive insensitivity to external stimuli before dying.

Mouse Lethality Bioassay

Lethality is quantified as the $LD_{50\%}$ caused by intravenously injecting 0.1–0.3 ml venom into the tail veins of female mice. Use groups of four mice at a time for each concentration of venom; repeat the assays several times. Be certain to inject appropriate control solutions. Observe the mice for 24 hr and determine the amount of venom which kills 50% of the mice.

ASSAY OF HEMOLYSIS ACTIVITY

COMMENTS

Hemolysis is a convenient assay for determining the cytolytic activity of venom. I recommend the following hemolytic assay because it allows for quantification by several different means and because it is easily standardized.

MATERIALS

Large male Sprague-Dawley or Wistar rats (300 g or larger) conveniently supply fresh amounts of red blood cells. The rats can be lightly anesthetized with diethyl ether in a large desiccator. Obtain blood using a 10-ml disposable syringe equipped with a 20-gauge, 1.5-in. needle and containing 500 units of heparin. Graduated, conical centrifuge tubes (12–15 ml), ice, and a refrigerated centrifuge (e.g., IEC PR-J or PR-2) equipped with swinging buckets are needed. Wash the red blood cells in isotonic saline buffered with tris (144 mM NaCl and 10 mM tris-HCl, pH 7.4). In addition, a constant-temperature water bath, spectrophotometer, and small, high-speed centrifuge capable of rapid acceleration and deceleration (e.g., Centrifuge Model 59, Fisher Scientific Company) are needed.

PROCEDURES

Preparing Red Blood Cells

Perform hemolysis reactions on washed rat red blood cells (rbcs). Draw about 5–6 ml of blood by cardiac puncture from large male rats lightly anesthetized with ether. Immediately transfer the blood to conical, graduated centrifuge tubes (12–15 ml) on ice; centrifuge them for 5 min at 1000g at 4°C. Remove the serum and white buffy layer by aspiration; suspend the resultant pellet of rbcs in 10 times its volume of anisotonic buffered saline in a 50-ml graduated centrifuge tube. Repeat the washing procedure twice and suspend the washed rbcs in from 5 to 8 times the volume of the pellet with isotonic buffered saline.

Standardizing Red Blood Cell Concentration

In order to relate the results of different hemolysis experiments it is necessary to standardize the concentration of rbcs used as follows: Using a siliconized glass pipet, dilute a 0.1-ml aliquot of the washed rbc suspension with 1.9 ml distilled water; mix and let stand for 5 min. Separate the resulting hemolysate from the red cell membranes by centrifuging at 5000g for 5 min. Read the absorbancy of the solution in the spectrophotometer at 570 nm. From this value, calculate the amount of isotonic saline that would have to be added to the stock rbc suspension such that a 1:20 dilution of this suspension with distilled water will result in a 100% hemolysate which will read 1.20 absorbancy units. This 1:20 dilution of the standardized stock suspension (about 12.5 v/v) is referred to as a 0.625% rbc suspension. Calculate the extent to which the stock rbc suspension is diluted as follows:

Let $O.D._1$ = absorbancy of a hemolysate prepared by diluting the original stock rbc suspension 1:20 with distilled water and thereby lysing all the rbcs

$O.D._2$ = absorbancy to which the hemolysate of the stock rbc suspension should read after lysing with 19 volumes of distilled water (i.e., 1.20 absorbancy units for all experiments)

$concn._1$ = number of rbcs per unit volume of original 1:20 suspension

$$= \frac{\text{total number of rbcs in original stock suspension}}{\text{volume of original stock suspension}}$$

concn.$_2$ = number of rbcs per unit volume of final (0.625%) suspension

$$= \frac{\text{total number of rbcs in final stock suspension}}{\text{volume of final stock suspension}}$$

number rbcs$_1$ = number rbcs$_2$, since the total number of rbcs remain the same because no rbcs are added or discarded.

Since O.D. is proportional to concentration, then O.D.$_1$ is proportional to concn.$_1$ and O.D.$_2$ is proportional to concn.$_2$. Therefore,

$$\frac{\text{O.D.}_1}{\text{O.D.}_2} = \frac{\text{concn.}_1}{\text{concn.}_2}; \frac{\text{O.D.}_1}{\text{concn.}_1} = \frac{\text{O.D.}_2}{\text{concn.}_2}; \frac{\text{O.D.}_1}{\text{rbc}_1/\text{vol}_1} = \frac{\text{O.D.}_2}{\text{rbc}_2/\text{vol}_2}$$

and (O.D.$_1$) (vol$_1$) = (O.D.$_2$) (vol$_2$) since, rbc$_1$ = rbc$_2$. Since O.D.$_1$ is measured and vol$_1$ known, then vol$_2$ can be calculated to give O.D.$_2$ equal to 1.20 absorbancy units (O.D.$_2$).

A 0.625% rat rbc suspension contains approximately 8×10^7 red blood cells/ml and will produce a hemolysate of 1.20 absorbancy units when completely hemolyzed. Accordingly, 1.00 absorbancy units is equal to 6.67×10^7 hemolyzed rbcs/ml.

Hemolysis Assay System

Carry out the hemolysis assays with standardized 0.625% red cell suspensions in an isotonic buffered saline. Both isotonicity and buffering capacity are to be maintained whenever materials are added to the suspending medium. Equilibrate the reaction mixture at 30° for 10 min before beginning the assay. After the reaction has been initiated, take 2- or 1-ml aliquots at timed intervals and centrifuge immediately at high speed (10,000g) for 2 min. Save a portion of the supernatant hemolysate to read on the spectrophotometer at 570 nm at a later time. As many as nine reactions including controls can be carried out simultaneously.

Mathematical Treatment of Hemolysis Data

Calculate the percentage of hemolysis of the red cells from the absorbancy readings of the hemolysates. Because 100% hemolysis is standardized to read 1.20 absorbancy units, the percentage of hemolysis of any hemolysate aliquot is calculated by dividing the measured optical density by

0.012. The data from the hemolysis reaction can be expressed as either "percentage of hemolysis" or "absorbancy at 570 nm." The data may be plotted against time (in minutes) on the abscissa of linear graph paper and gives a sigmoidal curve. Using data plotted in this manner the rates of hemolysis can be ascertained by either of two methods: the maximum slope of the hemolysis curve (expressed as percentage of lysis per minute or $O.D._{570/min}$) or the time for 50% hemolysis to occur (expressed as t_{50}).

As a general rule it is possible to determine whether the lytic agent is acting catalytically (e.g., as an enzyme) or stoichiometrically (e.g., as a detergent or channel former) by measuring the rates of hemolysis at different concentrations of the lytic agent and then arranging the data so that plots of the rate of lysis versus lysin concentration yield a straight line. If the rate of lysis increases along a straight line with a linear increase in lysin concentration, then the lysin is probably acting enzymatically (refer to Fig. 2 in Hessinger and Lenhoff, 1973). If the increase in the rate of lysis follows a straight line while the increase in lysin concentration increases logrithmically then the lytic action is probably the result of the formation of a fixed stoichiometric interaction between lysin and some membrane component(s) (e.g., refer to Fig. 4 in Martin and Padilla, 1971, and Fig. 2 in Pastor, 1973).

A second way of plotting the data has been described in detail elsewhere (Ikezawa, 1963, 1964). By using this method, it is possible to analyze the prehemolytic kinetics of the hemolysis reaction and thereby possibly determine some of the kinetic parameters that are more closely related to the mechanism of action of the hemolysin. Plots of the log percent of the red cell concentration ($\log C/C_o$) against time (minutes), where C_o is the original cell concentration and C is the cell concentration at time t, will yield a straight line for pseudo-first-order reactions. In such a plot there will typically be a prehemolytic or initial induction period before first-order kinetics begin, particularly if the time course plots are sigmoidal. The induction period or time it takes the hemolysis reaction to attain a first-order rate is defined operationally as the time interval between zero time and the intersection of the extrapolated first-order line to the time axis at $\log C/C_o$ equal to 1, corresponding to 0% lysis. Since lysis is a terminal osmotic event resulting from one or more prehemolytic events, the duration of the induction period can be a useful kinetic parameter for determining which of the reactants and conditions that affect the rate of lysis also affect the events of the induction period. These prehemolytic events might include the binding of the lytic agent(s) to the red cell membrane, their interaction with ionic cofactors, and any enzymatic and/or structural rearrangements in membrane components that result in an increase in membrane permeability. By systematically varying the concentrations of the reactants and the order in which they are added it is possible to determine which participate in the prehemolytic events and in what sequence they act.

Screening Chromatographic Column Elution Tubes for Hemolysis Activity

Disposable microtitration plates (V-shaped Microtiter Plates, #220-25, Cooke Engineering) can be used to screen the contents of column elution tubes for hemolysis activity. Put one drop (about 0.05 ml) of isotonic saline into each well. Next, take 25 μl from each elution tube to be tested and put into a separate well in a row along the length of the plate's edge. Use the Micro-Diluter (#220-30, 0.025-ml capacity) to mix the test solution with the saline and to transfer 25 μl of the 1:3 diluted tube sample solution from the first well to the well behind it (in the row along the width of plate's edge). Swirl the Micro-Diluter in the well to produce mixing and then transfer to the next well, carrying 25 μl of the 1:9 solution, and so forth. The result should be a series of dilutions of each test solution in the progression of 1:3, 1:9, 1:27, etc. Finally, add one drop of 1.25% rbcs (made up as 1 ml 12.5% stock rbcs in isotonic saline with 3 ml isotonic CaCl-tris, and 6 ml isotonic saline) to each well. After shaking gently, incubate the whole plate at 37°C for 60 min. Put the plate into the cold (4°C) to allow the cells to settle out for a few hours or overnight and then evaluate the data.

Use a grading system of 4, 3, 2, 1, and 0, where 4 = 100% lysis, 3 = 75%, 2 = 50%, 1 = 25%, and 0 = 0%. In this manner it is possible to screen 12 tubes per plate, each at different dilutions, and identify which tubes possess hemolytic activity and approximately to what extent.

MANOMETRIC ASSAY OF PHOSPHOLIPASE ACTIVITY

COMMENTS

Phospholipase A_2 is a common toxic component of many animal venoms, including those from snakes, spiders, and insects (Tu, 1977). Phospholipase A_2 is also the only known enzymatic activity of *Aiptasia* nematocyst venom where it functions as a component of the hemolytic system of toxins in that venom (Hessinger and Lenhoff, 1976). Although phospholipase A_2 from many venom sources has received much attention, as a class of enzymes they are not well understood. Of the various assay methods available I present only the manometric method in detail while also briefly considering the titrimetric and thin-layer chromatographic methods.

The manometric method is based upon the release of free fatty acids, which dissociate to give rise to hydrogen ions that combine with HCO_3^- to release CO_2. The evolution of CO_2 is followed manometrically. The advantages are that many samples can be assayed simultaneously, that kinetic studies can be performed, and that less specialized and less expensive equipment than the pH-stat are used. On the other hand there are several disadvantages: pH control is not good since the bicarbonate buffer is consumed in the evolution of the CO_2 gas; the operating pH range is limited to the buffering range of the bicarbonate buffer, from about pH 6 to 9; an intermittent rather than a continuous record of the individual reactions is obtained; and the method cannot distinguish between the different types of phospholipase activities (these would first have to be identified by thin-layer chromotography).

MATERIALS

Use a Warburg-type manometric respirometer. Supply the CO_2 component of the bicarbonate buffer from a tank of compressed 5% CO_2 and 95% nitrogen equipped with a two-stage regulator. To obtain pH values of 6.0, 7.0, 8.0, and 9.0, equilibrate the 5% CO_2 gas with reaction mixtures containing 0.66, 6.6, 66, and 660 mM bicarbonate, respectively. Emulsify the phospholipid substrate (e.g., egg yolk lecithin, grade II-E, Sigma Chemical Co.) with a detergent. Both nonionic detergents, such as Triton X-100 (Rohm and Haas) or Tween 25 (Mann Research Laboratories), and ionic detergents, such as deoxycholate, should be tried in various concentrations, although a 2:1 molar ratio of detergent to phospholipid is generally optimal (Denis, 1973).

PROCEDURES

Prepare the basic reaction mixture of 1.0 ml 2% L-α-lecithin, 0.5 ml 25% Tween 25, 0.5 ml 5.1% NaCl, 0.5 ml 0.03 M $CaCl_2$, and 0.5 ml 0.066 M $NaCO_3$ to give a calculated pH of 8.0 when equilibrated with 5% CO_2 and 95% N_2 gas mixture. Add Ca^{2+} last to prevent precipitation of $CaCO_3$. Lecithin appears to inhibit the precipitation of Ca^{2+}. Equilibrate the reaction flask of the Warburg respirometer containing 3.0 ml of basic reaction mixture mixture for 15 min with a flow of gas as 30°C and with a shaking rate of 120 oscillations/min. Add test solutions to the reaction mixture at zero time from the reaction flask sidearm and measure the evolution of CO_2 manometrically.

PRECAUTIONS

Control of the reaction mixture pH is complicated by two factors: First, the measured pH of the reaction system decreases 0.2–0.3 pH units from the pH calculated by the Henderson–Hasselbalch equation for various mixtures of bicarbonate and 5% CO_2. Second, the addition of some of the reaction mixture components to the bicarbonate buffer can lower the pH another 0.1–0.2 pH units.

Discussion of Titrimetric Method

The enzymatic release of fatty acids from phospholipids can be followed by titrating the released acids with a standardized alkali base solution. The milliequivalents of added base equal the milliequivalents of released fatty acid. Frequently a pH-stat is mechanically interfaced with a strip-chart recorder to provide a continuous record of the time course of the reaction. The advantages are that the reaction can be monitored both automatically and continuously. Furthermore, the pH-stat provides absolute control of the pH of the reaction system. The disadvantages are that the assay is not specific for just the A_2 type of phospholipase and that only one reaction at a time can be performed. For details, see Denis (1973).

Discussion of Thin-Layer Chromatographic Method

Use of this method permits identification of the lipid components of the reaction system whether they be reactants, products, or nonparticipants. Analysis of the results can indicate the type(s) of active phospholipases in the system. For complex mixtures of phospholipids, I recommend two-dimensional thin-layer chomatography (Hessinger and Lenhoff, 1976). For purified systhetic or natural phospholipids, one-dimensional chomatograms gives suitable separation of the substrates and products. One distinct disadvantage of this method for routine assays is that extraction of the phospholipids from the reaction system is required before the sample can be applied to the thin-layer plate. Bligh and Dyer (1959) describe a simple procedure. For complex mixtures and highly quantitative work, however, I prefer the method of Folch *et al.* (1957).

Another disadvantage of this method is that it is not well suited for kinetic studies, since individually timed samples must be extracted and chromatographed. To analyze the relative amounts of substrate and product, the extracted phospholipids are chromatographed and the lipid spots are visualized with iodine vapor, identified by comparison with standards, scraped off the plate, and collected into test tubes, where they are analyzed colorimetrically for total phosphorus by the method of Bartlett (1959).

EFFECT ON NEURAL ACTIVITY OF CRAYFISH VENTRAL NERVE CORD

COMMENTS

Measurement of the effects of venom components on the action potential conduction of the giant motor fibers of the crayfish is a particularly useful and repeatable way to study suspected neurotoxins. It appears that all well-studied neurotoxins from sea anemones act in basically the same fashion: They preferentially block conduction along crustacean axons by inhibiting the inactivation of the early, transient inward ("sodium") current (Narahashi et al., 1969; Hessinger et al. 1973; Rathmayer et al., 1975).

MATERIALS

Living and healthy crayfish (e.g., *Procamborus clarkii*) can be obtained commercially from North Carolina Biological Supply Co., Burlington, NC. A dissecting microscope is helpful, and dissecting equipment is needed. Construct a dissecting dish with a molded paraffin bottom into which the isolated nerve can be pinned and immersed in a physiological medium such as van Harreveld's solution (Van Harreveld, 1936). Use warmed petroleum jelly (Vaseline) contained in a 25-ml syringe to construct compartment bridges across the nerve in the dissecting dish. Employ glass microelectrodes filled with 3 M KCl for intracellular recordings with any single-beamed oscilloscope. Place the specimen and all electrical components, including a stimulator (e.g., Tetronix series 160), within a Faraday cage to eliminate interference from external electrical sources.

PROCEDURES

Chill the crayfish on ice for 15 min to slow down its motor activity. Submerge the animal in van Harreveld's solution before dissecting. Remove the ventral nerve cord carefully from the animal and pin it dorsal side up through the sixth abdominal and second thoracic ganglia. Secure the segment of nerve cord between the third and fourth abdominal ganglia to the dish bottom with tiny pins placed at the junction of the third and fourth ganglia and their first roots. Finally, carefully remove the connective tissue sheath covering the nerve cord between the third and fourth ganglia and expose the four giant dorsal fibers.

After the dissection and desheathing are completed, remove all fluid from the chamber except for the thin film clinging to the nerve cord. Quickly construct two Vaseline bridges across the cord anterior to the third abdominal ganglion, dividing the chamber into three separate compartments. Refill all three compartments with van Harreveld's solution. Adjust the amount of fluid in the most posterior compartment, which should contain the desheathed segment of nerve cord, to a predetermined volume of usually 0.5–1.0 ml. Place a stimulating electrode of platinum wire in the anterior and middle compartments and ground the posterior compartment.

Penetrate a single neuron in the desheathed region with a 3 M KCl-filled glass capillary electrode. You should find that single action potentials are evoked by brief (0.5 msec) square-wave pulses from the stimulator. Note and record photographically the normal action potentials (i.e., of the neuron in van Harreveld's solution alone). Gently add a measured amount of venom or toxic fraction in van Harreveld's solution to the fluid in the posterior compartment of the dish. After the venom is applied, record single action potentials at frequent timed intervals until the experiment is terminated. Record the resting potentials at the beginning and at the end of the experiments to determine if the passive properties of the nerve membrane have been affected by either the procedure or the venom. The venom-induced effects on crayfish axons typically include multiple depolarizations superimposed on prolonged action potentials and action potentials with two plateaus followed by irreversible nerve failure (Hessinger et al., 1973).

REFERENCES

Bartlett, G. R. 1959. Phosphorus assay in column chromatography. J. Biol. Chem. 234:466–468.

Bligh, E. G., and Dyer, W. J. 1959. A rapid method of total lipid extraction and purification. Can. J. Biochem. Physiol. 37:911–917.

Denis, E. A. 1973. Kinetic dependence of phospholipase A$_2$ activity on the detergent Triton X-100. J. Lipid Res. 14:152–159.

Folch, J., Lees, M., and Stanley, G. H. S. 1957. A simple method for the isolation and purification of total lipids from animal tissues. J. Biol. Chem. 226:497–509.

Hessinger, D. A., and Lenhoff, H. M. 1973. Assay and properties of the hemolysis activity of pure venom from the nematocysts of the acontia of the sea anemone Aiptasia pallida. Arch. Biochem. Biophys. 159:629–638.

Hessinger, D. A., and Lenhoff, H. M. 1976. Mechanism of hemolysis induced by nematocyst venom: Roles of phospholipase A and direct lytic factor. Arch. Biochem. Biophys. 173:603–613.

Ikezawa, H. 1963. The kinetic analysis of hemolysis by *Clostridium perfringens (Cl. welchii)* alpha-toxin (phospholipase C). *J. Biochem.* **54**:301–311.

Ikezawa, H. 1964. Comparative kinetics of hemolysis of mammalian erythrocytes by *Clostridium perfringens* alpha-toxin (phospholipase C). *J. Biochem.* **55**:217–224.

Martin, D. F., and Padilla, G. M. 1971. Hemolysis induced by *Prymnesium parvum* toxin: Kinetics and binding. *Biochim. Biophys. Acta.* **241**:213–225.

Narahashi, T., Moore, J. W., and Shapiro, B. I. 1969. *Condylactis* toxin: Interaction with nerve membrane ionic conductances. *Science* **163**:680–681.

Pastor, Z. 1973. Pharmocology and mode of action of prymnesin. In: *Marine Pharmocognosy* (D. F. Martin and G. M. Padilla, eds.), Academic Press, New York.

Rathmayer, W., Jessen, B., and Beress, L. 1975. On the effect of purified toxins of two sea anemones species (Coelenterata) on neuromuscular transmission in the cray fish. *Naturwissenschaften* **62**:538–539.

Shapiro, B. I. 1968. A site of action of toxin from the sea anemone *Condylactis gigantea*. *Comp. Biochem. Physiol.* **27**:519–531.

Tu, A. 1977. *Venoms: Chemistry and Molecular Biology*. Wiley, New York.

van Harreveld, A. 1936. A physiological solution for fresh water crustaceans. *Proc. Soc. Exp. Biol. Med.* **34**:428–432.

Part XI

Analytical Procedures

Special Techniques for Weighing Microgram Quantities of Tissue and Assaying Them for Enzyme Activities

Charles L. Rutherford

PURPOSE

To carry out biochemical analyses on single hydra or parts of an animal and to relate those measurements to the dry weight of the tissue analyzed. There are three essential steps: (1) the quick freeze-drying of the hydra; (2) the dissection and weighing of pieces of dry hydra tissue as light as 0.1 μg; (3) the biochemical assay of those dried tissues.

INTRODUCTION

Assays of parts of a single hydra should be useful when one needs to know the enzyme activity or substrate level of particular areas of the animal. Standard methods such as penetration of vital dyes or substrates are not always valid for hydra because of its limited permeability to ionic substances. In addition, if the living hydra is dissected into the desired parts of the animal before the assay, the simple act of dissection may alter the metabolism of the tissue. The methods I describe eliminate those difficulties.

These methods are adaptations to hydra (Rutherford and Lenhoff,

Charles L. Rutherford • Biology Department, Virginia Polytechnic Institute and State University, Blacksburg, Virginia .

1969) of the ultramicrobiochemical procedures developed by Lowry and Passonneau (1972) to assay vertebrate tissue. With hydra it is possible to freeze, dry, preserve, and analyze animals of desired physiological and developmental states.

FREEZE-DRYING HYDRA AND DISSECTING BITS OF TISSUE

COMMENTS

In order to maintain substrate levels present *in vivo*, hydra must be frozen as rapidly as possible. The method described allows this quick freezing without resulting in the contraction of the hydra. By freeze-drying and storing the animals at low temperatures under vacuum, the tissue can be maintained for long periods of time without loss of enzymes or labile substrates. In addition, the morphological integrity is retained so that precise cellular regions can be dissected. The method also allows the investigator to preserve the tissue from an experiment for subsequent analysis at a later time. The actual dissection is done freehand under a stereo microscope with implements constructed from readily available low-cost supplies. With practice, a single hydra can be dissected into 50–60 sections, while tentacles, hypostome, body, and basal disk region can be isolated at the first trial.

MATERIALS

Liquid Freon-12; dry ice; 1/4-in. Plexiglas; glass microscope slide; fast-freeze flask (Labconco No. 75410); freezer dryer (any manufacturer); vacuum vial (Virtis No. 10-159); freezer (preferably ultralow, -80°C); stereo microscope; radium foil (20 mm wide, 16 μCi/cm, Amersham/Searle Corp., Arlington Heights, IL 60005); and fiber optic illuminator (optional; Dolan Jenner Industries, Inc., Woburn, MA).

Microscalpels and Hair Points. Construct the microscalpel from a tiny section of razor blade attached to a 0.5-cm length of thin spring steel wire. Attach the steel wire to a 1-cm length of copper wire anchored in a wooden dowel rod. Construct hair points, of either human eyelash or cat hair, in a similar fashion, except cement the hair directly to the copper wire.

PROCEDURES

To freeze hydra, use liquid Freon-12 precooled in a dry-ice–acetone bath. Use a freezing chamber constructed from a 1×1×1/4-in. section of Plexiglas having a 1/2-in.-diameter hole in the center attached flat to a 1×1-in. section of a glass microscope slide. Place a single hydra in a drop of culture solution on the microscope slide in the center of the hole. After the hydra relaxes to its normal length, quickly pour the cold Freon over the entire holder; the hydra should freeze in less than 1 sec. Insert several of these holders with frozen hydra into a drying chamber. Lyophilize the sample overnight and store them at reduced pressure in the screw cap vials. Several hundred of these vials will conveniently fit into a divided storage box (Revco). Thus, with proper inventory control the animals from many experiments can be retained in a state in which further measurement of enzyme activities is possible.

On the day an assay is to be performed, remove the desired vial from the freezer and allow the contents to come to room temperature (approximately 30 min). Remove the specimen to be dissected from the vial and place it on black cardboard for examination under a stereomicroscope. Photograph the specimen if a permanent record of the experiment is desired. Place the specimen on a 4×4 in.-square stage. To control static electricity, suspend a 1/2-in.-square piece of radium foil directly above the dissecting surface. Bring a sample into focus at a magnification of 10–40× and at an illumination yielding maximum clarity. I recommend a fiber optic illumination because the flexible support rod can be positioned to detail critical dissections and, more importantly, because little heat is generated at the light source. Tape a 3-in.-square piece of aluminum foil to the front of the microscope to prevent the operator's breath from disturbing the sections. Cut the specimen freehand with the microscalpels while manipulating the tissue with hair points. To minimize tremor, press the side of the hand and fingers against the cutting surface. Touch the tip of the razor blade to the plastic surface to act as a pivot for the sectioning procedure. Make the cut by rocking the microscalpel slowly downward from the pivot. With some practice, sections 20 μm in diameter with a dry weight of 0.1 μg can be obtained.

CONSTRUCTION AND USE OF THE QUARTZ BALANCE

COMMENTS

The sections of tissue are next weighed on a quartz fiber balance (Fig. 1). Such balances are capable of far greater sensitivity than commercially available instruments. Although the balance appears to be fragile, if constructed as described herein, it will endure continuous usage for years.

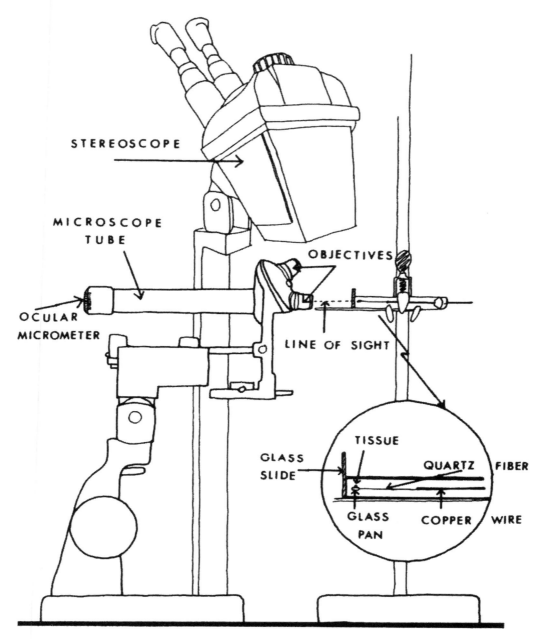

FIGURE 1. Lowry quartz fiber ultramicrobalance.

Moreover, once calibrated, the balances should show no detectable change in sensitivity for 5 years or more.

MATERIALS

Quartz fibers and glass rods (Amersil, Inc., Hillside, NJ 07205); gas–oxygen torch (Tescon Corp., Minneapolis, MN); copper wire (20 gauge); sealing wax; epoxy resin; 20-mm glass Petri dish; glass syringe (1–10 ml); radium foil; ocular micrometer (size will depend on sensitivity of the balance); stereomicroscope; p-nitrophenylphosphate (Sigma Chemical Co.); 50 mM carbonate buffer, pH 10.0; spectrophotometer.

PROCEDURES

The quartz fibers can be either purchased (to 3 μm diameter) or made by hand. I suggest making a number of fibers of varying diameters and storing them for later use. In a few hours a limitless supply of various fibers can be drawn out from a hot quartz rod for a fraction of the cost of purchase. I use the "slingshot" arrangement, as described in detail by Lowry and Passonneau (1972), for stretching a quartz rod into a fiber. Attach one end of the rod to a stationary mount and the other to a stretched rubber band. Bring the flame from a gas–oxygen torch to the rod. At the moment the quartz becomes fluid, the tension on the rubber band is released, thus stretching the rod into a fiber. Fibers of varying thickness can be made by altering the tension on the rubber band or by using different-size rods.

To prepare the fibers for the most sensitive balance, use the "draft" from the gas–oxygen torch to "pull" the fiber. Hold the rod lengthwise in the flame until a thin fiber forms. Continue to heat the fiber until the flow of warm air upward pulls the quartz into a fine quartz thread. An assistant can then capture the fine thread on a black cloth. Fibers of less than 0.2 μm can be made in this manner. Store the fibers taped at either end to the bottom of a 20-mm glass Petri dish.

Mount the fiber to a 2-in. section of 20-gauge copper wire. The length of the fiber will depend on the relative sensitivity of the balance. The balances we are currently using have sensitivities from 0.05 to 10 μg, with fibers ranging from 1 to 10 cm in length. Attach the fiber to the copper wire by either sealing wax or epoxy resin. The resin is polymerized by the heat from a fine-tipped soldering iron. To the free end of the fiber, attach a flat weighing pan made from thin fragments of a bubble blown from quartz tubing. Select the pans so that when applied to the fiber only a slight deflection will occur.

Attach the copper wire to the plunger of a glass syringe. Cut off the closed end of the syringe barrel and insert the plunger and attached fiber. The balance is then ready for permanent mounting on a balance support. Several supports have been described (Burt, 1966; Lowry, 1941; Lowry and Passonneau, 1972); construction of a support will depend upon the amount of use to be expected. We use two specially constructed rugged aluminum supports (details will be furnished upon request). With any support a sliding glass "door" in front of the cut end of the syringe barrel must be provided to prevent interference by air currents (Fig. 1). Finally, place a 1/4-in.-square section of radium foil in the balance to dispel electrostatic charges.

The resulting displacement of the fiber tip by the applied tissue section can be measured by an ocular micrometer. For most purposes a $1\times$ or $4\times$ objective is optimum, as higher powers require short working distances. For viewing the loading of the balance, I recommend the use of a second stereoscope set at a slight angle to the first.

Calibration of the Quartz Fiber Balance

Select the appropriate objective and eyepiece lense for the desired degree of magnification at the tip of the quartz fiber. Place a crystal of p-nitrophenol on the weighing pan and record the deflection. Select the range of crystal sizes and record the corresponding degree of tip displacement. Dissolve each separate crystal in 500 μl of 50 mM carbonate buffer, pH 10, and read the optical density of the solution at 400 nm using a spectrophotometer. The weights of the crystals can then be calculated from the optical density readings made with a p-nitrophenol standard solution. The extinction coefficient for the dye is 15,000 M^{-1}cm^{-1}. Calculate the sensitivity of the balances from the deflections and from the weights of the crystals.

Use of the Balance

The procedure for weighting tissue sections will depend on the acquired skill of the investigator. For the first few trials I recommend dissecting a single tissue section; place it on a 1×8-cm. piece of black cardboard for transporting it to the balance. "Zero" the balance by placing the pan image on a arbitrary scale marker on the ocular micrometer. Open the glass door and place the tissue section on the pan with a hair point. Close the door and measure and record the deflection of the fiber. Transport the cardboard and tissue section back to the dissecting area, where the assay will be performed. As one gains confidence with handling the microsections, several pieces of tissue can be aligned on the cardboard at once. If the sections are weighed and placed in the reaction vessels in order, as many as 50 sections can be handled at a single time.

PRECAUTIONS

I recommend that you dissect and weigh the dried tissues in a small room maintained at a low humidity. If the humidity is too high, the tissues may take up water, resulting in erroneous weighings and in the degradation of labile substrates within the tissue.

OIL WELL METHOD FOR ASSAYING ENZYME ACTIVITY

COMMENTS

While the dissection and weighing of tissue sections are unique to the micromethods, the actual assays of enzyme activity are in most cases simply the adaptation of large-scale assays to the microlevels. The primary adaptation to a microassay is a reduction in the size of the reaction volume. The extent of the reduction is dictated by the ratio of the blank value and the amount of product of an enzyme reaction. The methods to be described will enable you to assay enzymes in sections of tissue containing approximately 200 cells. The endogeneous level of many substrates, as well as enzymes with low activity, can be measured by utilizing an additional step of enzymatic cycling (Lowry and Passonneau, 1972; Rutherford, 1976). However, the latter techniques are beyond the limits of this discussion.

The methods used for enzyme assays utilize the native fluorescence properties of the pyridine nucleotides (Lowry *et al.*, 1957). Enzymes which require a pyridine nucleotide as a cofactor can be assayed in a single step. With the use of auxiliary enzymes most compounds of biological interest can be assayed by these methods. The reaction time and temperature must be rigidly controlled. Likewise, the reaction conditions must be shown to result in a maximum velocity of the enzyme and to support a linear rate of product formation during the time of incubation.

MATERIALS

Mineral oil; hexadecane; silicone liquid (Sigmacote, Sigma Chemical Co., Saint Louis, MO); substrates and cofactors for enzyme assays (various sources); Teflon; oil well racks (Teflon obtainable from Plywood and

Plastics, Inc., Richmond, VA 23230; or use microtest tissue culture plate No. 3034, Falcon, Oxnard, CA 93030); constriction pipets (H. E. Pederson, Copenhagen, V, Denmark; pipets holding less than 10 μl must be made by hand and calibrated as described by Lowry and Passonneau, 1972); plastic Petri dishes; fluorometer (for measuring pyridine nucleotides in a Farrand fluorometer use a Corning No. 5840 filter for the incident light and No. 4308 filter for the emitted light).

PROCEDURES

When an individual organism or sections of an individual organism are assayed, the reactions must be carried out under a hexadecane:mineral oil (3:7 v/v) mixture. The reaction vessel is a 4-mm well drilled into a $20 \times 120 \times 5$-mm Teflon block (Fig. 2). Use a flat-ended drill to produce a flat bottom well. A thin, translucent layer of Teflon remains at the bottom of the well, thus enhancing the visibility of small volumes of samples in the well.

Just prior to use, dip the constriction pipet to be used in the oil well procedure into Sigmacote while forcing air through the pipet. This process leaves a thin layer of silicone on the outer surface, thus preventing adhesion of small amounts of the reagent to the tip of the pipet. Add a small volume of reaction mixture to the bottom of the well. Pick up a whole organism or a small section with the hair points and add it directly to the reaction volume. This procedure guarantees maximum mixing of the reagents and the enzyme to be assayed. Incubate the oil well racks by placing them in plastic Petri dishes floating in a water bath. Stop the reaction by adding acid or alkaline reagents or by heating the well rack for 5 min at 100°C in an oven.

The procedure for isocitrate dehydrogenase will be described as an example of an enzyme assay in microquantities of tissue. Add the dry sections to 5 μl of a reaction mixture containing 0.1 M imidazole buffer (pH 6.5), 0.02% albumin, 1.0 mM MnCl$_2$, 1.5 mM NAD$^+$, 10 mM inorganic phosphate, 1 mM ADP, 5 mM sodium amytol, and 5 mM isocitrate. Incubate the reaction at 25°C for 60 min, and stop it by heating at 90°C for 10 min. The following conversion reaction occurs:

$$\text{isocitrate} + \text{NAD}^+ \rightarrow \alpha\text{-ketoglutarate} + \text{NADH}$$

When you are certain you have sufficient activity, remove the entire 5 μl reaction mixture and place it in 1 ml 50 mM carbonate–bicarbonate buffer (pH 10.0). Measure the fluorescence of these samples along with appropriate blanks and standards; calculate the specific activity based on the dry weight of the tissue assayed. If sufficient fluorescence over the blank value is not

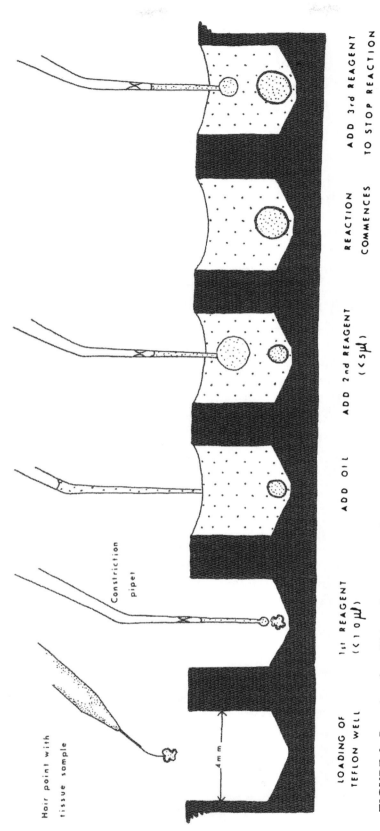

FIGURE 2. Procedure for addition of reagents to oil wells. Note: It is not absolutely necessary to add a final reagent to stop the reaction, as application of heat will do.

obtained by this direct assay, the NADH produced can be measured by one of the procedures of enzymatic cycling.

PRECAUTIONS

In principle, the microtechnique should present no more pitfalls than those encountered with less sensitive procedures. However, because the reaction mixtures are microscopic and, therefore, cannot be observed directly, the investigator must insure that each step of the procedure performs its intended function.

Some common errors encountered include:

1. Incorrect pH changes when acids or basic solutions are added to stop a reaction or destroy unreacted nucleotides.

2. An insufficient amount of one substrate or cofactor is added to the reaction mixture.

3. The amount of an enzyme added is not sufficient to convert all of the metabolite to a product in a given interval of time.

4. High blank values result from fluorescent contaminants in the reagents or in the tissue extract itself.

5. High blank values result from endogenous levels of substrates or enzymes.

While most of the pitfalls encountered in the microassays can be rather easily eliminated, it demands from the analyst some skill in recognizing where the problem exists and in adapting the procedure to the specific requirements of the assay.

ACKNOWLEDGMENTS. This research was supported by Grant Number AG0067, awarded by the National Institute on Aging, DHEW, and by Grant Number CA24150, awarded by the National Cancer Institute, DHEW.

REFERENCES

Burt, A. M. 1966. Modification of the Lowry quartz fiber "Fishpole" ultramicrobalance. *Microchem. J.* 11:18–25.

Lowry, O. H. 1941. A quartz fiber balance. *J. Biol. Chem.* 140:183–189.

Lowry, O. H., and Passonneau, J. V. 1972. *A Flexible System of Enzymatic Analysis.* Academic Press, New York.

Lowry, O. H., Roberts, N. R., and Kapphahn, J. L. 1957. The fluorometric measurement of pyridine nucleotides. *J. Biol. Chem.* 224:1047–1064.

Rutherford, C. L. 1976. Glycogen degradation during migration of presumptive cell types in *Dictyostelium discoideum*. *Biochim. Biophys. Acta.* **74**:179–222.

Rutherford, C. L., and Lenhoff, H. M. 1969. Enzymes of glucose catabolism in *Hydra*. II. Application of microfluorometric analysis to patterns of enzyme localization. *Arch. Biochem. Biophys.* **133**:128–136.

Chapter 50

Extracting and Characterizing Hydra RNA: Modifications to Allow Extraction of Undegraded Material in the Presence of High Levels of Degradative Enzymes

Georgia E. Lesh-Laurie, Joseph R. Voland, and Stephen S. Macintyre

PURPOSE

Because hydra is rich in degradative enzymes (i.e., nucleases and proteases), the application of conventional techniques for the isolation of macromolecules invariably results in the isolation of degraded material (Voland, 1975). We describe herein a modified phenol–chloroform procedure for the extraction of total RNA from *Hydra oligactis* which overcomes these difficulties.

INTRODUCTION

The procedure described below allows for the extraction of RNA from hydra at an efficiency comparable to that obtained employing a modified

Georgia E. Lesh-Laurie ● Department of Biology, Cleveland State University, Cleveland, Ohio. Joseph R. Voland ● Department of Pathology, University of California, San Diego, La Jolla, California. Stephen S. Macintyre ● Department of Anatomy, Case Western Reserve University, Cleveland, Ohio.

Schmidt–Thannhauser (Schmidt and Thannhauser, 1945) method (Voland *et al.*, 1977). Because our results show that the absorption patterns (A_{260}) generated using hydra RNA extracted by this method are similar to those of other organisms, and because molecular-weight determinations of the ribosomal fractions reveal hydra rRNAs to be distributed into weight ranges consistent with the rRNA's from other organisms (Stewart and Letham, 1973; Voland *et al.*, 1977), we conclude that the adverse effects of degradative enzymes have been minimized and that the extraction procedure does not modify the RNA (i.e., cause cross-linking or result in degradation).

Both sodium dodecyl sulfate and diethylpyrocarbonate are necessary for the extraction of undegraded RNA from hydra. If either of these materials is omitted, mostly degraded RNA is obtained. Bentonite, alternatively, is not essential to the extraction of undegraded hydra RNA; exclusion of bentonite from the homogenizing buffer, however, reduces the stability of the preparation. Regardless of the RNase inhibitors used, significant degradation of the RNA species is observed after a period of 1 month, even at 0°C. Hydra must be homogenized and the RNA extracted at 0°C. Hot-phenol (60°C) extraction procedures (Gregory and Lerman, 1964) yield degraded RNA.

MATERIALS

Reagents. Chloroform; diethylpyrocarbonate (Eastman Organic Chemicals, Rochester, NY); DNase (DNase I, RNase free, Worthington Biochemicals, Freehold, NJ); 95% ethanol; phenol (redistilled from commercial phenol); potassium acetate.

Buffers

RNA Homogenizing Buffer. Tris(hydroxymethyl)aminomethane (pH 7.0), 10 mM; 0.5% sodium dodecyl sulfate; 0.01% bentonite.

Tris Buffer. Tris(hydroxymethyl)aminomethane (pH 7.0), 0.01 M.

RNA Sample Buffer. Tris(hydroxymethyl)aminomethane (pH 7.8), 36 mM; 30 mM NaH$_2$PO$_4$; 10 mM EDTA; 0.2% sodium dodecyl sulfate; 7% sucrose.

DNase Buffer. Tris(hydroxymethyl)aminomethane (pH 7.4), 100 mM;

10 mM MgCl$_2$ · 6H$_2$O; 0.25% Mg-treated bentonite (bentonite equilibrated with 10 mM MgCl$_2$ · 6H$_2$O).

RNA Running Buffer (Loening, 1967). Tris(hydroxymethyl)aminomethane (pH 7.8), 36 mM; 30 mM NaH$_2$PO$_4$; 10 mM EDTA; 0.2% sodium dodecyl sulfate.

Other

The supplies necessary to extract hydra RNA include routinely available glassware, an apparatus for tissue homogenization, and a high-speed refrigerated centrifuge. Autoclave all glassware to destroy the ubiquitously occurring RNases. Fractionation of the extracted RNA requires the capability to perform either polyacrylamide gel electrophoresis (the method described below) or sucrose gradient analysis.

PROCEDURES

RNA Extraction and Purification

Place 50–200 hydra that have been fasted for 1 day in 4 ml of RNA homogenizing buffer (0°C) to which diethylpyrocarbonate has been added to give a final concentration of 10%. Homogenize the animals (0°C) with 10 vertical strokes in a glass tissue homogenizer utilizing a motor-driven Teflon pestle run for 1 min at high speed. Pour the homogenate into an autoclaved 30-ml centrifuge tube and rinse the homogenizer with 1 ml tris buffer. Add the rinse volume to the homogenate.

Mix the homogenate with an equal volume of phenol-chloroform (1:1 v/v) (Perry *et al.*, 1972). Shake the mixture vigorously for 30 sec and then agitate with a Vortex mixer at high speed for 1 min. Centrifuge the resultant mixture at 14,500g for 10 min at a running temperature of 0°C. Transfer the aqueous phase to an autoclaved 15-ml centrifuge tube with a Pasteur pipet. Add 0.1 volume potassium acetate (20% w/v) to the aqueous phase followed by two volumes of cold (−20°C) 95% ethanol. Cover the tube with parafilm, invert it several times to completely mix the ethanol and aqueous phases, and place it in a freezer overnight.

Following overnight precipitation, centrifuge the nucleic acids at 14,500g for 10 min. Pour off the ethanol and allow the pellet to dry until an ethanol odor is no longer detectable (about 30 min). Dissolve the pellet in 0.5 ml tris buffer and remove 0.05 ml of this solution for spectrophotometric analysis. Add potassium acetate and ethanol to the remainder of the solution, as described above, and allow the nucleic acids to precipitate for a minimum of 2 hr. Centrifuge the precipitated nucleic acids, remove the remaining supernatant, and allow the pellet to dry. Dissolve the dried pellet in 0.5 ml RNA sample buffer and store it at 4°C.

To determine the position of the DNA peaks on polyacrylamide gels, treat the final nucleic acid pellet with DNase. Precipitate the nucleic acids out of the sample buffer with ethanol, as described above. Dissolve pellet in 0.5 ml DNase buffer and add DNase I to give a final concentration of 10 μg/ml. Incubate the sample at 37°C for 1 hr, repeat the phenol–chloroform extraction to remove the DNase, and perform two ethanol precipitations to concentrate the RNA. Because this step adds the possibility of RNase contamination, discontinue it once you determine the position of the DNA peaks in the polyacrylamide gel.

Dissolve the material set aside for spectrophotometric analysis in tris buffer and determine its absorption at 260 nm. Using this procedure, an A_{260} reading of 24 is equivalent to 1 mg/ml of RNA.

RNA Fractionation

The extracted RNA can now be fractionated and examined on 6×95-mm or 6×65-mm polyacrylamide gels at acrylamide concentrations of 2.4% (95 mm) or 7.2% (65 mm). (For details of preparing gel, see Caston and Jones, 1972). Prerun the gels for 30 min in RNA running buffer before the sample is loaded. Load between 20–40 μg of RNA (as determined spectroscopically) on each gel; this amount contains sufficient RNA so that the peaks are easily recognizable. It also guards against overloading of the gel. Overloading in a gel can be easily perceived by the appearance of aggregate peaks and by a decrease in resolution; hence, run controls for overloading.

Separate the RNA species by electrophoresis at 50 V (7.5 mA/gel) for 2.5 hr (2.4%) or 1.5 hr (7.2%). Analyze gels in a recording spectrophotometer equipped with a linear transporter. We employ a Gilford Recording Spectrophotometer with scanning carried out at 260 nm at a scanning rate of 2 cm/min.

ACKNOWLEDGMENTS. We acknowledge support from a Denver M. Eckert grant for Cancer Research from the American Cancer Society, a Brown-Hazen grant from Research Corporation, a Graduate Alumni Fund grant-in-aid, and U.S. Public Health Service grant HD 00038 to Dr. J. Douglas Caston.

REFERENCES

Caston, J. D., and Jones, P. 1972. Synthesis and processing of high molecular weight RNA by nuclei isolated from embryos of *Rana pipiens. J. Mol. Biol.* **69**:19–38.

Gregory, G. P., and Lerman, M. I. 1964. Separation and some properties of distinct classes of newly-formed ribonucleic acid from animal cells. *Biochim. Biophys. Acta* **91**:678–680.

Loening, U. 1967. The fractionation of high-molecular-weight ribonucleic acid by polyacrylamide gel electrophoresis. *Biochem. J.* **102**:251–259.

Perry, R. P., La Torre, J., Kelly, D. E., and Greenberg, J. R., 1972. On the lability of poly(A) sequences during extraction of messenger RNA from polyribosomes. *Biochim. Biophys. Acta* **262**:220–226.

Schmidt, G., and Thannhauser, S. S., 1945. A method for the determination of desoxyribonucleic acid, ribonucleic acid, and phosphoproteins in animal tissues. *J. Biol. Chem* **161**:83–89.

Stewart, P., and Letham, D. 1973. *The Ribonucleic Acids.* Springer-Verlag, New York.

Voland, J. R. 1975. Biochemical interactions and morphogenesis in *Hydra.* Master's thesis, Case Western Reserve University, Cleveland.

Voland, J. R., Lesh-Laurie, G. E., and Macintyre, S. S., 1977. A procedure for the extraction and characterization of RNA from the freshwater cnidarian *Hydra. Comp. Biochem. Physiol.* **57 B**:203–208.

Chapter 51

Colorimetric Analysis for Protein of Hydra

Howard M. Lenhoff

PURPOSE

To determine the amount of protein in samples of hydra tissues from as few as three to five animals.

INTRODUCTION

In determining the specific activity of enzymes and of radioactive fractions, it is essential to know the protein content or the dry weight of the tissue fraction being analyzed. The following modification of the simple and sensitive colorimetric method of Lowry *et al.* (1951) serves admirably for hydra. One slight change needed for hydra is the addition of sodium hydroxide to hydrolyze the relatively insoluble nematocyst capsules.

MATERIALS

Prepare 500 ml of a "protein reagent" consisting of 0.06% sodium tartrate, 0.03% cupric sulfate, and 4% sodium carbonate as follows: To prevent precipitation of cupric carbonate, dissolve the first two reagents in

Howard M. Lenhoff ● Department of Developmental and Cell Biology, University of California, Irvine, California.

450 ml distilled water, slowly add and dissolve the powdered sodium carbonate, and bring the final volume to 500 ml with water. Prepare the diluted phenol (Folin-Colciateau) reagent (Fisher Scientific Co.) by diluting the purchased stock solution 1 part to 2 parts of distilled water just before using it. Store the stock phenol reagent at 4°C. To prepare a protein standard solution, dilute 1 ml of a stock solution of serum albumin calibrated at 10 mg/ml by Armour Pharmaceutical Co. (Scottsdale, AZ) with 250 ml of distilled water. Store the resultant solutions, which will contain 40 μg protein N/ml, at −25°C in 1.5-ml aliquots in plastic test tubes until needed.

Other materials needed are a spectrophotometer or a colorimeter fitted with a 650–nm filter, and a water bath set at 37°C (optional).

PROCEDURES

To each 0.5 ml of the sample (suspensions of finely homogenized or sonicated material, or soluble proteins) add 5 ml of the protein reagent. Mix and incubate them at room temperature for 1 hr or, to save time, at 37°C for 0.5 hr. At the conclusion of the incubation, add 0.5 ml of the diluted phenol reagent, mix thoroughly, and let the tubes sit for 20 min at room temperature. Determine the absorbance at 650 nm and subtract the absorption of a reagent blank consisting of 5.5 ml of the mixed reagent solutions and 0.5 ml of water.

Compare the measured absorbances to those obtained with standards made from the diluted calibrated protein. Because the plot of absorbance against protein is not completely linear, prepare a standard curve ranging from 4 to 20 μg protein N per tube. These can be prepared by using 0.1, 0.2, 0.3, 0.4, and 0.5 ml of the diluted protein with the difference in volume compensated by adding 0.4, 0.3, 0.2, 0.1, and 0 ml of water to the respective tubes.

COMMENTS

A variation of the above procedure is useful when dealing with pooled small pieces of special parts of the hydra, such as the tentacles, too small to homogenize into a fine suspension. In these cases, place the tissues in a test tube, remove as much culture solution as possible with a fine tapered eye dropper, add 0.5 ml of 1 N NaOH, and let the samples sit for 15 min. Then add 5 ml of the protein reagent and proceed as described above.

When first carrying out the analyses, it is best to make duplicates or even triplicates of the samples. With practice and familiarity with the tissues being analyzed, you should aim to adjust your sample size to about 10 μg protein N per 0.5 ml and use only four protein standards—one of 8 μg, two of 12 μg, and one of 16 μg.

REFERENCES

Lowry, O. H., Rosebrough, N. J., Farr, A. L., and Randall, R. J. 1951. Protein measurement with the Folin phenol reagent. *J. Biol Chem.* **193**:265–276.

Chapter 52

Determining Respiration and Oxygen Evolution of Green Hydra with the Rank Brothers Oxygen Electrode

Donald W. Phipps, Jr.

PURPOSE

To measure oxygen consumption or evolution by as few as 150 green hydra or oxygen evolution from isolated symbiotic algae in suspension.

INTRODUCTION

The Rank Brothers Oxygen Electrode is a simple water-jacketed polarographic oxygen electrode designed for monitoring oxygen concentration in volumes of solution ranging from 0.5 to over 5 ml. The device offers a rapid response time which is well suited to photosynthetic or respirometric measurements of small organisms such as hydra. A chart recorder may be coupled to the instrument for continued monitoring or easily determining rates of oxygen exchange.

The oxygen consumption of about 150 hydra may be measured by the following procedure. Measurement of total animal protein following respiration measurements allows calculation of specific respiration rates.

Oxygen evolution from isolated algal symbionts in suspension or from green hydra can be measured by slightly modifying the procedures for measuring oxygen consumption.

Donald W. Phipps, Jr. ● School of Life Sciences, University of Nebraska, Lincoln, Nebraska.

MATERIALS

Rank Brothers Oxygen Electrode (Rank Bros., Cambridge, England); chart recorder (optional); controlled-temperature water bath; calibrating oxygen meter (such as International Biophysics Corporation's dissolved oxygen and temperature monitor); magnetic stirrer and stir bar; air stone; aquarium pump or other source of air; 300-to 500-ml beaker; basket to hold animals (see text for description); M solution (Chapter 4); sodium dithionite.

For measuring oxygen production, in addition to the above materials, use the following: a slide projector; mirrors; collimating lens; neutral density filters; diaphragm; Plexiglas rod (5/8-in OD) machined to fit electrode chambers and polished at both ends to transmit light; ring stands; clamps.

PROCEDURES

Electrode Calibration

Connect the water bath to the chamber jacket and adjust it to maintain the desired temperature. Put 5 ml M solution into the chamber and start the stirring bar. Add a pinch of sodium dithionite crystals to the electrode chamber. The oxygen reading should fall at once to near zero. After the reading has stabilized add another small amount of dithionite. If no further decrease in the chamber oxygen reading is observed, adjust the zero point of the electrode. Place approximately 200 ml M solution in the beaker and stir at a moderate rate on the magnetic stirrer. Bubble air into this solution with the airstone at about 200–500 ml/min while monitoring the oxygen concentration with the calibrating meter. Allow the solution to saturate (about 8 mg oxygen liter^{-1} at 25°C). Flush electrode chamber with the air-saturated M solution and adjust the electrode sensitivity to indicate the correct oxygen concentration. Turn off the magnetic stirrer in the electrode chamber.

Oxygen Consumption

A basket is required to protect the hydra from the spinning stir bar in the electrode chamber (see Fig. 1). A suitable basket may be made from 0.003–0.005-in. cellulose acetate plastic and Dacron mesh (4 threads/mm) glued together with Duco Household Cement. Place 150 hydra in the basket, rinse them with 1.3 ml fresh M solution to remove debris, and insert the basket in the electrode chamber. Remove all bubbles from the chamber and seal it. Test to see that basket does not interfere with the stir bar. After 2 or 3 min, linear oxygen readings with time should be obtained. By noting the rate of

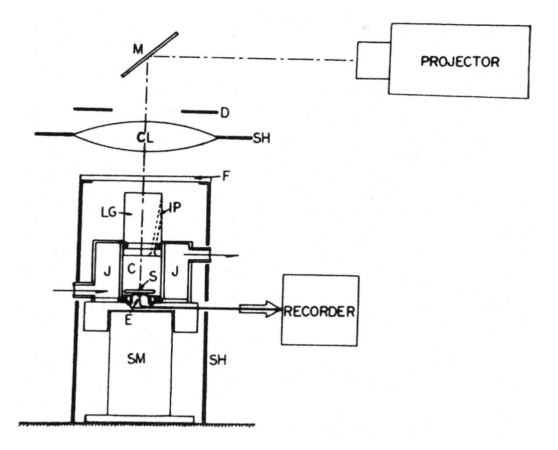

FIGURE 1. Schematic of experimental assembly for measurements of photosynthetic oxygen evolution in green hydra. (M) Mirror assembly. (D) diaphragm stop. (CL) collimating lens. (SH) cardboard light shields. (F) neutral density filter(s). (LG) light guide. (IP) injection port for introduction of isotopes, etc., (C) electrode chamber, (J) water jacket, (S) stir bar, (E) oxygen electrode, (SM) stirring motor assembly.

decrease in the chamber oxygen concentration and taking into account the chamber volume, the respiration rate of the hydra may be calculated. This may then be normalized by determining the protein content of the 150 animals.

Special Precautions for Measurement of Oxygen Consumption

Data should be taken from about 5–10 min of linear recording to determine respiration rates, but the oxygen concentration in the chamber should not be allowed to fall to near zero because the respiration rate of hydra decreases markedly at this point.

Fewer than 150 hydra may be used for measurements. To obtain a sufficient change in chamber oxygen concentration, smaller chamber volumes or longer recording times must be used. Very small chamber volumes lead to electrode instability. With such small volumes the oxygen consumption by the electrode itself may add significantly to that observed.

Prolonged incubation times may promote the growth of microorganisms carried over with the hydra. While these contribute only minimally to the oxygen consumption at first, after a few hours they may account for a large fraction of the respiration measured.

The Rank Brothers Electrode is not temperature compensated; thus, the temperature of the solution used for calibration must be close to the electrode temperature. If bubbles are present in the chamber, the equilibrium between gaseous oxygen in them and the dissolved oxygen in the chamber may mask or confuse the readings. Bubbles often cause electronic noise characterized by excessive shift and meter fluctuations.

Excessive noise in the recordings may also be caused by a bad electrode membrane. Replace membranes if addition of sodium dithionite fails to bring a rapid drop in the electrode reading, if there is excessive fluctuation in recordings, or if the electrode has gone unused for more than 5 days.

Finally, calibrating the electrode with another meter is necessary only if quantitative measurements of oxygen exchange are desired. Otherwise simply setting the zero level with dithionite is sufficient to set the electrode for determining relative amounts of oxygen exchange.

Oxygen Production

Assemble the apparatus shown in Fig. 1. Calibrate the oxygen electrode as previously described. Direct the light to the collimating lens with the mirrors so that a focused beam is produced which should fill the electrode chamber as much as possible. Remove the electrode from the beam and place a quantum sensor on the electrode stir motor. Place the Plexiglas light guide over the sensing element and set the top of the light guide at the same distance from the collimating lens as when it is in place on the electrode. Use the neutral density filters for coarse adjustment and the diaphragm for fine adjustment of the light intensity.

Use 150 hydra to measure photosynthesis of intact animals. Hold the hydra in a basket (Fig. 2) in the electrode as described previously. If isolated symbionts are used suspend them in 5 ml of an isolation buffer consisting of 100 mM K$_2$HPO$_4$/KH$_2$PO$_4$ buffer (pH 6.4), 1 mM CaCl$_2$, and 1 mM MgSO$_4$. Adjust the algal concentration to about 2×10^7 cells per 5 ml or about 0.01 mg chlorophyll per 5 ml. Seal the electrode chamber with the light guide. Bicarbonate or inhibitors may be added through the injection port drilled in the guide. Recording for 5–10 min in the light with an equal period

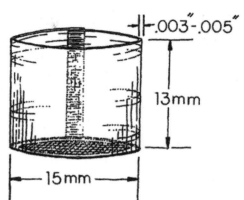

FIGURE 2. Basket used to hold hydra in oxygen electrode chamber. About 150 hydra will cover mesh area and be held away from stir bar during measurements.

in the dark should be sufficient. Subtract rates of dark respiration of whole hydra from their rates of oxygen evolution; light has not been found to substantially alter the rate of host respiration during the short times required for measurements, and the host respiration is a major source of oxygen consumption by the system in the light (Phipps and Pardy; 1982). Do not, however, subtract the respiration rates of the isolated algae from their rates of oxygen evolution, as in the light respiration in algae has been shown to be inhibited (Brown and Tregunna, 1967).

Rates of photosynthetic oxygen evolution may be normalized on a per-milligram hydra protein, per-milligram algal chlorophyll, or per-algal cell basis.

PRECAUTIONS

In addition to the precautions for oxygen consumption measurements, check the light intensity before each experiment. Projector lamps darken with use, causing a gradual decrease of intensity. Check the mirrors and lens frequently for proper alignment; clamp them securely during measurements.

REFERENCES

Brown, D. L., and Tregunna, E. B., 1967. Inhibition of respiration during photosynthesis by some algae. *Can. J. Bot.* **45**:1135–1143.

Phipps, Jr., D. W. and Pardy, R. L. 1982. Host enhancement of symbiont photosynthesis in the hydra-algae symbiosis. *Biol. Bull.* **162**:83–94.

Part XII

Symbiotic Relationships

Isolating Endosymbiotic Algae from
Hydra viridis

L. Muscatine

PURPOSE

To isolate endosymbiotic algae from host tissue in order to examine the characteristics and properties of those algae free of host tissue and to use the isolated algae in reinfection studies.

MATERIALS

Drive motor with screw chuck; tissue grinder (Potter-Elvehjem type, with Teflon pestle, 30-ml capacity); centrifuge; 10- to 15-ml conical, graduated centrifuge tubes; bolting cloth (35-μ mesh); and funnel.

PROCEDURES

Collect about 4500–5000 hydra from mass cultures, rinse them several times in culture solution, place in a chilled (5°C) glass tissue grinder, and adjust suspension volume to 1 ml. Pass a motor-driven teflon pestle through the suspension about 20 times. Pour the homogenate through fine-mesh bolting cloth to remove large particles and collect the filtrate in conical centrifuge tubes. Centrifuge at 1500g for 2 min and discard the turbid

L. Muscatine • Department of Biology, University of California, Los Angeles, California.

supernatant containing the bulk of the animal tissue debris. Resuspend the dark green pellet of algae in M solution and centrifuge several times over a 10-min period. Repeat until the supernatant is clear. Examine an aliquot of the algal pellet under the microscope at high magnification to determine the extent of contamination with animal tissue (e.g., count the relative number of menatocysts). Repeat the washing procedure until the contaminants are reduced to an acceptable level.

COMMENTS

The procedure is designed to isolate relatively clean algae gently and rapidly but not in high yields. Algae isolated in this manner show the usual normal range of photosynthetic products as determined by $^{14}CO_2$ tracer techniques. Algae exposed to media employed in more sophisticated fractionation and centrifugation techniques (i.e., SDS, sucrose gradients, etc.) should likewise be checked for photosynthetic efficacy.

REFERENCES

Muscatine, L. 1965. Symbiosis of hydra and algae. III. Extracellular products of the algae. *Comp. Biochem. Physiol.* 16:77–92.

Chapter 54

Preparing Aposymbiotic Hydra

R. L. Pardy

PURPOSE

To prepare and maintain strains of *Hydra viridis* free of their endosymbiotic algae.

METHOD I. GLYCEROL

INTRODUCTION

In this method, first described by Whitney (1907), experimental hydra are cultured in a medium containing glycerol. Under such conditions, the hydra gradually lose their algal endosymbionts and become "bleached."

MATERIALS

M solution (Chapter 4); 1% glycerol (v/v made up in M solution); Petri dishes; *Artemia* nauplii (Chapter 6).

PROCEDURES

Place 25–30 green hydra in 30–50 ml 1% glycerol solution. Feed the animals daily with *Artemia* nauplii and change the glycerol medium 2–3 hr postfeeding. After about a week on this regimen some of the animals will

R. L. Pardy ● School of Life Sciences, University of Nebraska, Lincoln, Nebraska.

become free of green symbionts. Place the white animals into glycerol-free M solution and maintain them on the daily feeding schedule. Some of these animals may turn green; discard them. Animals that are completely free of algae will give rise to clones of aposymbiotic hydra.

COMMENTS

The major drawbacks with the glycerol method involve the relatively long time required (several days to weeks) and its applicability to but one or two green hydra strains. The method is useful for producing partial apo-symbionts, especially with the Carolina strain of *H. viridis* (Muscatine and Lenhoff, 1965). Partial aposymbionts will eventually repopulate with algae if returned to glycerol-free M solution.

METHOD II. PHOTOBLEACHING

INTRODUCTION

Green hydra subjected to intense light while exposed to the photo-synthetic inhibitor 3-(3,4-dichlorophenyl)-1,1-dimethyl urea (DCMU) lose their algae within a day or two. The method appears to be effective with all strains of green hydra so far tested. (Pardy, 1976; Fracek and Margulis, 1979).

MATERIALS

M solution; 5×10^{-6} M DCMU prepared in M solution; 150-W reflector flood lamp (available at most hardware stores); cold platform or refrigerated water bath; 5-cm Petri dish.

PROCEDURES

Place 25–50 green animals in a Petri dish containing 25–30 ml of the DCMU solution. Set the dish with the animals on a cold platform maintained at 15°C. Suspend the reflector flood lamp 10–15 cm over the animals and keep the light on continuously throughout the bleaching process. Do not feed the animals, but change the DCMU solution daily.

With small animals (Florida and Carolina strains), aposymbionts should begin to appear after 24 hr. With larger animals (English and European strains) 36–48 hr may be required. Place bleached animals in fresh M solution and start feeding. More than 80% of the animals should remain algae-free and produce aposymbiotic progeny.

PRECAUTIONS

Because DCMU solutions lose potency after a few months, prepare them only in quantities needed to last a week of bleaching. Culture newly produced aposymbionts through three or four generations before using them in experiments to make sure that the bleaching process is complete.

METHOD III. TRIMETHORPRIM

INTRODUCTION

Jeon (1977) utilized an antibacterial drug, trimethoprim, which causes the green hydra to expel its symbionts. The method is fairly rapid, though the drug inhibits the animals' growth and appears to be toxic to smaller animals.

MATERIALS

M solution; trimethoprim (Calbiochem-Behring Corp. San Diego, CA 92112); Petri dishes.

PROCEDURES

Incubate green hydra in M solution containing 80 μg/ml trimethoprim for 7 days. Transfer the animals to M solution containing 200 μg/ml trimethoprim for 4–7 days. Feed the hydra daily throughout the treatment. The animals should become pale and free of algae in the lower portion of the body column and produce algae-free buds. So far the method has only been used successfully on the Carolina strain of *H. viridis*.

*METHOD IV. GAMMA IRRADIATION**

INTRODUCTION

Aposymbiotic hydra can be prepared by exposing animals to gamma rays. The treatment is effective for English and Swiss strains of *H. viridis* but not the nonbudding mutant strain of *H. viridis* (Lenhoff, 1965).

MATERIALS

60×15-mm plastic Petri dishes; "M" solution; ^{137}Cs-source gamma irradiator.

PROCEDURES

Select 10–20 24-hr fasted hydra from a logarithmically growing population and place them in a plastic Petri dish containing "M" solution. Irradiate the hydra at room temperature using 4–10 krad provided by the cesium source. Following irradiation culture the animals by routine methods.

Periodically examine the hydra for the presence of algae using a dissecting microscope at $20\times$. Use a white background and scan their bodies for traces of remaining algae. The animals should become pale within 14 days; most should be algae-free after a month of continuous culture and asexual reproduction. Those that remain algae-free can be cloned to establish aposymbiotic lines.

COMMENTS

Hydra (English and Swiss strains) receiving 4–6 krad become pale within 14 days following irradiation. During this time, animals continue to feed and reproduce asexually. At the end of 1 month of culture most of the animals are aposymbiotic. Hydra receiving 7–10 krad become pale within 7–10 days following irradiation. These animals, however, often are unable to eat and are depressed for several days. Very pale or completely bleached animals can be selected and cared for from these cultures.

* Patricia Novak, Department of Developmental and Cell Biology, University of California, Irvine, California.

PRECAUTIONS

Gamma irradiation may have varying effects on other strains and species of hydra (Fradkin *et al.*, 1978). The nonbudding strain mutant treated with 4–5 krad become pale within 2 weeks of treatment. At greater than 5 krad the animals start deteriorating and decompose 2–3 weeks after the treatment.

REFERENCES

Fracek, S., and Margulis, L., 1979. Colchicine, nocodazole and trifluralin: Different effects of microtubule polymerization inhibitors on the uptake and migration of endosymbiotic algae in *Hydra viridis*. *Cytobios* **25**:7–15.

Fradkin, M., Kakis, H., and Campbell, R. D. 1978. Effects of γ irradiation of hydra: Elimination of interstitial cells from viable hydra. *Radiat. Res.* **76**:187–197.

Jeon, K. W. 1977. A new method for obtaining aposymbiotic hydra using trimethoprim as a bleaching agent. **59**:255–258.

Lenhoff, H. M. 1965. Cellular segregation and heterocytic dominance in hydra. *Science* **148**:1105–1107.

Muscatine, L., and Lenhoff, H. M. 1965. Symbiosis of hydra and algae. II. Effects of limited food and starvation on growth of symbiotic and aposymbiotic hydra. *Biol. Bull.* **129**:316–328.

Pardy, R. L., 1976. The production of oposymbiotic hydra by the photodestruction of green hydra zoochlorellae. *Biol. Bull.* **151**:225–235.

Whitney, D. D. 1907. Artificial removal of the green bodies of *Hydra viridis*. *Biol. Bull.* **13**:291–299.

Chapter 55

Introducing Symbiotic Algae into Aposymbiotic Hydra

R. L. Pardy

PURPOSE

To introduce symbiotic algae into aposymbiotic hydra as a means for studying the biology of host–symbiont reassociation. With slight modification, this method may be modified to inject reagents, isotopes, or other kinds of particles into the hydra's enteron (gut).

MATERIALS

Pasteur pipets; glass capillary tubes, inner diameter 1 mm, outer diamter 1.5 mm; Bunsen burner; Tygon tubing, inner diameter 1/16 in., plastic Petri dishes (10 cm); dissecting microscope; Parafilm; suspension of algal symbionts; microinjection pipet (see below); aposymbiotic hydra.

PROCEDURES

Constructing a Microinjection Pipet

Attach a 30-cm length of small-bore Tygon tubing to a mouthpiece, such as a Pasteur pipet. Draw a piece of capillary tubing out to a fine, slender point

R. L. Pardy ● School of Life Sciences, University of Nebraska, Lincoln, Nebraska.

using a small flame. The point should be small enough so that it can be readily slipped through the hydra's mouth yet not so small as to allow leakage. Insert the micropipet into the end of the Tygon tubing. It should be possible to draw up and expel algae using gentle suction or air pressure through the mouth piece.

Injecting Aposymbiotic Hydra

About an hour before injection (or even the night before) transfer 24-hr fasted aposymbiotic hydra into a clean Petri dish. Allow the animals to settle and attach to the bottom of the dish. It is essential that the hydra attach as it is nearly impossible to inject hydra that are floating free in the medium. Using a clean Pasteur pipet transfer a dense slurry of algae from the centrifuge tube (Chapter 53) to a square of Parafilm where the suspension will "bead up." Cover the drop with the lid of a small Petri dish to prevent the cells from drying. Using the injection apparatus, slowly draw up some of the suspension into the microinjection needle. Under the dissecting microscope locate an attached hydra; with the tip of the needle gently prod the base of the hydra, making it contract into a spherical shape. Insert the needle through the hydra's mouth and slowly expel algae into the enteron. Continue expelling the slurry until the animal begins to inflate. At this point stop injecting. Wait a few seconds and then slowly withdraw the needle. The animal's mouth will usually close after the tip is completely withdrawn.

Following a successful injection leave the hydra undisturbed for several hours; then gently transfer them to fresh medium. After about 5 hr the animals should regurgitate the excess, unincorporated algae. Examine injected hydra with the dissecting microscope to see if there is any green tinge in the host's gastric region. The green color indicates that the hydra have taken up some of the symbionts. Feed the animals daily 24 hr after injection. within a week the hydra should be completely populated with the algae symbionts.

REFERENCES

Pardy, R. L., and Muscatine, L. 1973. Recognition of symbiotic algae by *Hydra viridis*. A quantitatve study of the uptake of living algae by aposymbiotic *H. viridis*. *Biol. Bull.* 145:565–579.

Pool, R. R., Jr. 1979. The role of antigenic determinants in the recognition of potential algal symbionts by cells of *Chlorohydra*. *J. Cell Sci.* 35:367–379.

Chapter 56

Measuring Number of Algal Symbionts in *Hydra viridis*

R. L. Pardy

PURPOSE

To determine the number of symbiotic algae living within individual digestive cells, in an intact hydra, or in a population of hydra.

METHOD I. IN INDIVIDUAL CELLS

INTRODUCTION

This method makes use of the maceration technique of David (1973, Chapter 20) and is useful for estimating the algal population in either whole or parts of hydra (Pardy, 1974) and for determining the rate or degree of symbiont uptake by aposymbiotic animals (Pardy and Muscatine, 1973; Pool, 1979). The maceration method applied to a single green hydra yields a cell suspension containing approximately $1.3–1.5 \times 10^5$ digestive cells, a number which is optimum for counting algae in cells.

R. L. Pardy ● School of Life Sciences, University of Nebraska, Lincoln, Nebraska.

MATERIALS

M solution (Chapter 4); maceration fluid (Chapter 20); 37% formalin; Pasteur pipets; small vials (3–5 ml); hemacytometer; 1-ml measuring pipets; compound microscope (phase optics helpful but not necessary).

PROCEDURES

Put about 20 hydra in a vial and remove the culture medium, leaving the animals clustered in a small drop. Add 0.9 ml maceration fluid. after 10 min tap or flick the bottom of the vial with a finger to disrupt the hydra's tissues. Add 0.1 ml formalin to the cells. After a few minutes gently shake the vial to disperse the cells and transfer a few drops of suspension to the hemacytometer with a Pasteur pipet. Identify the digestive cells (Chapter 1) by finding a elongated cells having numerous green endosymbionts. Use the hemacytometer grids as guides for examining the suspension systematically.

PRECAUTIONS

Sources of error arise from incomplete maceration of the animal tissue or rupture of digestive cells. Tentacles are particularly difficult to macerate. The nutritional status of the animals seems to affect maceration: animals that have just been fed have digestive cells that rupture easily; starved animals require prolonged exposure to the maceration fluid (several hours to overnight) to cause adequate separation of cells. Under any condition the cells are fragile; handle them with care. Avoid violent pipeting. Finally, it is possible to mistake cell inclusions for symbiotic algae. Under phase optics, well-fed hydra have digestive cells with refractile particles that are greenish and are roughly the same size as the symbionts. These inclusions are not green when the digestive cells are viewed with bright-field illumination.

METHOD II. FROM KNOWN NUMBERS OF HYDRA

INTRODUCTION

This method is useful for determining the total number of symbionts in a specific population of green hydra or in a single animal. It is well suited for analyzing the growth kinetics of the algal symbionts (Pardy, 1974).

MATERIALS

Hemacytometer; volumetric flask (2–5 ml); Pasteur pipets; serological pipet (red cell); compound microscope; M solution (Chapter 4).

PROCEDURES

Prepare isolated symbiotic algae by homogenizing a known number of green hydra as described (Chapter 53). Following the final wash, resuspend the algal pellet in a small volume of M solution. Transfer this suspension to a 2- or 5-ml volumetric flask and adjust the volume with M solution. Alternatively use a red-cell serological pipet for preparing a known dilution of symbionts. Apply a drop of the diluted cell suspension to the hemacytometer and wait at least 3 min to allow the cells to settle onto the counting grid. Count the number of cells and calculate the concentration of the symbionts in the original suspension. Since the number of hydra homogenized is known, you can estimate the average number of symbionts per individual hydra.

PRECAUTIONS

Using this method it is possible to determine the number of symbionts in as few as five animals. The reliability of the estimate diminishes, however, as the number of animals homogenized decreases. The accuracy of the method depends upon completely homogenizing the animal tissue, completely and accurately resuspending the symbionts in a known volume, and accurately identifying the symbionts under the microscope. Freshly fed animals possess algae-like particles that may confuse the count. These are kept to a minimum by not using fed animals or by washing the isolated symbionts with a 1% solution of SDS (sodium dodecyl sulfate) before resuspension.

*METHOD III. FLUOROMETRIC ESTIMATION OF NUMBERS OF ALGAL SYMBIONTS IN GREEN HYDRA**

INTRODUCTION

This technique takes advantage of the high degree of fluorescence emitted by chlorophyll molecules excited by ultraviolet light. In practice, first prepare a standard curve relating fluorescence to numbers of algae. This

* With R. H. Meints, School of Life Sciences, University of Nebraska, Lincoln, Nebraska.

curve can be used for estimating the number of algae in a sample having an unknown number of cells.

MATERIALS

Fluorometer, Turner model III (Turner Associates, Palo Alto, CA 94303) equipped with a No. 110-853 excitation source, a No. 5-60 primary filter, a No. 2-64 secondary filter, and a red-sensitive photomultiplier with a 2-R surface. Other instruments may be suitable if they emit excitation radiation at 390–460 nm and are sensitive to fluorescent radiation at 665 nm. Hemacytometer; Pasteur pipets; measuring pipets; fluorometer cuvettes (quartz *not* necessary); 5-ml test tubes; absolute methanol; centrifuge tubes; clinical centrifuge; compound microscope.

PROCEDURES

Standard Curve

Prepare a standard curve relating number of algae to fluorescence. Use a suspension of algae (Chapter 53) quantified by means of a hemacytometer. Using this stock suspension of algae, prepare a series of dilutions ranging from approximately 5×10^2 to 2×10^5 cells/ml in centrifuge tubes. Centrifuge the suspensions for 2–3 min at about $1000g$ (the highest speed on a clinical centrifuge is sufficient). Discard the supernatent layer and resuspend the cells in a known volume of methanol. Extract the cells for a minimum of 0.5 hr at 4°C in the dark. Read the extracts in the fluorometer and plot fluorometer units against cell number.

Estimating the Number of Symbionts in a Single Hydra

Pipet a single hydra into a 5-ml test tube. Using a Pasteur pipet remove as much of the culture medium as possible, leaving the hydra behind. Add a known volume of absolute methanol and extract the animal in the dark at 4°C. After a minimum of 0.5 hr transfer the extract to a cuvette and record the fluorometer reading.

PRECAUTIONS

The amount of methanol used in extraction depends upon the size of the fluorometer cuvettes; nonetheless, this amount must be standardized. As the amount of chlorophyll per symbiont may vary depending upon conditions under which the hydra were maintained, it may be necessary to construct a series of standard curves for analysis of symbionts obtained under various experimental conditions. Finally, in some instances the intensity of fluorescence may exceed the capacity of the instrument. If so, neutral density filters or attenuation slits (Meints and Pardy, 1980) may be used as an alternative to diluting the sample.

REFERENCES

David, C. N. 1973. A quantitative method for maceration of *Hydra* tissue. *Wilhelm Roux Arch. Entwicklungsmech. Org.* 171:259–268.

Pardy, R. L. 1974. Some factors affecting the growth and distribution of the algal endosymbionts of *Hydra viridis. Biol. Bull.* 147:105–118.

Meints, R. H., and Pardy, R. L. 1980. Quantitative demonstration of cell surface involvement in a plant-animal symbiosis: Lectin inhibition of reassociation. *J. Cell. Sci.* 43:239–251.

Pardy, R. L., and Muscatine, L. 1973. Recognition of symbiotic algae by *Hydra viridis*. A quantitative study of the uptake of living algae by aposymbiotic *H. viridis. Biol. Bull.* 145:565–579.

Pool, R. R., Jr. 1979. The role of antigenic determinants in the recognition of potential algal symbionts by cells of *Chlorohydra. J. Cell Sci.* 35:367–379.

Chapter 57

Measuring *in Vivo* Translocation of Reduced Organic Carbon Compounds from Endosymbiotic Algae to Hydra

L. Muscatine

PURPOSE

To measure the movement of materials from autotrophic endosymbionts to their heterotrophic hosts. The usual approach is to label the autotroph by exposing the intact association (i.e., the green hydra) to $^{14}CO_2$ and then to assay the heterotroph for the appearance of fixed ^{14}C (Cernichiari *et al.*, 1969; Eisenstadt, 1971; Smith, 1974).

MATERIALS

Tissue grinder (Potter-Elvehjem type, with Teflon pestle 15-ml capacity); 10- to 15-ml conical, graduated centrifuge tubes; 25-ml Erlenmeyer flasks; centrifuge; irradiance source (40-W fluorescent lights are sufficient); scintillation counter; culture solution, $Na_2^{14}CO_3$ (New England Nuclear, 10–20 mCi/mmol).

L. Muscatine ● Department of Biology, University of California, Los Angeles, California.

PROCEDURES

Place 50–100 green hydra in 3 ml M solution in a 25-ml flask. Introduce 20–50 mCi of isotope, mix gently, and seal the flask. Incubate the flask in light at 18°C for about 2 hr. Remove the hydra and wash them through three changes of fresh, unlabeled culture solution to remove most of the unused isotope. Transfer the hydra to a tissue grinder, adjust the volume to 0.5 ml, and disrupt them gently to obtain a uniform homogenate. Several plunges of the pestle is usually sufficient. Transfer the homogenate to a centrifuge tube and centrifuge for 1 min at 400g to get a pellet of algae (and nematocysts). Draw off and save the supernatant. Resuspend the algae and repeat the centrifugation step until a clear supernatant is obtained. Combine and centrifuge all supernatants at 1500g to pellet any contaminating algae in the supernatant "animal" fraction. Decant the supernatant and combine the pellets. Adjust the supernatant ("animal") and pellet ("algae") fractions to known volumes, take aliquots of each, acidify each aliquot with a drop of 0.2 N HCl to remove remaining $^{14}CO_2$, and assay them for radioactivity. From the counts obtained, compute as follows:

$$\frac{\%\ ^{14}C\ \text{translocated}}{\text{to animal cells}} = \frac{(^{14}C\ \text{in animal tissue})}{(^{14}C\ \text{in algae} + ^{14}C\ \text{in animal tissue})} \times 100$$

COMMENTS

It is advisable to practice separating animal and algae fractions using unlabeled hydra. For dark controls, use hydra maintained in dark during the incubation period and then treat them as described above; separate the algae from the animal fraction in dim light. Alternatively, the aposymbiotic hydra may be incubated with the isotope. In either case, determine the specific activity of label picked up by the hydra (i.e., cpm/unit animal tissue) by measuring radioactivity and total protein. Compare these data to similar data for green hydra animal tissue from experiments carried out in the light. The extent of heterotrophic ^{14}C fixation can then be ascertained. Failure to completely remove unused $^{14}CO_2$ is a serious source of error. If necessary, warm the slightly acidified samples and, in a hood, expose them to a gentle airstream for 10–15 min.

Contamination of animal tissue by labeled algae is also a serious source of error. It may be corrected by a somewhat tedious procedure. Pass the animal tissue fraction through a Whatman GF/C filter. Extract the filter with 100% acetone and estimate total chlorophyll (chl) a by the method of Jeffrey and Humphrey (1975). Repeat this procedure with equal aliquots of an algal pellet to estimate chl a and ^{14}C content. Once the ratio of ^{14}C to chl a is known for the pellet, estimate the ^{14}C in algae contaminating the animal fraction as follows:

$$\frac{(^{14}C \text{ algal pellet})}{(\text{chl } a \text{ algal pellet})} = \frac{X}{(\text{chl } a \text{ in animal fraction})}$$

where $X = {}^{14}C$ due to contaminating algae. Usually, 30–40% of the total ^{14}C fixed is translocated, mostly as maltose-^{14}C.

REFERENCES

Cernichiari, E. C., Muscatine, L., and Smith, D. C. 1969. Maltose excretion by the symbiotic algae of *Hydra viridis. Proc. R. Soc. B* **173**:557–576.

Eisenstadt, E. 1971. Transfer of photosynthetic products from symbiotic algae to animal tissue in *Chlorohydra viridissima.* In: *Experimental Coelenterate Biology* (H. Lenhoff, L. Muscatine, and L. V. Davis, ed.), University of Hawaii Press, Honolulu, pp. 202–208.

Jeffrey, S. W., and Humphrey, G. F. 1975. New spectrophotometric equations for determining chlorophylls a, b, c_1 and c_2 in higher plants, algae, and natural phytoplankton. *Biochem. Physiol. Pflanz.* **175**:191–194.

Mews, L. K. 1980. The green hydra symbiosis. III. The biotrophic transport of carbohydrate from alga to animal. *Proc. Roy. Soc. Lond. B* **209**:377–401.

Smith, D. C. 1974. Transport from symbiotic algae and symbiotic chloroplasts to host cells. *Symp. Soc. Exp. Biol.* **28**:485–520.

Chapter 58

Spectrophotometric Assay
for Maltose

That T. Ngo, Jeanne Ivy, and Howard M. Lenhoff

PURPOSE

To quantify spectrophotometrically maltose secreted by isolated endo-symbiotic algae *in vitro*.

INTRODUCTION

Endosymbiotic zoochlorellae of *Hydra viridis* differ from free-living chlorellae in that they synthesize and secrete the disaccharide maltose into their environment (Muscatine, 1965). Furthermore, the zoochlorellae of hydra secrete maltose *in vitro* for at least 24 hr, and the maximal secretion occurs at pH 4.0 (Cernichiari *et al.*, 1969).

The assay is based upon the colorimetric measurement of the H_2O_2 produced stoichiometrically from maltose by the following series of re-actions:

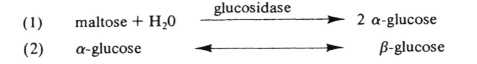

$$(1) \quad \text{maltose} + H_2O \xrightarrow{\text{glucosidase}} 2 \ \alpha\text{-glucose}$$

$$(2) \quad \alpha\text{-glucose} \longleftrightarrow \beta\text{-glucose}$$

That T. Ngo, Jeanne Ivy, and Howard M. Lenhoff ● Department of Developmental and Cell Biology, University of California, Irvine, California.

(3) β-glucose $\xrightarrow{\text{glucose oxidase}}$ $H_2O_2 + \delta$-gluconolactone

(4)   chromagens $+ H_2O_2 \xrightarrow{\text{peroxidase}} H_2O +$ color

MATERIALS

Hydra viridis; Petri dishes; micropipets, 25 and 50 μl; fluorescent light (ca. 33 W); water bath; magnetic stirrer; Millipore filter (HA 0.45 μm, 13 mm); Millipore filter holder; spectrophotometer; Maertin's solution (62.5 mg/liter, $Ca(NO_3)_2 \cdot 4H_2O$, 12.5 mg/liters $MgSO_4 \cdot 7H_2O$, 19 mg/liters K_2HPO_4, with its pH adjusted to 6.9 with 1 N HCl; McIlvaine's buffer (0.1 M citric acid-disodium phosphate, pH 4.0; sodium phosphate buffers, pH 6.5 and 7.0; α-glucosidase, glucose oxidase peroxidase and maltose (Sigma Chemical Co.); 3-dimethylamino benzoic acid (Eastman Kodak Co.); 3-methyl-2-benzothiazolinone hydrazone hydrochloride (Aldrich Chemical Co.).

PROCEDURES

Isolate endosymbiotic algae (Chapter 53) from 1.5 ml chilled packed hydra (Chapter 9) and suspend them in 2 ml Maertin's solution diluted 1:1 with 0.001 M McIlvaine's buffer. Place the suspended algae in a Petri dish set 2.5 in. under a fluorescent light. Stir the suspension gently using a magnetic stirrer.

To initiate the secretion of maltose, add 2 ml 0.1 M McIlvaine's buffer, pH 4.0, to the algae suspension. Remove 50-μl aliquots of the suspension at 5-min intervals and, to stop maltose secretion, mix them with 50 μl 0.5 M sodium phosphate buffer, pH 7.0, and place them in an ice bath.

To 1-ml portions of the chilled suspension, add 25 μl α-glucosidase (i.e., ca. 1 unit) and incubate the solution for 30 min at room temperature. Then, to each solution to be assayed, add in rapid succession: 0.33 ml 4m M 3-dimethylamino benzoic acid, 0.33 ml 80 μM 3-methyl-2-benzothiazolinone hydrazone hydrochloride monohydrate, and 0.33 ml of an enzyme solution containing 1000 units of glucose oxidase and 300 units of peroxidase in 100 ml 0.1 M sodium phosphate buffer, pH 6.5.

Incubate the mixed solutions at 37°C for 30 min, remove the algae by filtering it through a Millipore filter, and read the absorbance at 590 nm.

Compare the absorbance with a standard curve obtained using solutions of maltose ranging from 2 to 20 μM.

COMMENTS

The algae are removed from the incubation mixtures in order to get stable absorbance readings. Maltose secretion by the isolated zoochlorellae, which is negligible at pH 7.0, can be reinitiated by resuspending the algae in fresh pH 4.0 buffers. The isolated algae can be stored overnight at 4°C in sodium phosphate, pH 6.5, and initiate maltose secretion again for at least another 24 hr.

REFERENCES

Cernichiari, E., Muscatine, L., and Smith, D. C. 1969. Maltose excretion by the symbiotic algae of *Hydra viridis*. *Proc. R. Soc. B* **173**:557–576.

Muscatine, L. 1965. Symbiosis of hydra and algae. III. Extracellular products of the algae. *Comp. Biochem. Physiol.* **16**:77–92.

Ngo, T. T., and Lenhoff, H. M. 1980. A sensitive and versatile chromogenic assay for peroxidase and peroxidase-coupled reactions. *Anal. Biochem.* **105**:389–397.

Part XIII

Methods for Epizootilogical Research with Hydras

Chapter 59

Experimental Methods for Epizootilogical Research with Hydras

Alan E. Stiven

PURPOSE

To present culture and analytical methods for research on hydras and their associated ectoparasitic fauna, with special emphasis on the use of the hydra–*Hydramoeba* system as a model for epizootilogical investigations. I use the term *epizootic* to characterize the dynamics of infectious disease in host populations (Tanada, 1963).

INTRODUCTION

Several species of hydra have been reported infected by the parasite *Hydramoeba hydroxena* (Entz). Such infections move rapidly through natural hydra populations and often lead to extinctions of the host populations particularly in late summer (Bryden, 1952). The parasite is cosmopolitan in its distribution, having been reported repeatedly from Europe, Asia, and North America (Stiven, 1973).

In experimental epizootilogical research, the epiootic can be compartmentalized into a variety of interacting and interdependent biological and environmental variables. The causes of outbreaks in host populations are often found within the complexity of the host–pathogen interaction, and an

Alan E. Stiven ● Department of Biology 046A, University of North Carolina, Chapel Hill, North Carolina.

understanding of host resistance, pathogen infectivity, rates of population infection, and many other biological aspects is essential.

Hydra represents an excellent biological analog in epizootiology (Stiven, 1973) for many of the same reasons that popularized its use in developmental biology and ecological research (Slobodkin, 1964). One prime reason is its ease of mass culture as the host organism. Its population growth properties are directly tied to food intake and temperature (Stiven, 1964). Small or large populations of hydra can be replicated, infected, and counted with ease. An infective agent such as the parasitic *Hydramoeba* can also be grown on hydra in mass culture. Individual or large numbers of amoebae can be manipulated and counted with only the aid of a dissecting microscope. Of special significance, several species of hydra exist which are differentially susceptible to the hydramoeba attack, thus providing the basic material for creating mixed species host "populations" with varying levels of resistance Stiven, 1971).

METHOD I. CULTURING STOCKS OF HYDRAMOEBA

MATERIALS

Make up culture solution by adding 20 ml of a stock solution (20 g $NaHCO_3$ and 10 g EDTA dissolved in a liter of tap water) to 1 gal tap water (Loomis, 1953). Other hydra media utilizing distilled or deionized water (e.g., Muscatine and Lenhoff, 1965) are not suitable for culturing hydramoeba. *Hydramoeba* can often be obtained from pools or lakes in late summer by removing some vegetation from the littoral zone. Place it in an aquarium and look for infected hydra attached to the vegetation.

COMMENTS

Use both *Hydra pseudoligactis* and *Hydra viridis* for continuous culture of the amoeba, with the two hydra species sometimes cultured mixed, and sometimes separately. *Hydra viridis* is more resistant to amoeba infection; thus the infection can be maintained for a longer period of time before it becomes necessary to subculture a few heavily infected hydra into a new hydra culture. Hydramoebae quickly attach to the more susceptible *H.*

pseudoligactis; on the death of the host, more than 100 amoebae are produced a few days later.

Clones of other species of hydra, as well as the albino green hydra, can be used as hosts for infection experiments with *Hydramoeba*. The most susceptible species are *H. pseudoligactis* and *Hydra oligactis*. Next in susceptibility is the normal green hydra (*H. viridis*). Its albino form is slightly more susceptible (Stiven, 1971). *Hydra littoralis* (those originally obtained from pools near Ithaca, N.Y.) is essentially immune; hydramoebae attach to them but do not increase in number while there. Eventually they detach and die in the absence of a more suitable host.

PROCEDURES

Maintain cultures of both host and parasite in finger bowls at room temperature (20°–25°C) and natural day length. Initiate new infected cultures in finger bowls periodically by adding to separate hydra cultures a few heavily infected hydra. Feed the hydra with *Artemia* nauplii and clean, noninfected stock cultures of hydra daily according to standard procedures (Chapter 8). Feed and change the culture water of infected cultures every 2 days. Examine the infected cultures periodically for level of infection by examining at 120–250 power (see Method II). Change the culture dishes containing infected hydra at least once a week and even more frequently depending upon build-up of slime and the stage of the infection and frequency of feeding. Subculture these injected animals to new hydra cultures as soon as the infected hydra are reduced to small "stubs."

PRECAUTIONS

Keep the glassware for feeding and transferring hydra separate for uncontaminated hydra cultures and for infected cultures.

Keep "insurance cultures" of several hydra species and the hydramoebae in a refrigerator at about 5°C. Green hydra survive without feeding for 1–2 months at such a temperature. Hydramoebae will remain attached to hydra for at least a month, apparently causing little damage to them. The hydramoebae do not multiply at this low temperature. Culture water need not be changed periodically in these insurance cultures if just a few individual hosts are maintained in the covered finger bowl. Specimens of *H. pseudoligactis* do not survive as long as green hydra at 5°C.

METHOD II. INFECTION EXPERIMENTS WITH INDIVIDUAL HYDRA

COMMENTS

The rate of population growth of *Hydramoeba* on an individual hydra reflects both the degree of virulence of the parasite and the level of resistance or susceptibility of the host. The instantaneous growth rate of the amoeba can be assessed by initially infecting a single host by one or more amoebae.

PROCEDURES

To determine the instantaneous growth rate of the hydramoeba population on a single host, place a single hydra in each of the 1-ml depressions of a nine-spot depression plate and observe them under a dissecting microscope. Expose the host for a few hours to several infective (proteus type) amoebae from the stock culture. The amoebae should quickly move onto the tentacles and body column (Fig. 1A); control the initial number by varying exposure time or by carefully dislodging excess amoebae with an eyedropper that is drawn out so the bore is just slightly larger than the body of the parasite (about 50 μm). Record daily the increase in number of the amoebae on the surface of the individual hosts. The hydra should become covered with amoebae, and the host should eventually die (Fig. 1B). Some amoebae may detach and will be found on the substrate.

On susceptible hosts, amoeba population growth during the first few days should be exponential (Stiven, 1973), and the rate of increase of the amoeba can be calculated using the exponential growth equation

$$N_t = N_o E^{rt}$$

where N_t is the number of amoebae at time t, N_o is the initial number of amoebae, and r is the instantaneous growth rate. This rate can be calculated by a linear regression fit of the $\log_e$ of numbers against time, or by a two-data-point equation

$$r = (\log_e N_2 - \log_e N_1)/(t_2 - t_1)$$

where N_2 is the number of amoebae at some later time t_2 and N_1 is the number of amoebae at some earlier time t_1. It is important to repeat these

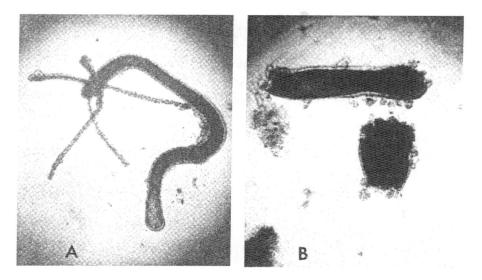

FIGURE 1. Photographs of *H. hydroxena* on the surface of hydra. (A) Hydramoebae become attached to the tentacles and the body surface during early stages of infection. (B) Hydramoebae increase in number over the hydra surface (may also be found in the gastrovascular cavity) and eventually cause disintegration of the hydra.

hydra infections under specified experimental treatments to compute means and variances of the instantaneous growth rates.

The geometric growth model can also be used to calculate the doubling time (t_D) for the hydramoeba population:

$$t_D = 0.6915/r$$

Time sequence histological data of the host–parasite system can also be obtained from infected hosts using the cultures. Current histological information on the mode of attack of the amoeba and the breakdown of the ectoderm and mesoglea is generally sketchy.

COMMENTS

Host mortality can be assessed by measuring the mean time of death of individual hosts initially infected with a specified number of amoebae, or by use of the survivorship curve if the times of death are spread out over an extended period.

PROCEDURES

Establish infections in individual hosts contained in separate dishes (such as nine-spot depression plates). Sufficient numbers (e.g., 20) of hosts should be used to calculate appropriate means and variances of the time of death. If the distribution of the times of death is skewed, a transformation (such as log) may be necessary to normalize the data before calculating the means.

In more resistant host species (e.g., *H. viridis*) the time of death among individual hosts is quite variable, and it may be advantageous to utilize the survivorship curve method. The survivorship curve method involves recording the number of animals that die as evidenced by disintegration over a period of time, starting with at least 20–25 hosts (the cohort) infected in the same manner. If a plot of the log of the number of survivors against time is linear, the use of least-square regression procedures will yield a value for the slope which is the instantaneous mortality rate.

Another variable that can be extracted from the survivorship curve is the time at which 50% of the population has died. This measurement can then be treated as a random variable, replicated, and compared with the results from different experimental treatments.

Use appropriate statistical procedures for contrasting the slopes of regression lines or mean times of death to compare differences due to species, initial infection levels, age of host, and such environmental conditions as temperature and pH.

METHOD III. EXPERIMENTALLY INFECTING POPULATIONS OF HYDRA

COMMENTS

Experiments involving large numbers of susceptible hosts require much more time to carry out. When a single infected host is placed in a susceptible population of, for example, 100 or more individuals, the hydramoebae from the inoculant cause new infections until eventually all or most of the susceptible individuals are infected. The rate at which the hydra population becomes infected follows the typical epizootic wave or curve (Bailey, 1957), which usually reaches a peak when about half the population becomes infected and drops to zero if all are infected. A curve describing the cumulative number (or the proportion of the total initial host population) of infections over a period of time is often sigmoid, and we find the logistic model (Stiven, 1964, 1973) to represent this process. You can calculate the initial instantaneous infection rate by fitting the logistic model to either numbers or proportion of hydra infected. This rate is an excellent measure characterizing the response of the population host–parasite system to many experimental ecological treatments (e.g., variations in host density, initial infection, and temperature) (Stiven, 1964).

PROCEDURES

To manipulate host population density, vary the number of hosts, the size of the container substrate, or both. We have worked with host densities as high as $12/cm^2$ by using 668 amoebae in a culture dish containing $55.7 \ cm^2$ of bottom substrate. Densities around 2–6 hosts/cm^2 are easier to set up, replicate, and count. To set up experiments varying the size of initial infection, you can either vary the number of hydramoebae on a single host inoculant or vary the actual number of infected host inoculants. Maintain population culture dishes in moist chambers in incubators. The culture dishes should be level to prevent disproportionate accumulations of detached amoebae.

PRECAUTIONS

One problem often encountered with dense populations of hydra is the tendency of some hosts to detach from the dish and to float. If a proportion of the host population is floating, the effective host density is accordingly changed. Lower these individuals to the substrate and remove the bubble by the dexterous use of a finely tapered eye dropper.

It is important not to feed the hydra population when using a more susceptible hydra species. The epizootic process is clearly disrupted by the mechanics of feeding and cleaning the hydra cultures, and you may lose significant numbers of detached amoebae. It is conceivable, on the other hand, that you may lower the level of resistance of the hydra population through starvation, although we have found this not to be the case in small host populations, where the infection process is quickly completed.

On the other hand, feed the hydra periodically if your experiment requires the population of hydra to increase in number. If constant densities of host populations are desired throughout the experiment, it is sometimes advantageous to use recently detached buds as the host individuals because they are of uniform size and if unfed will not bud before the epizootic is completed.

METHOD IV. ANALYSIS OF EPIZOOTICS IN POPULATIONS OF MULTIPLE SPECIES

The analysis of epizootics in multiple species systems might be used as model for exploring problems of community level resilience to pertubations, and the effects of first-order interactions among species on the epizootic process. Such can be achieved by using a variety of different hydra species (as well as the albino *H. viridis*). Each species or form possesses a different level of resistance to the hydramoeba and gives us a unique set of hydra host populations that can be combined in a variety of different proportions to yield host "communities" with varying levels of overall resistance (Stiven, 1971). These synthetic communities can be easily constructed using unfed, newly dropped buds (to eliminate reproduction) from the different species. The introduction of an inoculant and the subsequent monitoring of the numbers of new infectives in each species population should be carried out as described in a single species population experiments (see Method III).

METHOD V. OTHER PROTOZOANS EPIZOOTIC ON HYDRAS

Two other protozoans epizootic on hydra have been described, yet little appears known about their individual effect and their parasitic nature. Practically nothing is known of their interactions and synergistic relationships with the host. The ciliate *Trichodina pediculus* has often been reported occurring on hydra, but seems to be only an obligatory commensal (Fulton, 1923). Another ciliate, *Kerona pediculus*, has frequently been described as a harmful ectoparasite on hydra (Yeatman, 1965), although Coleman (1966) describes the *Kerona*–hydra association as obligate commensalism with neither host nor hypotrich damaged by the association. Applying the methods for hydramoebae described in this article to these protozoa should prove of interest.

ACKNOWLEDGMENTS. Research supported by grants from the National Science Foundation.

REFERENCES

Bailey, N. T. J. 1957. *The Mathematical Theory of Epidemics*. Hafner, New York.

Bryden, R. R. 1952. Ecology of *Pelmatohydra oligactis* in Kirpatricks Lake, Tennessee. *Ecol. Monogr.* 22:45–68.

Coleman, D. C. 1966. The laboratory population ecology of *Kerona pediculus* (O.F.M.) epizoic on *Hydra* spp. *Ecology* 47:703–711.

Fulton, J. F. 1923. *Trichodina pediculus* and a new closely related species. *Proc. Boston Soc. Nat. Hist.* 37:1–30.

Lenhoff, H. M., and Loomis, W. F. 1961. *The Biology of Hydra and Some Other Coelenterates*. University of Miami Press, Coral Gables, Fla.

Loomis, W. F. 1953. The cultivation of *Hydra* under controlled conditions. *Science* 117:565–566.

Muscatine. L., and Lenhoff. H. M. 1965. Symbiosis of hydra and algae. I. Effects of some environmental cations on growth of symbiotic and aposymbiotic hydra. *Biol. Bull.* 128:425–424.

Slobodkin, L. B. 1964. Experimental populations of *Hydrida. J. Am. Ecol. Suppl.* 33:131–148.

Stiven, A. E. 1964. Experimental studies on the epidemiology of the host parasite system, hydra and *Hydramoeba hydroxena* (Entz). II. The components of a simple epidemic. *Ecol. Monogr.* 34:119–142.

Stiven, A. E. 1971. The spread of *Hydramoeba* infections in mixed hydra species systems. *Oecologia* 6:118–132.

Stiven, A. E. 1973. Hydra-hydramoeba: A model system for the study of epizootic processes. *Curr. Top. Comp. Pathobiol.* 2:146–212.

Tanada, Y. 1963. Epizootiology of infectious diseases. *Insect Pathol.* 2:423–463.

Yeatman, Harry C. 1965. Ecological relations of the ciliate *Kerona* to its host *Hydra. Turtox News* 43:226–227.

Part XIV

Electrophysiology and Behavior

Chapter 60

Recording Electrical Activity

Robert K. Josephson and Norman B. Rushforth

PURPOSE

To record spontaneous electrical potentials, to monitor transepithelial potentials, and to measure conduction velocity in the column of hydra.

METHOD I. SPONTANEOUS POTENTIALS

INTRODUCTION

The first successful electrical recordings from hydra (Passano and McCullough, 1962, 1963, 1964, 1965) were made with glass capillary microelectrodes of the sort commonly used for intracellular recording. Because they are much easier to use, suction electrodes made from glass tubing or from drawn plastic tubing have supplanted capillary microelectrodes for recording spontaneous potentials from hydra. Spontaneous electrical activity can also be monitored by measuring current flow around a hydra restrained in a tube.

Robert K. Josephson ● School of Biological Science, University of California, Irvine, California. Norman B. Rushforth ● Department of Biology, Case Western Reserve University, Cleveland, Ohio.

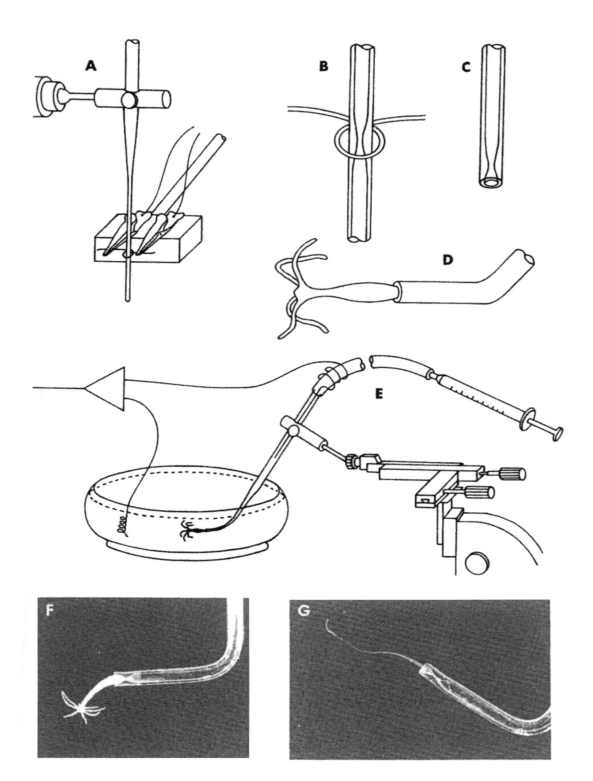

GLASS SUCTION ELECTRODES

Manufacture and Use

The preparation of a glass suction electrode (Josephson, 1967) is illustrated in Fig. 1. Make the electrode from glass tubing that has an internal constriction near the tip, which results in a bell-shaped opening. For use with whole hydra, make the inner diameter at the tip 0.1–0.6 mm, the internal diameter of the constriction 0.05–0.15 mm, and the constriction about 0.5 mm from the open end. These electrodes can also be used to record from single, isolated tentacles (Rushforth and Burke, 1971). For use with single tentacles, make the internal diameter of the open end about 0.1 mm, with the other dimensions reduced accordingly. Attach the electrode to a syringe by flexible plastic tubing. Make electrical contact with the fluid within the electrode by inserting a chlorided silver wire through the wall of the plastic tubing into the end of the glass electrode. Wrap the silver wire several times around the outside of the plastic tubing and glue it in place with epoxy cement. Fill the electrode with culture solution to the internal silver wire and lightly suck a hydra, or an isolated tentacle, into the open end of the electrode. For whole animals it is most convenient to attach the electrode to the base of the hydra so the animal sits with its base in the bell-shaped opening. Record electrical potentials between the silver wire within the electrode and a coil of chlorided silver wire in the bathing solution. Exert as little suction as possible on the hydra; excessive suction distorts the normal pattern of spontaneous potentials and leads to atypical behavior (Rushforth, 1971). Animals under light suction sometimes pull their base out of the electrode, ending the recording, but more often animals stay in an electrode for hours or days. Measurements are usually terminated by the impatience of the investigator rather than by the recalcitrance of the hydra.

FIGURE 1. A glass suction electrode for recording spontaneous activity from hydra. (A) Make a constriction in a piece of drawn glass tubing by heating a loop of Nichrome or platinum wire which surrounds the tubing. Heat the wire by AC current. Fine control of the current and therefore the temperature of the coil can be obtained by using a 6- or 12-V filament transformer to supply current to the coil and powering the transformer from a line voltage rheostat (0–110 V or 0–220 V). (B) As the glass heats, its inner walls flow together to form a constriction. (C) Score the tubing just below the constriction with a diamond and break it at that point. Fire polish the end in a microflame to give a bell-shaped opening with smooth edges. (D) A hydra in an electrode. (E) The recording setup. Mount the electrode in a manipulator. Attach a syringe to the electrode by flexible tubing to provide suction to hold the preparation in place. Record potentials between a chlorided silver wire inserted through the wall of the flexible tubing into the lumen of the electrode and a second chlorided silver wire in the bath surrounding the animal. (F and G) Photographs of a hydra and a single tentacle in suction electrodes.

Behavior of Hydra on the Electrode

With a little care, you can hold a hydra in a suction electrode so that its behavior apears normal. The animal should feed, and in long-term experiments produce buds. In the terminal stages of budding, just prior to detachment of the bud, electrical potentials from a bud can be recorded in attenuated form from the base of the parent. The pattern of contraction pulses (CPs) from a bud appears to be independent from that of a parent, but the relation between parental and filial electrical activity has yet to be studied in detail. You may observe overt behavior of the hydra with a dissecting microscope while recording its electrical activity. To correlate behavior with electrical activity, it is convenient to manually record behavioral events with a telegraph key aranged to deflect the trace on one channel of a penwriter that is also displaying electrical events on another channel.

Problems Caused by Electrode Impedance

In any recording system some fraction of the voltage signal occurs as a voltage drop along the electrode, so the effective input to the first stage of amplification is less than the source voltage. The effective input signal to the recording amplifier, V_i, is given by

$$V_i = V_s \times [R_a/(R_e + R_a)]$$

where V_s is the potential at the tip of the electrode, R_a is the input resistance of the amplifier, and R_e is the electrical resistance of the electrode. Hydra culture solution (Chapter 4) is quite low in ions and therefore a poor electrical conductor. The electrical resistance of the glass suction electrodes used with whole hydra is 5–20 MΩ. Because of this high resistance, there can be severe attenuation of the signal along the length of the electrode unless amplifiers with moderately high input impedance are used. Signal attenuation may not be important if one is interested only in the pattern of activity, but it must be considered when evaluating the amplitude of recorded responses. Threading a fine silver wire down the lumen of the electrode to the constriction reduces the electrode resistance to 6 MΩ or less. The reduced electrode resistance reduces electrical interference and inherent noise and makes it possible to use amplifiers with relatively low input impedance without severely attenuating the signals of interest.

FLEXIBLE PLASTIC ELECTRODES

Suction electrodes made from drawn plastic tubing have proven extremely useful for recording from the surface of hydra and many other coelenterates (e.g., Josephson, 1965, 1966; Mackie and Passano, 1968). To prepare flexible suction electrodes, heat a piece of Tygon or polyethylene tubing, 1–5 mm in diameter, over a tiny flame and pull it, just as one pulls thin glass tubing from larger glass tubes. Construct an appropriate microburner by mounting a 20-gauge hypodermic needle on the end of the flexible gas line. The working temperature range for plastic tubing is small, and it usually takes practice before one can pull the tubing to appropriate length and thickness. If the plastic is not sufficiently hot it breaks rather than elongates, and if just a bit hotter the plastic chars and bursts into flame. Cut the drawn portion of the tubing transversely with a razor blade where it is of appropriate diameter to produce a smooth opening. Be certain to attach the electrode to a manipulator so its tip can be placed at the desired locus for recording. To do this conveniently, mount a length of glass tubing in a manipulator and attach the drawn plastic tubing as a replaceable tip on the end of the glass tubing. Electrical contact with the electrode lumen and suction are produced as with the glass suction electrodes described above.

Plastic suction electrodes are particularly useful for multichannel recordings. Several electrodes can be placed on a single animal for comparison of activity at different sites. Fine plastic suction electrodes have considerably higher electrical resistance than do the glass suction electrodes, and amplifiers with high-input resistance should be used with drawn plastic electrodes.

MONITORING EXTERNAL LONGITUDINAL CURRENT

Taddei-Ferretti *et al.* (1976) have developed a promising technique for recording endogenous activity from hydra. These workers recorded potentials from a hydra sucked entirely into a polyethylene tube of 0.5 mm internal diameter (see also Taddei-Ferretti and Cordella, 1975, 1976). They filled the tube with culture solution and entirely immersed it in solution except for the ends of the tube which remained above. A small hole in the side of the tube, made with a pin, gave electrical contact between the lumen of the tube and the outer solution. The hydra was positioned in the tube so that a desired part of the column lay adjacent to the hole. Potentials were recorded between the ends of the tube or between either end and the culture solution surrounding the tube; in the latter configuration, the potential recorded is that

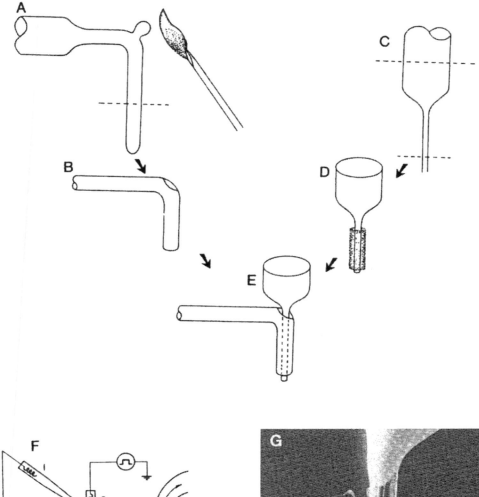

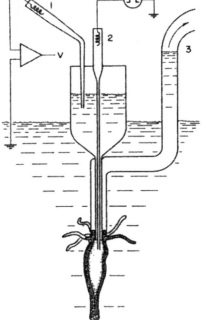

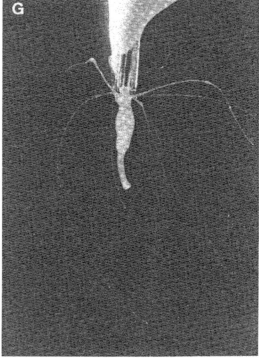

between the end of the tube and the tube lumen at the transverse hole. The potentials recorded are equal to the longitudinal current flow in the solution surrounding the animal times the longitudinal electrical resistance of the fluid pathway. Thus this method allows measurement of the longitudinal current flow surrounding the animal. The results obtained with this technique are unexpected; for example, bursts of contraction pulses are often preceded by large, slow changes in external longitudinal current, and the direction of current flow can be different at the two ends of the animal.

METHOD II. TRANSEPITHELIAL POTENTIALS

The transepithelial potential of hydra can readily be measured by inserting a glass capillary microelectrode through the body wall into the lumen of the gut (Macklin, 1967, 1976; Josephson and Macklin, 1969), but the animal often pulls off the electrode or tears its tissue against the electrode during spontaneous contractions. Thus, this method is unsuitable for long-term recordings. By using the holder illustrated in Fig. 2, it is possible to monitor transepithelial potential for long periods. In addition, with this holder the enteron of the animal can be perfused and electrical current passed across the body wall while measuring the transepithelial potential (Josephson and Macklin, 1969; Macklin and Josephson, 1971).

The holder consists basically of two concentric glass tubes. The inner diameter of the outer tube is approximately 0.7 mm at the tip, and the radial distance between the inner and outer tubes is about 0.15 mm. Hold the hydra in the space between the two tubes by slight suction. To create the suction which holds the animal in place, use a syringe attached to the outer tube by flexible tubing. The inner tube passes through the wall of the outer tube and

FIGURE 2. A holder for recording transepithelial potentials from hydra. (A) Heat a piece of drawn glass tubing and bend it to a right angle. Seal the thin end of the tubing. Heat the outer edge of the angle in a microflame and blow a small bubble in the tubing at that point. (B) Break off the bubble and file its edges with a fine sharpening stone to produce a hole in the convex side of the angle. (C) Make a funnel-shaped cup from a second piece of drawn tubing by scoring and breaking the tubing above and below the drawn portion. (D) Dip the thin part of the cup in molten wax. The wax layer on the cup keeps the two parts of the holder concentric during final assembly. (E) Insert the cup into the outer tube and fix it in place with epoxy cement. The cement used should be quite viscous or it will flow into and occlude the annulus between the two tubes. After the epoxy has set, remove the wax by dipping the end of the holder into warm xylene. (F) The recording setup. Record transepithelial potentials between the cup and the outer bathing solution. Current can be passed through the body wall using a long, thin electrode inserted through the cup into the enteron. The voltage (1) and current (2) electrodes are chlorided silver wires in glass tubes containing 1–2 M KCl in 2% agar. Apply slight suction to the outer tube of the holder (3) to keep the hydra in place. (G) A hydra on a holder.

then expands to form a small cup. The fluid-filled inner tube serves as an electrical conductor to the enteron and as a pathway for introducing a current electrode or a perfusion pipet into the enteron.

The assembly of the hydra holder is illustrated in Fig. 2. Fill the inner tube and cup with culture medium before mounting the animal on the holder. Grasp the hydra lightly by the tentacles with fine forceps and gently pull the mouth over the end of the inner tube which protrudes slightly beyond the orifice of the outer tube. Carefully suck the animal into the space between the tubes. The tentacles are sometimes damaged while the animal is placed on the holder; otherwise the animal is uninjured and appears normal when released. While it is on the holder, the animal's mouth is held open and the tissue about the mouth is somewhat compressed. This stress alters the pattern of spontaneous activity; thus this type of holder is not recommended for monitoring spontaneous electrical behavior of hydra.

METHOD III. INTRACELLULAR RECORDING

Intracellular recordings give information on the excitable properties of nerve and epithelial cells most directly. Successful intracellular recording requires virtual elimination of relative movement between the electrode and the impaled cell. The difficulty in immobilizing hydra tissue has greatly impeded investigations using microelectrodes to record from hydra, but some partial successes have been achieved. Macklin (1967) used glass capillary electrodes to determine the voltage profile across the body wall of hydra. The potential increased in several discrete steps as the electrode was advanced through the body wall. Kass-Simon (1976) and Kass-Simon and Diesl (1977) have recorded potentials from dissociated epithelial and nerve cells of hydra and from epithelial cells of intact, nerve-free hydra; nerve-free animals (Chapter 36) were used because they do not contract spontaneously (Campbell *et al.*, 1976). The reported membrane potentials are small, 2–25 mV, which may be a consequence of cell damage during electrode insertion. Intracellular recording is almost certain to be an important technique for investigating excitability in hydra when the technical problems are better resolved.

METHOD IV. MEASURING CONDUCTION VELOCITY

The conduction velocity of a propagated wave is usually measured as the distance between two recording sites along the pathway divided by the time increment between the appearance of homologous portions of the wave at the two sites. For example, the conduction velocity of an axon is given by the ratio of the distance between two pairs of recording electrodes and the delay between the appearance of the spike peak (or onset) at the two recording sites. Unfortunately a pulse recorded from two suction electrodes on hydra is often sufficiently dissimilar in appearance at the two sites that it is not obvious which portions of the two recorded responses are really homologous (Josephson, 1967). This dissimilarity makes it difficult or impossible to determine the temporal delay between equivalent portions of the response at the two recording sites.

Conduction velocity can also be determined with a single recording channel if one varies the site of pulse initiation. As a stimulating electrode on the column is moved toward the recording site, the latency between the stimulus and the recorded response decreases; and as the stimulating electrode is moved away from the recording site, the latency increases. Assuming that the pulse initiation time at the stimulating electrode is independent of stimulus location, the change in distance between the stimulating and recording electrodes divided by the corresponding change in response latency gives the conduction velocity. This method avoids the difficulty introduced by dissimilarity in pulse shape at two recording sites. Pulses propagated in the same direction to a single recording electrode are sufficiently similar in shape, no matter where the pulses are initiated, that the latency to an identifiable portion of the response wave form can be measured and used to determine conduction velocity.

PROCEDURES

The following procedure has been used to measure the conduction velocity of CPs in the column of hydra (Josephson, 1967; Campbell *et al.*, 1976). Hold a hydra suspended between two recording electrodes, one on the hypostome and the other on the base. Allow the hydra to elongate maximally. Adjust the position of the electrodes to take up any slack in the column, and measure the length of the column with an ocular micrometer. This length is termed the working length. Place a stimulating electrode on the column at varied positions to initiate CPs, allowing the column to relax to the working length before each stimulus. Photograph, from an oscilloscope screen, the CPs recorded from both the basal and hypostomal electrodes. Measure the photographed responses to determine the latency between each shock and an identifiable point on the evoked CP, perhaps most usefully the positive peak

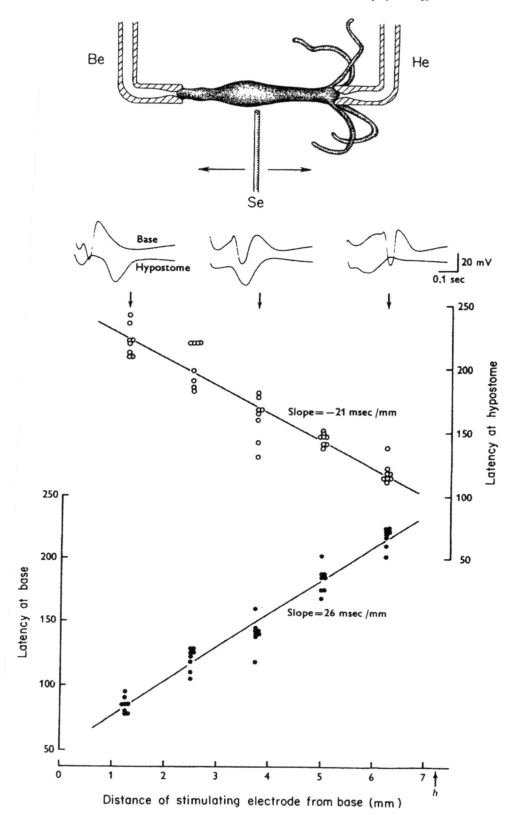

Slope = −21 msec /mm

Slope = 26 msec /mm

Distance of stimulating electrode from base (mm)

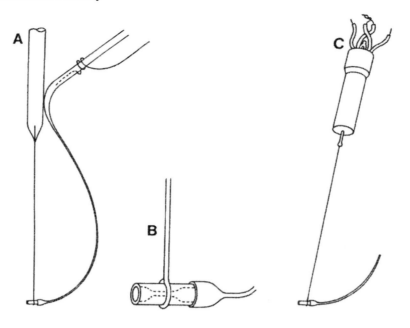

FIGURE 4. (A) One way to mount a suction electrode so that it is compliant and can move with a contracting animal. Suspend a glass electrode tip attached to a length of drawn plastic tubing from a length of thin wire held in a manipulator. (B) Details of the electrode tip. The wire is fixed to the glass tip with epoxy cement. (C) If the wire is attached to a sensitive transducer rather than directly to a manipulator, the arrangement in (A) can be used to measure column contraction. When this arrangement was first used (Josephson. 1967). the most appropriate transducer was a vacuum tube device (RCA 5734) shown in the figure. Now semiconductor transducers are available that would be more suitable (information available from Aksjesels-kapet Mikro-Elektronikk, 3191 Horten, Norway; and Endevco Co., San Juan Capistrano, CA 92675).

of the CP (see discussion in Josephson, 1967). Plot these latencies as a function of the distance between the stimulating and the recording electrode (Fig. 3). The conduction velocity is the reciprocal of the slope of the least-squares regression line of this plot.

FIGURE 3. Measuring conduction velocity of CPs in the column of hydra. Suspend a hydra between two suction electrodes (top of figure) and stimulate the column at varied positions with a stimulating electrode (Se). The stimulus to response latency at the basal and hypostomal electrodes (Be and He) varies systematically with the position of the stimulating electrode (insets below the diagram of the stimulated animal). Plot the latencies of potentials recorded at the base and hypostome as a function of the position of the stimulating electrode as in the lower portion of the figure (from Josephson, 1967). Obtain conduction velocities from the slopes of the resulting least-squares regression lines.

COMMENTS

If you use rigid glass suction electrodes in determining the conduction velocity, adjust the distance between the electrodes continuously as the animal contracts spontaneously or in response to stimuli; otherwise the hydra often pulls out of one of the two recording electrodes. The procedure can be made a little less trying for the experimenter, and probably for the hydra as well, if one of the two recording electrodes is compliant so that it follows the movement of the contracting animal. Ideally the electrode should move freely when the animal contracts yet keep the column under slight tension so as to pull out the column during relaxation. One arrangement for doing this is shown in Fig. 4. Cut off the tip of a glass electrode and insert it into the end of a length of drawn plastic tubing. Attach the electrode tip to the end of a length of thin, springy wire, the other end of which is mounted in a manipulator used for positioning the electrode. With very thin and therefore very flexible plastic tubing, the electrical resistance of the fluid-filled portion of this electrode is quite high, 200–400 MΩ, and very high impedance amplifiers are necessary.

ACKNOWLEDGMENTS. Preparation of this chapter was supported by NSF Grant BMS 75-09530 to RKJ and NIH Grant MH 10734 to NBR.

REFERENCES

Campbell, R. D., Josephson, R. K., Schwab, W. E., and Rushforth, N. B. 1976. Excitability of nerve-free hydra. *Nature (London)* **262**:388–390.

Josephson, R. K. 1965. Three parallel conducting systems in the stalk of a hydroid. *J. Exp. Biol.* **42**:139–152.

Josephson, R. K. 1966. Neuromuscular transmission in a sea anemone. *J. Exp. Biol.* **45**:305–320.

Josephson, R. K. 1967. Conduction and contraction in the column of *Hydra. J. Exp. Biol.* **47**:179–190.

Josephson, R. K., and Macklin, M. 1969. Electrical properties of the body wall of *Hydra. J. Gen. Physiol.* **53**:638–665.

Kass-Simon, G. 1976. Coordination of juxtaposed muscle layers as seen in *Hydra.* In: *Coelentrate Ecology and Behavior* (G. O. Mackie, ed.), Plenum Press, New York, pp. 705–714.

Kass-Simon, G., and Diesl, V. K. 1977. Spontaneous and evoked potentials from dissociated epithelial cells of *Hydra. Nature (London)* **265**:75–77.

Mackie, G. O., and Passano, L. M. 1968. Epithelial conduction in hydromedusae. *J. Gen Physiol.* **52**:600–621.

Macklin, M. 1967. Osmotic regulation in *Hydra*: Sodium and calcium localization and source of electrical potential. *J. Cell. Physiol.* **70**:191–196.

Macklin, J. 1976. The effect of urethan on *Hydra. Biol. Bull.* **150**:442–452.

Macklin, M., and Josephson, R. K. 1971. The ionic requirements of transepithelial potentials in *Hydra*. *Biol. Bull.* **141**:299–318.

Passano, L. M., and McCullough, C. B. 1962. The light response and the rhythmic potentials of *Hydra*. *Proc. Natl. Acad. Sci. U.S.A.* **48**:1376–1382.

Passano, L. M., and McCullough, C. B. 1963. Pacemaker hierarchies controlling the behaviour of *Hydras*. *Nature (London)* **199**:1174–1175.

Passano, L. M., and McCullough, C. B. 1964. Coordinating systems and behaviour in *Hydra*. I Pacemaker system of the periodic contractions. *J. Exp. Biol.* **41**:643–664.

Passano, L. M., and McCullough, C. B. 1965. Coordinating systems and behaviour in *Hydra*. II. The rhythmic potential system. *J. Exp. Biol.* **42**:205–231.

Rushforth, N. B. 1971. Behavioral and electrophysiological studies of hydra. I. Analysis of contraction pulse patterns. *Biol. Bull.* **140**:255–273.

Rushforth, N. B., and Burke, D. S. 1971. Behavioral and electrophysiological studies of hydra. II. Pacemaker activity of isolated tentacles. *Biol. Bull.* **140**:502–519.

Taddei-Ferritti, C., and Cordella, L. 1975. Modulation of *Hydra attenuata* rhythmic activity: Photic stimulation. *Arch. Ital. Biol.* **113**:107–121.

Taddei-Ferretti, C., and Cordella, L. 1976. Modulation of *Hydra attenuata* rhythmic activity: Phase response curve. *J. Exp. Biol.* **65**:737–751.

Taddei-Ferretti, C., Cordella, L., and Chillemi, S. 1976. Analysis of *Hydra* contraction behaviour. In: *Coelenterate Ecology and Behavior* (G. O. Mackie, ed.), Plenum Press, New York, pp. 685–694.

Chapter 61

Bioassay for, and Characterization of, Activators and Inhibitors of the Feeding Response

Howard M. Lenhoff, Wyrta Heagy, and Jean Danner

PURPOSE

To describe conditions of the bioassay and the means for quantifying the potency of activators and inhibitors of the feeding response.

INTRODUCTION

The feeding response of hydra, i.e., the process in which food or food extracts stimulate the bending of the tentacles toward its mouth and the subsequent act of opening that mouth (Ewer, 1947; Loomis, 1958), is used as an accurate means for determining the structure–activity relationships of a chemical activator with its complementary receptor on the cell surface (Heagy, 1977; Lenhoff, 1981).

In hydra the feeding activator is the reduced tripeptide GSH (Loomis, 1955). We find that by using hydra grown under rigorously controlled conditions, by developing a simple and sensitive bioassay, and by applying

Howard M. Lenhoff ● Department of Developmental and Cell Biology, University of California, Irvine, California. Wyrta Heagy ● Department of Microbiology, University of Massachusetts, Amherst, Massachusetts. Jean Danner ● Biochemistry Section, NIOSH, Morgantown, West Virginia.

principles regarding the interactions of enzymes with their substrates and competitive inhibitors, it is possible to determine subtle differences in the shape and structure of GSH analogs while they are at the receptor site. In addition, because of the extreme sensitivity of hydra's GSH receptor–effector system to foreign substances in the environment, it is possible to determine the degree to which those substances affect the hydra by measuring the degree of the feeding response.

MATERIALS

The basic experimental test solution is composed of 10^{-3} M $CaCl_2$, 10^{-4} M NaCl, and 10^{-3} M of a buffer, such as histidine, imidazole, or tris (hydroxy) aminomethane, depending upon the pH desired. In addition to the typical normal glassware, other materials needed are a thermocouple to measure temperatures in small volumes; a temperature regulator (e.g., Haake, Inc.); containers to carry out the assay, such as a Maximov tissue culture depression slide with a cavity 36 mm in diameter and 5 mm deep, or a block of plastic containing a series of four 3-ml wells, each seated within an enclosed insulation well through which water of a constant temperature can be pumped; a binocular dissecting microscope; and at least five stopwatches. For your control activator, prepare a stock solution of 10^{-3} M GSH (Sigma Chemical Co.) and dilute aliquots 1/100 in the basic test solution immediately before using it. Use monosodium glutamic acid as a control competitive inhibitor.

COMMENTS

The feeding response induced by GSH or by other activators is a complex behavioral phenomenon consisting of a number of easily recognizable steps (Lenhoff, 1961). To quantify the bioassay, however, we measure only one of them, one that can readily and objectively be determined using a low-power binocular dissecting microscope. That measurement consists of noting the initial time that the mouth opens (t_i)in response to the activator, and the time and the mouth finally closes (t_f); the difference $t_f - t_i$, i.e., the duration of mouth opening, is a reliable measure of the feeding response, from which a number of constants can be calculated.

In order to get such reliable results, it is essential to use hydra that are approximately of the same developmental and nutritional state and that have been maintained uncrowded for 1–2 days in a solution of known composition free of added potassium ions. For the most accurate results, control the temperature and buffer the test solution.

PROCEDURES

Preparing the Hydra for the Bioassay

Remove from the mass cultures (Chapter 8) hydra that have been fasted for 1 day. Clean them free of debris and maintain the clean animals in a flat glass tray at densities of no more than 2000–3000 per 1500 ml of a solution of 10^{-3} M $CaCl_2$ and of 10^{-4} M $NaHCO_3$ adjusted to pH 7.0–7.5.

Conditions of the Bioassay

In each depression of a Maximov tissue culture slide, or assay wells of the insulated plastic block, place 2 ml of a solution containing the substance to be tested dissolved in the basic test solution buffered at the desired pH. For your trial assays, use 10^{-5} M GSH. Allow the temperature to equilibrate and set the wells on the stage of a binocular microscope set at about 15–20X magnification. Take five of the 2- to 3-day fasted hydra, each of almost the same size and pigmentation and having one new bud, rinse them together three times in 30-ml portions of the basic test solution and transfer them in one drop of liquid into the well containing the solution to be tested. At that moment start a stopwatch and, while observing the animals through the microscope, mark down the instant that each mouth actually opens (t_i) and closes (t_f). Under optimal conditions and depending upon the experimental conditions and the species of hydra used, the mouths will usually open within 20–60 sec and close after 20–30 min. Therefore, you can set up three to five experiments at a time, but stagger the times you start each experiment at about 5-min intervals. An example of how the hydra appear at various times during the feeding response to GSH is illustrated in Fig. 1.

Expressing the Data of the Bioassay

Express the magnitude of the feeding response as the average time $t_f - t_i$ during which the mouths of the five hydra remain open to an activator (e.g., GSH) under the conditions of the experiment. Examples of measurements taken with *Hydra littoralis* at four different pH values with 10^{-5} M GSH in histidine buffer are shown in Tables I and II. Note that although more variation is observed in the t_i measurements, they are small compared to

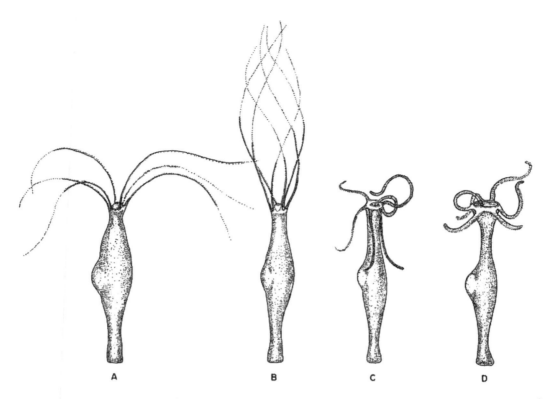

FIGURE 1. Stages in the feeding response to reduced glutathione. A hydra in the absence of GSH is shown in (A); the mouth is closed, and the tentacles are outstretched and relatively motionless. After the addition of GSH, the tentacles first begin to writhe and sweep inward toward the central vertical axis of the animal (B). Next, the tentacles bend toward the mouth, and the mouth opens (C). Shown in this composite drawing (C) are the various positions that a tentacle takes before contracting. These movements, culminating in mouth opening, usually all take place within half a minute. (D) shows how a hydra looks during the greater portion of the feeding response, its mouth open wide and the tentacles in various phases of contraction. Frequently, the tips of the tentacles are observed within the hydra's mouth, as shown in (C) and (D).

TABLE I. Measurements for t_i

pH		t_i (min)				Mean $t_i \pm$ S.D. (min)
5.41	0.30	0.48	0.52	0.52	0.53	0.47 ± 0.10
5.8	0.40	0.57	0.63	0.68	0.98	0.65 ± 0.21
5.9	0.30	0.32	0.34	0.42	0.43	0.37 ± 0.06
6.51	0.22	0.32	0.35	0.52	0.55	0.39 ± 0.14

TABLE II. Quantification of Feeding Response Based on $t_f - t_i$ Measurements

pH			t_f (min)			Mean $t_f - t_i \pm$ S.D.[a] (min)
5.41	39.75	39.83	39.87	40.20	40.63	39.59 ± 0.32
5.81	39.00	39.55	39.73	40.10	42.85	39.59 ± 1.31
5.93	39.00	39.05	39.72	40.52	44.73	40.15 ± 2.41
6.51	30.97	31.17	31.33	32.18	33.00	31.34 ± 0.72

[a] The t_i values used to calculate $t_f - t_i$ were those from Table I.

those of the overall $t_f - t_i$ measurements. In some cases, however, such as at suboptimal concentrations of GSH or in the presence of a competitive inhibitor of glutathione, you will find that the hydra either will not open their mouths or will take up to 6 min to do so. In these cases, the standard deviation will be large relative to $t_f - t_i$. Nonetheless, express data of this type similarly as $t_f - t_i$) during which the mouths of all five hydra tested remained open regardless of the number that respond positively. For example, if hydra

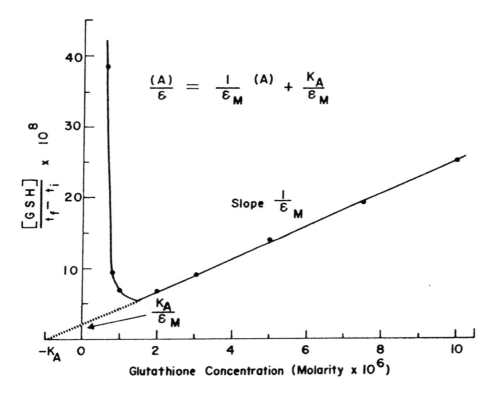

FIGURE 2. Determination of K_A and E_M by the modified Lineweaver–Burk plot. The assay involved the use of $t_f - t_i$ measurements.

numbers 1 and 2 do not open while hydra numbers 3, 4, and 5 open their mouths for 6, 9, and 13 min, respectively, then record the average t_f as

$$(0 + 0 + 6 + 9 + 13)/ 5 = 5.6$$

not as

$$(6 + 9 + 13)/ 3 = 9.3$$

Calculation of Activator Potency

Calculate the potency of activators by using a plot which takes into account the $t_f - t_i$ values measured at different activator concentrations. Figure 2 gives an example of a typical plot using $t_f - t_i$ values taken at a range of concentrations of GSH. The formula

$$\frac{(A)}{E} = \frac{1}{E_M} (A) + \frac{K_A}{E_M}$$

defines the curve: (A) refers to concentration of the activator; E, to the effect measured, i.e., $t_f - t_i$; E_M, to the maximum effect, i.e., the longest $t_f - t_i$ measured under the given conditions; and K_A, to the activator constant. From Fig. 2, you can see that it is possible to measure both E_M and K_A from the E data calculated at various (A)s. The derivation of this equation is presented elsewhere (Lenhoff, 1965, 1968, 1969).

The K_A value represents the potency of the activator; the lower the K_A the more effective the activator. This value is analogous to the K_M of an enzyme. Like the K_M, it is a property of the receptor and is a constant. Like the K_M, it represents the concentration of activator inducing a half-maximal response; for this reason, and to avoid possible confusion with enzymes, the K_A can also be called C_{50} (i.e., concentration of activator stimulating a 50% response). And, like the K_M, it represents the affinity of the receptor and the activator for each other: the lower the K_A, the lower the affinity. In addition, you can determine the pKs of ionizable groups at the receptor site that are affected by the binding of the activator by determining the K_A for the activator over a wide range of pH values (Lenhoff, 1969).

The E_M value is analogous to the V_M of an enzyme. Accordingly, it is not a constant of the receptor, but rather it represents the number of receptor–effector systems in a hydra available to be activated. Hence, you will find that under a particular set of conditions that the E_M will vary significantly. On the other hand, the K_A will not.

Calculation of Potency of Competitive Inhibitors

Competitive inhibitors (antagonists) are substances that are structurally similar to activators (agonists) so that they will bind to the receptor but will not activate it. Such binding, however, occupies space on the receptors and prevents activators from occupying the receptor site. Because both the competitive inhibitor and activator molecules are in equilibrium with the receptors, the competitive inhibitors can be made to occupy proportionally fewer receptor sites by increasing the concentration of the activator. The degree to which the activator is able to occupy more sites depends upon the K_A of the activator and the potency of the inhibitor.

This potency, called I_{50}, denotes the concentration of the competitive inhibitor that can lower by 50% the response stimulated by $2 \times 10^{-6}\ M$ GSH in the basic assay solution buffered by histidine at pH 6.2. The effect $(t_f - t_i)$ elicited by a $2 \times 100^{-6}\ M$ GSH was selected to represent a 100% response in this assay, because under basic assay conditions, $2 \times 10^{-6}\ M$ GSH elicits about a half-maximal feeding response. Hence, any increase in the concentration of an inhibitor will lead to an observed decrease in $t_f - t_i$. If, on the other hand, you use a concentration of GSH that would activate a near maximal $t_f - t_i$, then the competitive effects of the inhibitor will be less perceptible unless you use extremely large concentrations of inhibitor.

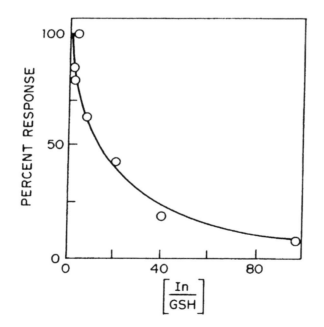

FIGURE 3. Quantification of inhibitory action of glutamate (see text).

To measure the I_{50} of a particular competitive inhibitor, follow the same basic procedures used to carry out the assay for an activator. Prepare every test solution so that it contains $2 \times 10^{-6} M$ GSH dissolved in the basic assay solution, and from 0 up to $10^{-2} M$ of inhibitor depending upon its potency. Add five hydra and record the t_i and t_f values as you do for quantifying activators. Usually around six different concentrations of inhibitor will suffice. Record the $t_f - t_i$ for $2 \times 10^{-6} M$ GSH in the absence of inhibitor as 100% activation, and all other $t_f - t_i$ measurements as a proportion of the 100% activation. Plot the percentage of activation values on the ordinate and the ratio if the concentration of inhibitor to GSH on the abscissa. A typical result for a good "high potency" inhibitor, glutamic acid, is illustrated in Fig. 3. To calculate the I_{50}, determine from your plot the concentration of inhibitor allowing a 50% activation to occur. From Fig. 3, the I_{50} for glutamic acid is $10^{-4} M$.

Testing Potency of Cell Poisons (Noncompetitive Inhibitors) Using the Competitive Inhibitor Assay

General cell poisons, such as Cu^{2+}, or other materials toxic to hydra (e.g., methyl phenyldiazenecarboxylate) (Lenhoff *et al.*, 1969) usually have a profound and immediate effect on hydra by inhibiting the feeding response noncompetitively, i.e., the inhibition is not reversed by added GSH in the medium.

To use hydra as a test for substances presumed to be cell poisons, simply incubate the hydra for varying times (e.g., 1–30 min) in the basic assay solution containing a known concentration of the compound in question. Rinse the animals with fresh basic assay solution at the end of the incubation period and measure for $t_f - t_i$ using those treated hydra in the basic assay solution containing $2 \times 10^{-6} M$ GSH. If the treated animals respond less than do nontreated animals, then you can conclude that the tested substance is a noncompetitive cell poison. Express potency as the concentration of inhibitor reducing the feeding response induced by $2 \times 10^{-6} M$ GSH by 50% after the test hydra have been sitting in a solution of that substance for 5 min.

PRECAUTIONS

Each specie of hydra responds differently to feeding activators. *Hydra littoralis* give the most reliable results and respond best at 22° C. *Hydra attenuata* also give easily measurable responses, but we recommend that you carry out the experiments at 29°C because at lower temperatures the t_f values range over 40 min, thereby making measurements very tedious. Other species, such as *Hydra pirardi*, may respond to GSH for as long as 100 min at 22°C. *Hydra viridis* gives such a small visual mouth opening response that it is difficult to record it. A number of hydra tend to close and open their mouths a number of times at the end of an extended response, or during an experiment carried out at low temperatures (4–15°C); in those cases, record all t_f and t_i values and calculate the total time that the mouths remained open during the experiment.

Potassium ions greatly inhibit the feeding response, and the inhibition can be reversed by placing the hydra in a potassium-free solution for a few hours (Lenhoff, 1965). The magnitude of the response is greatly affected by a number of other ions, such as Mg^{2+}, Na^+, and H^+. Hence, take care to use only the purest of salts and water for these experiments.

Finally, when working with such a sensitive phenomenon with whole animals, you will sometimes find unexplicable variations in the behavior of the animals. Therefore, we find it useful and recommend to you while quantifying one activator or inhibitor to run all experiments and controls during the same day using hydra from the same mass culture dish.

REFERENCES

Ewer, R. F. 1947. On the function and mode of action of nemotocysts of *Hydra*. *Proc. Zool. Soc. London* 117:365–376.

Heagy, W. 1977. Glutathione Receptor of Hydra: Structure-Activity Relationship. Doctoral dissertation, University of California, Irvine.

Lenhoff, H. M. 1961. Activation of the feeding reflex in *Hydra littoralis*. I. Role played by reduced glutathione and quantitative assay of the feeding reflex. 45:331–344.

Lenhoff, H. M. 1965. Some physiochemical aspects of the macro- and micro-environments surrounding hydra during activation of their feeding behavior. *Amer Zool.* 5:515–524.

Lenhoff, H. M. 1969. pH profile of a peptide receptor. *Comp. Biochem. Physiol.* 28:571–586.

Lenhoff, H. M. 1981. Biology and physical chemistry of feeding response of hydra. In: *Biochemistry of Taste and Olfaction* (R. H. Cagan and M. R. Kare, eds.), Academic Press, New York, pp. 475–497.

Lenhoff, H. M., and Bovaird, J. 1961. Action of glutamic acid and glutathione analogues on the hydra glutathione-receptor. *Nature (London)* 189:486–487.

Lenhoff, H. M., Kosower, E. M., and Kosower, N. S. 1969. Hydra as a biological amplifier for testing the thiol agent azoester. *Nature (London)* 224:717–718.

Loomis, W. F. 1955. Glutathione control of the specific feeding reactions of hydra. *Ann. N.Y. Acad. Sci.* 62:209–228.

Index

Acid fuchsin, 129
Acontia thread, 332
Acrolein, 89, 90
Acrylamide gel, 337–338
    separation gel, 337
    stacking gel, 337
Activation of head, defined, 313
Activation-inhibition model, 246–249
    chi-square distribution, 247
    gradient, 248
    level, 247–248
    log-linear model, 246
    optimization method, 248
    profile, shape of, 247–249
    test, statistical, 246–247
Activator, 311
    of feeding response, 443–451
    of head, 313
    potency, 447–449
Activity, electrical, 429–441
    conduction velocity, 436–439
    potential
        spontaneous, 429–435
        transepithelial, 435–436
    recording, intracellular, 436
Advantage of hydra in experiments, 3
Aggregate, 261–268
    development from, 251–259
    from nitrogen mustard treatment, 261–268
    into pellet, 254–257
Aiptasia pallida, see Sea anemone
Aldehyde, fixation by, 88–91

Alga, endosymbiotic, 388–411
    introducing into hydra, 399
    isolating
    maltose secretion by, 411
    measuring numbers by
        fluorometric estimation, 403–404
        growth kinetics, 402–403
        maceration technique, 401–402
        removing from hydra, 393
Ammonium alum, 128
Amputation and regeneration, 218
Analytical procedures, 361–387
Anchistropus sp., 18
Anesthesia, 97, 122
Aniline blue, 129
Antibiotics, 79–81, 212
Araldite for embedding specimen, 88–92
Artemia salina, 39–46
    cyst, 39–46
        and bacteria, 41
        decontamination, 41
        and fungi, 41
    food for hydra, 39–46
    hatching
        apparatus, 43
        method, 42–44
        by bubbling, 42, 44
        by floating, 42
    hatching solution, 41–42
    incubation, 44
    larva, axenic, 39–46
    nauplii, 2, 39–46, 54, 213, 306, 393, 419

453

Artemia salina, nauplii (*cont.*)
  harvesting method, 44–46
Autofluorescence, 134, 136
Autoradiography, 155, 162
  of cells, 155
  of ectoderm, 119
  of whole mounts, 205
Autotomy, 349
Axenic hydra, 79–83
  and antibiotics, 79–81

Bacteria as contaminants of hydra, 41, 189,
    257, 366
  growth, excessive, 287
  see also Axenic
Basal cell, 14
Basal disk, *see* Foot
Basement membrane, mammalian, 327
Battery cell, 9
Behavior, 429–451
Bellows of camera, 144
  calculation for length, 144
Bentonite, 374
Biebrich scarlet, 128
Bioassay, 349, 445–447
2,5-Bis(4′-aminophenyl-1′)-1,3,4-oxiazole,
    158
Bis-benzimide trihydrochloride pentahydrate
    (Hoescht *33258*), 132
BOA, *see* 2,5-Bis(4′-aminophenyl-1′)-1,3,4-
    oxiazole
Body
  column, 7
  morphogenic gradient of, 234
Bouin fixative, 122, 124, 126, 129
Brine shrimp, *see Artemia salina*
Budding, 1, 7, 10, 299
  inhibition, 314
  rate, 52, 68, 70
Buffers, listed, 374–375
n-Butyl alcohol, 342, 344

Capsule, 11
  of nematocyst, 2, 177, 335–339
Carbon
  colloidal, 132
  compound, organic, and translocation into
      hydra, 407–409
Carbon dioxide, radioactive, 193–195
6-Carboxyfluorescein, 133
  method, 137–138

6-Carboxyfluorescein (*cont.*)
  photobleaching with, 139
Cell, 9–14
  basal, 14
  cloning, 262, 264
  composition, 290–291
  counting chamber, 178, 251
  cycle
    analysis, 157–163
    doubling time, 158
    G2-phase, 160–161
    kinetics, 157
    S-phase, 159–160
    time, 158–159
  dissociation, 153, 263
  ectodermal, 9, 10
  endodermal, 9, 10, 14
  interstitial, 11–14, 291–294
    absence of, 295–302
    eliminating, 299–304
    lineage, 11–14
    and nitrogen mustard, 299–302
  glandular, 14
  lineage
    epitheliomuscular, 9–11
    interstitial, 11–14
  loss, monitoring of, 285–286
  mucous, 14
  of muscle mat, 9
  of nerve, 295–297
  types, 2, 5–14
  zymogen in, 14
  see also individual cell types
Chimera formation, 273–277
Chi-square distribution, 247
  test for, 312
Chlorella, endosymbiotic, 411
  see Alga, endosymbiotic
Chloroform, 374, 375
Chlorohydra sp., 22–24
Cinclide, 332
Cleaning hydra, 81–82, 253
Clone-forming cell, assay for, 264
Clorox, 106
Cnidoblast, *see* Nematoblast
Cnidocil, *see* Nematocyte
Cnidocyte, 12
Coelentron, 5
Colchicine, 167, 258, 281–287, 295–303
  and cell disappearance, 285
  double treatment, 284–286

Colchicine (*cont.*)
single treatment, 282, 284
Collecting specimens, 17–18
Column, 6
twisted mutant, 214, 216
Computer algorithm, hill-climbing, 246
Conduction velocity
of axon, 437
of propagated wave, 436
recorded, 437
Contamination, *see* Bacteria, Parasites
Copper, as cell poison, 450
Counting cells, *see* Quantification
Crab, *see* Fiddler crab
Crayfish, 348, 356–357
desheathing, 357
dissection, 357
nerve failure, irreversible, 357
Culturing hydra, 17–83
large numbers, 53–62
medium, 29–34
contaminants, 29
ingredients, 31–33
phenol red, 35–37
pure water, 30–31
tray method, 54–60
vertical plate method, 54–56, 60–62
Cytology, quantitative, 153–186
cell cycle analysis, 157–163
maceration technique, 153–156
mitotic index, 165–168
numbers of
nematoblasts, 169–182
nematocysts, 169–182
nematocytes, 169–182

DAPI, *see* 4,6-Diamidino-2-phenylindole-2-
hydrochloride
Dehydration, 98
Desmosome, 1, 9, 12, 21, 172, 173, 217
Detergent
Nonidet P-*40*, 328
Sarkosyl NL-*97*, 328
Development from aggregated cells, 251–259
4,6-Diamidine-2-phenylindole-2-
hydrochloride, 132
carcinogenic, 135
method, 135–136
Diadumene, *see* Sea anemone
3-(3,4-dichlorophenyl)-1,1-dimethylurea,
394

Diethylpyrocarbonate, 374, 375
Differentiation, sexual in hydra, 71–77
by carbon dioxide tension, 73–74
factors affecting, 71–72
by feeding schedule, 75–76
by temperature drop, 77
by temperature rise, 72–73
3-Dimethylamino acid, 412
Dimethylsulfoxide, 132
Disadvantage of using hydra in experiments,
2
Disk, basal, *see* Foot
Disk electrophoresis, 336
apparatus, 336
stock solutions, 336
Dissociating into cells, 153, 263
medium for, 153, 257
Dithioerythritol, 335
Dithiothreitol, 338, 335
DMSO, *see* Dimethylsulfoxide
DNA
bacterial, 189
content of hydra, 162
and hydroxyurea, 292
DNase, 374, 376
Doubling time of cells, 32, 158 *see* Growth
Dye, *see* Stain

Ecology dish, 263
Ectoderm, 5, 108, 138, 267–271
autoradiography, 119
and carbon particle, 183
-endoderm chimera, 273–277
formation, 268
isolation, 267–271
by mechanical method, 269–270
by perfusion method, 269
Egg, 8
hatching time, 214
stimulating formation, 71
Ehrlich's hematoxylin stain, 124, 125, 128
Electrode, 429–433
Electron microscopy
scanning, *see* Scanning electron microscopy
transmission, 87–94
preparation for, 87–90
Electrophoresis on acrylamide gel, 338
Electrophysiology, 429–451
Embedding specimen, 88, 89, 92, 123–124
Endoderm, 5, 138, 267–271
-ectoderm chimera, 273–277

Endoderm (*cont.*)
  formation, 268
  isolating, 267–271
  peeling off, 270
Endosymbiont, *see* Alga, endosymbiotic
  autotrophic, 407
Enteron, 101
  see Coelenteron
  surface, 109
Enzyme assay, 361–371
  oil-well method, 367–377
Eosin, 123, 128
Epidermis, 5
Ethanol, 117, 118, 122, 123, 128, 174, 198,
  199
Epizoötological research, 417–425
Evans blue, 132, 133, 136
  carcinogenic, perhaps, 137
Everting whole hydra, 270
Extrusion mechanism for nematocyst, 331

Fast green stain, 127
Feeder-layer technique, 261
Feeding
  forced, 304
  pipet, 288
  radioactive tissue, 194–195
  response, 443–451
    activator, 443–451
      potency, 447–449
    bioassay for, 443–451
    inhibitor, 443–451
      competitive, 448–450
      noncompetitive, 451
    and potassium ion, 450
    quantification, 447
Ferric alum, 127
Ferritin, 105
Feulgen stain, 124, 125, 127, 162, 166
  method described, 127
  and mitotic cell, 118–119
  reagent, 162
Fiddler crab, 342, 345, 348
Film, photographic, 146, 147
Filter, micropore, 197–198, 205–206
Fixative, 87–90, 107, 121–129, 166, 174
Fluorescent microscopy, 133
Fluorometer, 404
Foot (basal disk), 6–9, 231
  activator
    assay, 316–318

Foot (basal disk), activator (*cont.*)
    defined, 318
    purification, 323
  formation
    activation, 238–241, 243
    frequency of, 232, 234, 236
    inhibition, 238–241, 243
      gradient, 244–245
    optimization of activation–inhibition
      level, 244–251
    uncertainty, statistical, 241–247
  inhibitor, 318
    assay, 319
    defined, 318
    purification, 323
  sectioning, 124
Formalin, 402
Forced feeding, 304
Fractionation of tissue, 197–203
Freeze-drying, 362–363
Freeze-etching, 105–115
Freeze-fracture, 105–115
Fructose-1,6-diphosphate, 305–307
Fungus, 41

G2-Phase, 160–161, 291
Gastric cavity, 5
Gastrodermis, 5
Gentamicin, 257
Glass needle, 225–227
Glass suction electrode, 431–432, 439
Gluconic acid, 412
Glucose oxidase, 411
Glucose oxidase and peroxidase, 412
Glucosidase, 412
Glutaraldehyde, 89, 90, 96, 106
Glutathione, 195, 269, 446
  and mouth-opening, 269
Glutinant
  stereoline, 12
  streptoline, 12
Glycerol, 128, 332, 393–394
Gonad development, 213
Gonocyte, meiotic, 14
Gradient, morphogenic, 234
Grafting, *see* Transplantation
  dish, 225–226
  tissue, 1, 2, 225–233, 274, 299, 301
Granule, intramembranous, 110, 111, 114
Green hydra, *see* Hydra
Growth

Growth (*cont.*)
  count, 49–50
  curve, 158
  rate, 32, 47–52
    calculation, 51
    clonal, 48–52
    doubling time, 32, 158
    precautions, 51–52
Gut, 5
  see Coelenteron, Enteron

Hair point, 362
Handling hydra, 17–83
Hatching time of egg, 214
Head, 6, 7, 231, 311
  activation–inhibition model, 238
    defined, 313
    gradient, 233, 235
    optimization level, 244–251
    uncertainty, statistical, 241–247
  activator
    assay
      fast, 313–314
      standard, 321–313
    purification, 321, 323
  formation, frequency of, 232, 234,
    236, 238
  inhibitor
    assay
      alternative, 315–316
      standard, 314–315
    defined, 315
    purification, 323
  reduced, 231
Heidenhain Susa fixative, 125
Hemacytometer, 404
Hematoxylin, 128, 166
  Ehrlich's, 124, 125
  iron, 124–127
Hemolysis
  assay, 349–353
  curve, 352
  data, plotted, 352–353
  microtitration, 353
  percentage of, 352
  plotting data, 352–353
  spectrophotometry of, 351
  treatment, mathematical, 351–353
  see Rat red blood cells
Hexadecane, 368
Histology, 87–140

Hoechst *33258*, 133–135
  carcinogenic, 134
Hydra, epithelial, 281
  cloning, 286
  culturing, 287–290
  definition, 287
  feeding technique, 288, 289
    by force, 288–290
  formation, 287
    by colchicine, 287
    by gamma-irradiation, 287
    by inbreeding, 287
  inserting shrimp into, 288
  maintaining, 290
  mouth-opening, 288
Hydra, green
  oxygen evolution, 383–387
  photosynthesis, 386
  respiration, 383–387
Hydra species, 19–28
  H. americana, 23, 25
  H. attenuata, 22, 26, 154, 175, 235,
    281–286, 292, 295–297, 299, 304,
    312, 450
  H. braueri, 23, 25
  H. canadiensis, 25
  H. carnea, 23, 26, 27
  H. cauliculata, 23, 26, 27
  H. circuminata, 25
  H. fusca, 25
  H. hadleyi, 22–24
  H. hymanae, 22–25
  H. littoralis, 23, 27, 31, 32, 235–237,
    336–337, 341–346, 419, 445
  H. magnipapillata, 26, 211, 213, 281
  H. minima, 23, 25
  H. oligactis, 23–26, 267, 373
  H. ovata, 25
  H. parva, 25
  H. pirardi, 26, 299, 450
  H. pseudoligactis, 23–26, 267, 299, 329,
    418, 419
  H. robusta, 25, 26
  H. rutgerensis, 23, 26, 27
  H. stellata, 25
  H. utahensis, 23, 25
  H. viridis, 22, 154, 213, 244, 247, 267,
    281, 295–297, 329, 394–396, 411,
    412, 418, 419, 450
  H. viridissima, 22–24
  H. vulgaris, 23, 26, 27

Hydra species (*cont.*)
  criteria for identifying, 19
  literature on systematics, 20
  see specific aspects of hydra
Hydramoeba hydroxena, 18, 417–418
  growth, 420–421
  host mortality, 421
  hydra system, 417
  infection rate, 423
  stock culture, 418–419
  survivorship curve method, 422–423
Hydranth, 5, 6
  count of, 49–50
Hydroxyurea, 281, 291–294
  and cell population, 293
  and DNA, 292
Hypostome, 5, 6, 92, 100, 102, 112, 113,
    124, 231

Immunofluorescence, indirect, 138–139
Immunoglobulin (goat anti-mouse), 133
Inbreeding, 287
  depression, 2, 3
  sexual, 211–221
  see Mutant
India ink marker, 183–186, 274
Infection, bacterial, *see* Bacteria
Inhibition, *see* Foot, Head
Injecting hydra, 189, 400
Interference microscopy, 119
Iron hematoxylin stain, 124, 125, 127
Irradiation
  gamma-ray, 287, 303–304, 396
Isocitrate dehydrogenase, 368
  microassay for, 368
Isorhiza, 217
  atrichous, 12, 173
  holotrichous, 12, 173
Isotope technique, 189–203

Kerona pediculus, 18, 424

Labeling
  double, 160
  by feeding, 193
  by injection, 193–196
  radioactive, 158–159, 189–207
  with $^{14}CO_2$, 196
N-Lauroyl sarcosine, 328
Lavdowsky's fixative, 118, 119, 122, 124,
    166

Lead nitrate stain, 171–176
  preparation, 172, 174
L-α-Lecithin, 354
Leeuwenhoek, Anthony van, 1
Lethality
  bioassay, crustacean, 348–349
  LD_{50}, 349
Light microscopy, 117–130
Log-linear model, 246
Lyophilization, *see* Freeze

M solution, 31
Maceration technique, 153–156, 166, 401
  autoradiography, 155
  counting cells, 154–155
  fixative, 153
  for single cells, 153–156
  solution for, 153, 402
  staining, 156
Macrophotography, 143–149
Maertin's solution, 412
Magnesium uranyl acetate, 89
Mallory's triple stain, 124, 125, 129
  one-step method, 129
Maltose
  of alga, endosymbiotic, 411
  assay, spectrophotometric, 411–413
McIlwaine's buffer, 412
Medium, *see* Culture solution
Membrane, 110, 111
Mercaptoethanol, 335, 338
Mesolamella, 2, 5, 102, 103, 112–114, 186,
    281
  isolation, 327–329
  properties, 327–329
  sticky, 328
Mesoglea, *see* Mesolamella
Methanol, 318, 321, 404
3-Methyl-2-benzothiazolinone hydrazone
    hydrochloride, 412
Methylene blue staining, 131
  of nematocyst, 119
Methylphenyldiazenecarboxylate, 450
Methylsalicylate, 123
Metridium sp., *see* Sea anemone
Microassay, 367
  precautions, 370
Microelectrode, glass capillary as, 429–432,
    435
Microinjection pipet, 399–400
Micropipet, 184

Microscalpel, 362
Microscopy
  bright field, 181
  electron, 87–104
  fluorescent, 133
  interference, 119
  light
  phase, 169, 251
  polarization, 119
  scanning electron, 95–104
  transmission electron, 87–94
Microtitration
  dilution, 353
  plate, 353
Microtubule, 1, 2
Mineral oil, 368
Mitosis
  duration, 161
  index, 161, 165–168
  labeled as a technique, 160–161
Mitotic index, 161, 165–168
  defined, 165
  for growth estimation, 165
  and growth rhythm, 167
Morphogen, 311–324
  assay, biological, 312–318
    for activator, 312–314, 316–318
    for inhibitor, 314–316, 318
  purification on column, 318–323
Morphogensis, 311–324
  control, chemical, 311–324
Morphology, 5–14
Mount, whole, 117–120, 166–167, 174–175
Mouse, 345
  CAF strain, 342
  lethality bioassay, 349
  LD_{50}, 349
  liver, radioactive, 195
  tissue, radioactive, 195
Mouth, 7
  -opening, 269, 288
Muscle mat, 9
Mutant, 211–221
  cell types in altered proportions, 215, 219
  developmental, 211
  inbred, 211–221
  male, sterile, 270
  maxi, 214
  mini, 214
  multiheaded, 215–216
  nematocyst-deficient, 215, 217

Mutant (cont.)
  regeneration-deficient, 215
  twisted column, 214, 216
Mycostatin, 212
Myoneme, 102, 103, 112, 114

Narcosis, see Anesthesia
Nauplii, see Artemia salina
Neck, 6, 7
Nematoblast, 11, 160, 219, 291–294, 299, 300
  lead nitrate-thioacetic acid stain, 171–176
  and microtubule, 2
  numbers of, 169–182
Nematocyst, 24, 90, 91, 96, 98, 108, 304, 305, 327–387
  assay for
    hemolysis, 349–353
    lethality, 348–349
    phospholipase, 353–355
  capsule, 2, 177, 335–339
  composition, 337–338
  discharged, 331–333
    mechanism for, 331
  dissolution, 337
  examination, 20–21
  extrusion, 331
    medium for, 331
  isolation, 327–328
  isorhiza, holotrichous, 21
  number, 169–182
  properties, 327–387
  in sea anemone, 331–333
  suspension, 176–178
  in tentacle, 217
  thread protein, 335
  toxin, 331
  type
    desmoneme, 21
    isorhiza
      atrichous, 21
      holotrichous, 21
    photomicrograph, 170
    stenotele, 21
  undischarged, 331–333
  venom, 341, 347–358
Nematocyte, 12, 162, 219, 301, 305–307
  on body column, 179–181
  and interference microscopy, 119
  and microscopy, bright-field, 181
  numbers, 169–182

Nematocyte, numbers (*cont.*)
    reduced, 305–307
    suspension, 176–178
    in tentacle, 176–178
    and toluidine-blue stain, 179
Nembutal, 122
Nerve
    cell, 13, 295–297
    net, 14
Neubauer cell counting chamber, 178, 251
Neuron, sensory, 13
Neutral red, 131
Nile blue sulfate, 131, 132
Nipple, 7
Nitrogen mustard, 258, 261–268, 275–276,
        299–302
    and cell cycle, 299–302
    precautions, 277
    treatment, 276

Oöcyte, 8, 14
Oögonium, 14
Operculum, 108
Optimization method, 244
Orange G, 129
Osmium tetroxide, 344
    dangers of, 345
Ovum, 14
Ovary, 7
Oxygen
    consumption measured, 383–386
    electrode, 383
        calibration, 384
        chamber, 387
        instability, 386
    evolution, 386–387
        of green hydra, 383–387
    and photosynthesis, 386

Paraffin, 121, 133
Paraformaldehyde, 89, 90, 97, 106
Parasites of hydra, 18
    *see also Anchistropus, Hydramoeba,
        Kerona, Trichodina*
Peduncle, 6, 7
Pelmatohydra oligactis, 32
    P. pseudoligactis, 32
Penicillin G, 212
Phagocytosis, 183, 300
Phase microscopy, 169, 251
Phenol, 374

Phenol (*cont.*)
    -chloroform extraction of RNA, 373–377
Phenol red, 35–37
Phospholipase
    assay
        manometric, 353–355
        titrimetric, 355
    carbon dioxide release, 354
    thin-layer chromatography, 355–356
    in venom, 353
Phosphorus method, 356
Phosphotungstic acid, 129
Photobleaching, 394–395
Photography, *see* Macrophotography
Photoöxidation, 338
Photosynthesis of green hydra, 386
Phototaxis, 18
    in an eyeless animal, 1
Physalia sp. venom, 347
Poisson distribution, 264
Polarization microscopy, of muscle process,
        119
Polyethylene needle, 190–191
Polyp, 5, 68, 69
Pore, aboral, 7
Portugese man-of-war, *see Physalia* sp.
Potassium ion, and feeding response, 450
Potassium acetate, 374–376
Potential
    spontaneous, 429–435
    transepithelial, 435–436
Procamborus clarkii, see Crayfish
Procedures, analytical, 361–387
Pronematocyst, 11
Protein
    analysis, colorimetric (Lowry *et al.*),
        379–381
Protozoön, 257, 263
Pyridine nucleotide fluorescence, 367

Quantification (numbers), 175
    and feeding response, 447
    pipetimetric, 64–65
    turbidimetric, 64
Quartz fiber ultramicrobalance, 363–367
    calibration, 366
    precaution, 367
    use, 366
Quartz filter, 365

Radioactive hydra, 193–196

Radioactivity
   assay, 199, 202
   calculation, 200, 202
   percentage, 202
Radioautography, *see* autoradiography
Rat red blood cell, 349
Razor blade fragment as knife, 226, 228
   holder for, 228
Reaggregation, 299, 301
Red blood cell
   absorbancy unit, 351
   hemolysis, 349–353 *see* Hemolysis
   preparation, 349, 350
   standardizing, 350–351
   washing, 350
Reflex camera, 144
Regeneration, 1, 299
   after amputation, 218
Relaxant, 122
Reproduction, asexual, 1, 53
Respiration of green hydra, 383–387
Rifampicin, 212, 257, 282, 288
RNA, 373–377
   buffer, 374
   electrophoresis, 376
   extraction by phenol-chloroform, 373–377
   fractionation, 87, 88, 376
   purification, 375–376
   ribosomal, 374
RNase, 375

Scanning electron microscope, 95–104
   resolution, 95
   x-ray microanalysis, 95
Schiff reagent, 119, 127
Sea anemone, acontiate, 331–333
   Aiptasia pallida, 332, 333, 347, 353
   Diadumene sp., 332
   Metridium sp., 332
   nematocyst venom, 347
   neurotoxin, 356
   sodium current, 356
Sectioning hydra, 123–124
SEM, *see* Scanning electron microscopy
Separation gel of acrylamide, 337
Sesame oil, 344
Sexually differentiated hydra, 71–77
   methods for, 73–76
Shock, electric, 306
   chamber for, 307
Size of hydra, 67–70

Sodium cacodylate, 89, 90, 106, 171
Sodium citrate, 332
Sodium dodecyl sulfate, 374, 403
Sodium pentobarbital, 106
Sodium thiosulfate, 300
Solutions, culture, 30–31
Species of *Hydra*, *see* *Hydra* species
Specimen chamber, 147–148
   for photography, 148
   for shock, electric, 307
Spermatid, postmitotic, 14
Spermatocyte, 14
Spermatogonium, 14
Spermatozoa, 14
S-phase of cell cycle, 159–160, 291
Spurr's embedding medium of low viscosity, 88
Square wave
   pulse, 357
   stimulator, 306
Squash preparation, 336–337
Stacking gel of acrylamide, 337
Staining, 88, 124–125
   maceration for, 156
   procedures, 118
   of tissue, 174
   vital, 1, 131–140
     by feeding
       colloidal carbon, 132
       colored food, 131
       fluorescent dye, 132
Stains
   acid fuchsin, 129
   aniline blue, 129
   Biebrich scarlet, 128
   eosin, 123, 128
   Evans blue, 132, 133, 136, 137
   fast green, 127
   Feulgen, 118, 162
     application, 118–119, 124–125, 127, 166
   fluorescent, 132
   hematoxylin, 124, 125, 128, 166
   India ink, 274
   iron hematoxylin, 124–127
   lead nitrate, 171–176
   Mallory's triple, 124, 125, 129
   methylene blue, 119, 131
   neutral red, 131
   Nile blue sulfate, 131, 132
   orange G, 129

Stains (cont.)
  phenol red, 35–37
  thiolactic acid lead, 119, 171–176
  toluidine blue, 118, 124, 125, 129, 179,
    180
  see also Dye
Stalk, 6
  see Peduncle
Stenotele, 12, 21, 172, 173, 178, 217
  dissolution, 337
  reduction in number, 306
Stereoline glutinant, 12
Streptoline glutinant, 12
Streptomycin, 265
Succinoxidase inhibitor, 341–346
Susa fixative, 122
Symbiont, green alga, 394, 401–405
Symbiosis, 388–413

Taeniola, 9
Tannic acid, 92
Teflon block, 368
Tentacle, 7, 231
  isolation, 176–177
  whorl, 6
Testis, 7, 81
  induce formation, 71
Theca, 8
Thioglycolate, 335, 338
Thiolactic acid lead staining, 171–176
  of nematoblast, 119
Thiol solution, 336, 337
Thymidine, labeled, 132, 158–162
  injected into hydra, 189
Tissue
  chimera, preparation of, 275–279
  culturing stem cells, 261–266
  dissociation, 154, 251–259
  ectoderm, 267–271
  endoderm, 267–271
  enzyme assay, 361–271
  grafting, 1, 2, 225–233, 274, 299, 301
  layer, viable
    separating, 267–271
  maceration, 153–156
  manipulation, 225–279
  microgram quantities, weighed out,
    361–371
  organization, 225–279
  pieces of, 155
  radioactive, 193–196

Tissue, radioactive (cont.)
  fractionation, 197–203
  regeneration, 1
  transplanting, 225–249
Toluidine blue stain, 118, 124, 125, 129,
    179, 180
  and interstitial cell, 118
Track plate, nuclear, 205, 206
Transection, 81–82
Translocation, of reduced organic carbon
    compounds, 407–409
Transplantation
  axial, 231
  experiments, 235–236
  of foot, 231
  of head, 231
  lateral, 230, 231
  property, intrinsic, 234
  quantitative interpretation, 233–249
Tray method for culturing hydra, 54, 56–60
  cleaning, 56–58
  feeding, 56
  precaution, 59–60
Treatment, chemical, 258
Trembley, Abraham, 1
  Mémoires(1744), 1
Trichloracetic acid, 198–199
Trichodina pediculus, 424
Trimethoprim, 395
t-Test, 312
TX, see 6-Carboxyfluorescein

Uca pugilatov, see Fiddler crab
Uncertainty, statistical, 241–248
Urethane, 122, 174

Vital staining, 131–140
  review of, 131–132
  see also Dye, Stain
Van Harreveld solution, 356
Variable, redundant, 245
Vertical plate method for culturing hydra,
    54–56, 60–62
  care of tank, 61
  feeding, 61
  precaution, 61–62
  seeding, 60
Villus, endodermal, 11
Volvent, 12

Warburg flask, 194

X-ray microanalysis, 95
Xylene, 117, 118

Zenker fixative, 122
Zymogen, 14